NEUROSECRETION

IV. International Symposium on Neurosecretion
IVe Symposium International sur la Neurosécrétion

Strasbourg 25-27 Juillet 1966

Editor

F. Stutinsky

With 87 Figures

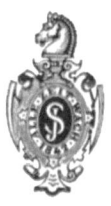

Springer-Verlag Berlin · Heidelberg · New York 1967

ISBN-13: 978-3-642-87611-0   e-ISBN-13: 978-3-642-87609-7
DOI: 10.1007/978-3-642-87609-7

Title-No. 1438

In Memoriam Ernst A. Scharrer

1905—1965

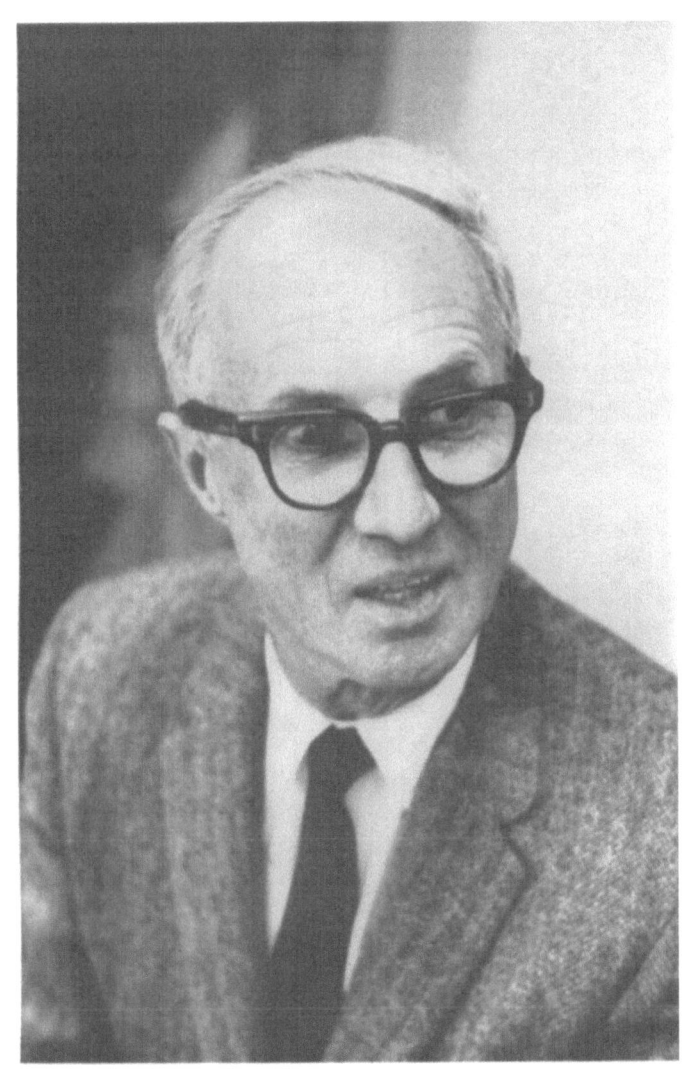

Ernst Scharrer

Avant-Propos

Le IVe Symposium sur la Neurosécrétion à Strasbourg, succède à celui de Naples (1953), de Lund (1957) et de Bristol (1961). Ceux qui ont assisté aux réunions précédentes ne manqueront pas de noter que d'importants changements sont intervenus depuis la dernière rencontre. Certaines figures familières et amies sont absentes. Il nous manque surtout l'un des créateurs de ces réunions: son amitié, son jugement, son intelligence pénétrante et sa vaste expérience nous ferons cruellement défaut. Mais, ERNST SCHARRER a cependant participé à la mise au point de ce 4e Symposium. Il y a plus de deux ans déjà — car cette réunion devait avoir lieu plus tôt — il me conseillait de l'organiser sur le modèle des Laurentian Conferences. Il était d'avis que pour éviter une réunion trop chargée qui ne laisse pas assez de temps pour la discussion, il fallait limiter le nombre et le temps des exposés: c'est ce que nous avons essayé de faire.

Un deuxième caractère distingue cette rencontre des précédentes. Un coup d'oeil sur le programme de ces journées permet de noter que les titres des rapports sont plus éclectiques et embrassent un champ plus large. Je voudrais brièvement justifier cette extension de nos préoccupations.

Depuis la réunion de Bristol d'une part, depuis le 4e Symposium d'Endocrinologie Comparée de Paris d'autre part, il apparaît que nous avons de plus en plus de difficultés à définir et à délimiter le concept de neurosécrétion. C'est un vieux problème qui resurgit à chacune de nos réunions. Il paraissait assez simple et facile à résoudre tant que l'on se bornait à n'envisager que le système hypothalamo-neurohypophysaire. La définition qui se dégageait des discussions du Symposium de Naples en 1953, était claire: la cellule neurosécrétrice était une cellule nerveuse contenant des granules élaborés, ayant un prolongement axonal qui ne formait de synapses, ni avec d'autres neurones, ni avec d'autres organes effecteurs et dont le produit de sécrétion, de nature hormonale, passait dans les capillaires, au niveau d'organes «neuro-haemaux», terme auquel je préfere, en ce qui concerne les Vertébrés, celui de système ou d'organe «neuro-glio-vasculaire». Je crois, en effet, que le rôle de la glie a été trop négligé dans les phénomènes qui nous interessent. La définition à laquelle je viens de faire allusion, est celle de SCHARRER et c'est celle à laquelle j'ai toujours apporté mon adhésion.

Cependant, les résultats des études ultrastructurales, la découverte des fibres à catécholamines dans l'éminence médiane incitent à nous demander si la définition ci-dessus englobe tous les faits actuellement connus.

Ainsi, la définition s'applique bien, en ce qui concerne la présence des granules et leur destinée vasculaire, aux fibres de l'éminence médiane contenant des catécholamines; mais il ne s'agit plus là d'hormones, mais de médiateurs chimiques.

De plus, il semble que des fibres neurosécrétoires authentiques peuvent se terminer sur des cellules glandulaires (dans le lobe intermédiaire par ex.) ou sur des cellules gliales, voire épendymaires.

La distinction entre fibre nerveuse végétative «banale» et fibre nerveuse végétative «spécialisée», je veux dire neurosécrétoire au sens classique du terme, devient donc au moins à la limite, de plus en plus arbitraire. Il me paraît donc nécessaire que ceux qui s'interessent à la fibre neurosécrétoire, s' intéressent aussi à la fibre nerveuse végétative en général et y appliquent d'une manière convergente des méthodes morphologiques, physiologiques et biochimiques. Ce sont ces considérations qui, à mon sens, justifient certains titres de ce programme, qui, à première vue, paraissent sans rapport étroit avec la neurosécrétion.

Nous sommes également confrontés avec le difficile problème des «releasing-factors» qui sont probablement de nature peptidique. D'une manière générale, sauf peut-être chez le Cobaye, nous n'avons aucune idée où ils sont élaborés et surtout si leurs cellules d'origine se confondent ou non avec des cellules neuro-sécrétrices déjà inventoriées.

Enfin, une question non moins troublante pour le concept classique de la neurosécrétion est posé par la zone hypophysiotrope hypothalamique de Halász qui, comme on le sait, est seule à conserver aux cellules basophiles des implants hypophysaires une structure normale. Cette zone, dont les trophines ne peuvent agir que par diffusion, ne correspond à aucun groupement cellulaire connu, ni à aucune structure nerveuse définie.

Il ne s'agit là que de quelques problèmes parmi beaucoup d'autres posés par la définition classique de la neurosécrétion. J'espère que nos rapporteurs et les discussions qui suivront leurs exposés fourniront des réponses au moins à certaines de nos questions.

Un certain nombre de nos collègues n'ont pas pu assister à la réunion, les uns, comme les Professeurs HELLER et M. THOMSEN, empêchés par la maladie, les autres comme les Docteurs ANGEL, DA LAGE, HERMAN, FARNER, HILD, JOHANSON, KLEIN, MARTIN, OLSON, RODECK, SACHS, SEITE, STAHL, E. THOMSEN, ZERBIB, nos collègues hindous, australiens, japonais, pour des raisons matérielles. JASINSKI, VIGH et TEICHMAN n'ont pas obtenu de visa.

Avant de terminer, je voudrais remercier tous ceux qui m'ont aidé matériellement à mettre sur pied cette réunion, en particulier tout le personnel de mon laboratoire et celui de l'Institut de Zoologie, mais une mention spéciale revient cependant au Professeur FOLLENIUS qui a été la cheville ouvrière de cette organisation.

Enfin, j'exprime ma plus vive gratitude à Monsieur le Professeur VIVIEN, Doyen de la Faculté des Sciences, d'avoir bien voulu présider la séance inaugurale de ce IVe Symposium sur la Neurosécrétion, et de nous avoir obtenu, de la Faculté des Sciences et du Conseil de l'Université de Strasbourg, de substantielles subventions.

Strasbourg en février 1967   F. STUTINSKY

Contents – Table des matières

Errata

page 43: ligne 1 et 1ère ligne de la légende:

lire: periodique

au lieu de: périodique

page 48: ligne 17:

lire: intermedia

au lieu de: intermédia

page 152: la légende de la figure 5 doit être modifiée de la façon suivante:

"The values for μMO_2 in buffer given on the ordinate should read 1, 2, 3, 4, 5 instead of 10, 20, 30, 40, 50. The rates indicated for O_2 uptake should read .07/min, .116/min, .033/min, and .083/min, instead of .7/min, 1.16/min, .33/min, and .83/min, respectively."

page 168: ligne 27:

lire: 3,4-dihydroxyphenylalanine

au lieu de: 3,4-dihydroxypehnylalaninc

pape 173: ligne 34:

lire: prolactin

au lieu de: prolaction

Discours Inaugural

de Monsieur le Professeur J. Benoit

Professeur au Collège de France (Paris), Président d'Honneur du Symposium

Monsieur le Doyen,
Monsieur le Président, Mes chers Collègues,
Mesdames, Mesdemoiselles, Messieurs.

Je veux tout d'abord exprimer ma vive reconnaissance à Monsieur le Professeur Stutinsky, Organisateur et Président de ce Symposium sur la Neurosécrétion, qui me fit l'amitié de m'inviter et de me prier d'y prendre la parole en qualité de Président d'Honneur.

Quand je prononce le mot de Neurosécrétion, un nom me hante: celui de l'éminent biologiste qui en eut, le premier, la notion claire; qui, le premier, conçut son énorme importance en Physiologie: Ernest Scharrer. Oui, au-delà de la peine que je ressens, que nous ressentons tous d'être maintenant privés de lui, je ne puis me défendre de l'impression qu'il est cependant aujourd'hui parmi nous, tant nous avons été habitués, dans les précédents Colloques, à le voir s'imposer au centre des problèmes et des discussions, tant nous savons que − seul d'abord, puis aidé par sa chère épouse − il avait forgé et développé ce concept essentiel de fonction endocrine de cellules nerveuses.

Son œuvre est trop importante pour que je ne veuille pas rendre aujourd'hui, brièvement, un hommage particulier au grand découvreur que fut Ernest Scharrer.

Né à Münich en 1905, Ernest Scharrer fit ses études de Médecine dans sa ville natale. Nommé assistant en 1928 à l'Institut de Zoologie de l'Université de Münich, il fit en 1929−1930 un stage d'une année, comme Sterling Fellow, à l'Osborn Zoological Laboratory de l'Université de Yale, à New Haven. Retournant en Allemagne, il fut successivement Assistant de Zoologie à l'Université de Vienne pendant un an, chercheur à l'Institut psychiatrique (section de Pathologie nerveuse) à Münich pendant deux ans, puis Chargé de la direction de l'Institut Neurologique à l'Université de Francfort sur le Main, à l'âge de 28 ans. Quatre années plus tard, en 1937, réprouvant les agissements hitlériens, il décida de quitter son pays et se rendit aux Etats-Unis. Fellow Rockfeller au département de Neuroanatomie, à Chicago en 1937, à New-York à l'Institut Rockefeller en 1938, il fut nommé en 1940 Assistant Professor of Anatomy à l'Université de Cleveland, puis Associate Professor à l'Université de Denver de 1946 à 1954, et enfin − et ce fut son dernier poste − Professeur titulaire d'Anatomie à l'Albert Einstein College of Medicine à New-York en 1955.

Ses affectations successives, comme l'énoncé de ses différents travaux, montrent que Scharrer a presque exclusivement consacré son activité scientifique à l'étude du système nerveux et en particulier du diencéphale.

Sa première publication date de 1928. Elle reprend, d'un point de vue différent, une belle expérience de von Frisch, qui, en 1911, avait constaté que les chromatophores du vairon, aveuglé par énucléation des deux yeux, répondaient encore à la lumière, lorsque celle-ci était dirigée sur le diencéphale. Scharrer choisit un autre test: le réflexe conditionné par l'association nourriture-lumière. Il put établir que la sensibilité de la peau n'entre pas en ligne de compte, que l'éclairement du diencéphale déclenche le réflexe, que ce dernier est diminué ou supprimé lorsque le poisson a subi la destruction plus ou moins complète du diencéphale, et enfin que, dans ce dernier, le noyau préoptique est très richement vascularisé et que ses neurones contiennent de très volumineuses vacuoles colorables par l'érythrosine, le bleu de toluidine ou l'orange G. Et Scharrer émet l'idée que ce noyau peut être une *glande à sécrétion interne, en relation avec l'hypophyse*. Sans doute Speidel décrivit-il en 1919, — et Scharrer le rappelle —, de semblables volumineux neurones glandulaires dans la moelle épinière de plusieurs poissons. Mais, en émettant l'hypothèse que l'origine du réflexe: lumière-nourriture est vraisemblablement située dans l'hypothalamus et aurait pour siège, à l'échelle cellulaire, les neurones glandulaires endocrines du noyau préoptique, c'est bien Scharrer qui met le premier en place, dans le chapitre encore brumeux de l'histophysiologie nerveuse, le concept de neurosécrétion. Il fonde son assertion sur des observations histologiques de plus en plus nombreuses qu'il étend des Poissons aux Amphibiens, aux Reptiles, aux Mammifères, et enfin à l'Homme, dans un travail qu'il publie avec Gaupp en 1933. En 1933 également, songeant à une expérience de Trendelenburg qui avait, en 1928, observé chez le Chien que l'hypophysectomie faisait monter dans le tuber le taux de l'adiurétine, Scharrer eut l'intuition que la neurosécrétion pourrait peut-être expliquer le diabète insipide. Mais les idées de Scharrer ne sont pas acceptées au début. Malgré ses travaux précis, qu'il accomplit seul, puis avec divers collaborateurs, dont le plus précieux et le plus fécond fut sans nul doute sa femme, Madame Berta Scharrer (qui étudiera avec soin la neurosécrétion chez les Invertébrés) la notion de Neurosécrétion et de «glande diencéphalique», deux termes créés par Scharrer, se heurtent presque pendant de nombreuses années à diverses objections. On se refuse à croire que des éléments de l'organisme aussi hautement différenciés, aussi nobles que les cellules nerveuses puissent jouir d'une fonction «glandulaire», considérée jusqu'alors comme de qualité inférieure. Certains notent d'autre part que le concept de neurosécrétion (sécrétion d'origine nerveuse) s'oppose à celui de neurocrinie (sécrétion endonerveuse) défendue par R. Collin. On objecte encore l'absence de preuves expérimentales du rôle physiologique des neurones neurosécrétoires, et surtout, on relève les difficultés de détection histologique, par les techniques courantes, du neurosécrétat et de son transit le long des neurites. C'est alors que Bargmann découvre, en 1949, les propriétés tinctoriales de la coloration de Gomori à l'hématoxyline chromique-phloxine. Grâce à cette technique, la détection des grains de neurosécrétion et leur migration le long de ce que Bargmann appelle la «voie neurosécrétoire hypothalamo-hypophysaire» est devenu aisée. Les doutes se lèvent définitivement. On accepte enfin le concept neurosécrétoire, produit terminal, si j'ose dire, sur les plans intellectuel et moral, du génie de Scharrer, de sa tenacité et de sa foi dans la théorie qu'il a créée. De tous côtés, les travailleurs s'intéressent à ce problème. Des centaines, des milliers de publications paraissent, relatives à maintes espèces des diverses classes de Vertébrés et des Invertébrés. L'année 1953 paraît favorable à ERNEST et BERTA SCHARRER pour organiser un Symposium sur la neurosécrétion à Naples. Qui parmi ceux qui eurent le privilège d'y prendre part n'évoquera l'importance scientifique de cette rencontre, laquelle suggéra cette paraphrase d'un mot historique: «plus tard, en rappelant cette réunion mémorable, qui consacre l'existence d'une science nouvelle, je pourrai dire avec fierté: j'y étais». Et qui ne se souvient du climat sympathique qui imprégna les réunions et le déroulement du symposium dans son entier ? Cela est en moi un souvenir vivace et a présenté un tel agrément et – souvenezvous! – une atmosphère aussi charmante, atmosphère qui était bien créée – c'était manifeste, sensible – par la personnalité généreuse des deux organisateurs, Madame et Monsieur SCHARRER, par leur gentillesse, leur exquise amabilité pour tous les participants. Madame SCHARRER me permettra de souligner ici, à côté des qualités intellectuelles de son mari, ses qualités morales, de bonté, d'altruisme, de dévoue-ment aux nobles causes; ses qualités d'enthousiasme et d'amour de la science qu'il servait; ses qualités humaines en un mot qui donnèrent un éclat particulier pendant sa trop courte existence, à sa personnalité officielle de savant telle qu'elle apparaissait dans ses publications, dans son enseignement, dans les réunions scientifiques.

J'ai parlé du premier Symposium qui s'est tenu à Naples. Un deuxième Sym-posium eut lieu à LUND en 1958, un troisième à Bristol en 1961, auxquels il ne m'a pas été possible, malheureusement, de me rendre. Et nous assistons au 4ème, ce qui prouve que le mouvement imprimé par les SCHARRER aux fervents de la Neurosécrétion continue à se développer dans les meilleures conditions.

Outre la reconnaissance que nous ressentons tous envers Monsieur et Madame SCHARRER pour les Symposia dont ils ont eu l'idée, nous devons leur exprimer aussi notre gratitude pour la revue Bibliographia Neuroendocrinologica qu'ils ont bénévolement fondée et que nous connaissons tous. Ayant eu l'occasion de m'inté-resser, il y a quelques années, aux difficultés de la documentation actuelle et aux remèdes qu'on pourrait lui apporter, j'ai cité, dans mon adresse présidentielle au Congrès International de Biologie cellulaire, à Providence, en 1964, le cas de cette revue comme celui d'une des initiatives les plus utiles pour l'information scienti-fique. Que devant chaque grand problème, devant des parties assez bien délimitées des Sciences biologiques, d'autres chercheurs aient le courage et le dévouement qu'ont eu les SCHARRER, une solution partielle très efficace sera trouvée aux pro-blèmes difficiles de la bibliographie actuelle.

Je vous ai parlé de quelques travaux de SCHARRER au début de sa carrière scientifique. Je ne puis m'étendre sur les autres. Je me reporterai seulement à l'une des remarques conclusives qu'il rédigea après le dernier Symposium de Bristol. S'élevant contre la tendance de quelques auteurs d'étendre le concept de cellule neurosécrétoire à toutes les cellules nerveuses, SCHARRER définit avec précision les attributs propres de la cellule neurosécrétrice: elle possède des granules carac-téristiques; elle n'est pas en jonction synaptique avec d'autres neurones ou organes effecteurs; son axone se termine sur un espace sanguin où se déverse son matériel neurosécrété et l'hormone ou les hormones qu'il contient. Les cellules nerveuses dites «classiques», au contraire, ont pour fonction essentielle de transmettre des

1*

impulsions nerveuses et s'acquittent de cette tâche grâce à des mécanismes humoraux dont les effets se limitent aux synapses.

Depuis cette réunion de Bristol en 1961, les recherches à l'échelon cytologique et même moléculaire ont fait de nouveaux progrès; nos connaissances des mécanismes de synthèse et de libération, ainsi que des modalités d'action des médiateurs monoaminergiques, par exemple, se sont notablement approfondies. Comme par le passé, les travaux concernant les Invertébrés ont apporté une contribution non négligeable à ces résultats. Mais d'autres recherches sont venues jeter des ponts entre les deux modes de neurosécrétion que séparait Scharrer: la neurosécrétion «excrétée» dans la circulation et la neurosécrétion des médiateurs du système nerveux central. L'histophysiologie a multiplié les observations de concomitances entre des phénomènes endocriniens liés à la neurosécrétion classique, et la présence ou l'activité de vésicules identifiées comme monoaminergiques.

Parallèlement, des recherches ont jeté quelque lumière sur les relations existant entre la neurosécrétion de transmetteurs hypothalamohypophysaires spécifiques et des structures hypothalamiques non neurosécrétoires au sens strict, mais chargées des fonctions neuroendocriniennes de contrôle et qui semblent intervenir en modifiant, ou en modulant, les synthèses neurosécrétoires.

Peut-être y aurait-il lieu d'atténuer quelque peu l'utile distinction établie par Scharrer? Les recherches sur la neurosécrétion rendront sans doute de plus en plus sensible le lien entre le neurosécrétat et les monoamines, les secondes jouant dans la synthèse, ou le transport, ou la libération du premier, un rôle capital dont les modalités sont encore imprécises. Les exposés et les contacts que nous permettra le présent Symposium apporteront sans doute des réponses à quelques-unes de ces questions.

Au seuil de ce Symposium, je veux, au nom de tous, exprimer dès maintenant au Professeur Stutinsky et à ses Collègues, nos vifs remerciements pour la peine qu'ils ont déjà prise à organiser cette réunion, dont je suis sûr qu'elle sera un succès et fera utilement progresser nos connaissances de la Neurosécrétion, prise en soi, ainsi que dans son cadre naturel, la Neuroendocrinologie.

The Hormonogenic Properties of Neurosecretory Cells

H. A. BERN

Department of Zoology and its Cancer Research Genetics Laboratory,
University of California, Berkeley

Recently KNOWLES and I (1966) presented an extended concept of neuro-secretion, which recognized the endocrine role of neurosecretory cells as deriving not only from their directly hormonogenic contribution but also from their indirect control of endocrine tissues by functional contacts between neurosecretory nerve fibers and endocrine cells (quasi-innervation) (see also BERN and KNOWLES, 1966). This consideration represented a continuation of the efforts at reestimating the concept of neurosecretion already begun two years ago in Paris by ERNST SCHARRER (1965). The aim of the present paper is to consider some aspects of the hormonogenic properties of neurosecretory neurons – the specializations related to their functioning as endocrine gland cells. The neuronal properties of these cells and their implications will be considered by KNOWLES in the following paper (KNOWLES, 1967).

Inasmuch as the material treated herein will in good part appear in a critique already in press (BERN, 1966), it will be presented in the form of an expanded abstract, with only the minimum essential citations.

1. Unreliable Nature of Light-Microscope Evidence for Neurosecretory Activity. A wide variety of structures in neurons will convey to cells staining properties, including affinities for the so-called neurosecretion stains, which will simulate the cytological picture characteristic of well-established neurosecretory cells. Organelles such as lysosomes and mitochondria, lamellar systems, pigmented globules, lipofuscins, crystalline arrays of virus particles, heavy glycogen deposits, can all mimic secretory inclusions. Vesicular structures associated with the nervous system of invertebrates may have a prominent neuroglandular appearance but can often be shown to be sensory organs. For example, the epistellar body of octopod molluscs and the parolfactory vesicle of decapod molluscs have both proved to be photoreceptors, characterized by rhabdome organization and rhodop-sin (NISHIOKA, YASUMASU, and BERN, 1966; NISHIOKA et al., 1966). The so-called follicle gland of gastropod molluscs also may be a sensory structure, although a glandular function remains possible in addition (SIMPSON et al., 1966).

These specialized neurons and nervous structures may be of equal or greater significance than the occurrence of neurosecretory cells. Students of neurosecretion are in a particularly favorable position to make such findings of general neuro-biological importance, but they need continue to be cautious in order to avoid misinterpretation of various neurocytological specializations as evidence for neurosecretory activity.

2. Significance of the Elementary Neurosecretory Granule in the "Diagnosis" of Neurosecretion. There is considerable evidence that the typical elementary granule (1000—3000 Å, membrane-limited, electron-dense) may be associated in some cases with neurotransmitter agents (as in leeches and gastropods). Accordingly, the granules may be present when neurosecretion is absent. Studies of the tetrapod neurohypophysis reveal an important difference between the median eminence (axons containing mostly small vesicles) and the pars nervosa (axons containing typical neurosecretory granules); thus, neurosecretion may be present when the typical granules are absent. Whatever else the small vesicles may represent in the median eminence, at least some of them are the morphological representation of neurosecretory material of hormonal significance. Future studies are needed to characterize chemically the significance of median eminence fiber inclusions, keeping in mind the evidence for both peptide and monoamine adenohypophysis-influencing factors.

3. Synthetic and Granule-Forming Properties of Neurosecretory Cells. The standard picture of the production of protein-secreting granules, with synthesis of the "raw material" by the endoplasmic reticulum and its "packaging" by the Golgi apparatus, has been applied to the neurosecretory cell. More recent electron-microscope visualizations indicate that small vesicles originating from the Golgi apparatus may themselves transform into elementary neurosecretory granules at some distance from their point of origin. Larger vesicles may also fill the cytoplasm of neurosecretory cells and later acquire electron density. More important than these qualifications regarding the role of the perikaryon is the increasing evidence for local production of neurosecretory vesicles and granules by organelles: lamellar and tubular systems, in the preterminal and terminal regions of the axon. The entire neurosecretory neuron is presently best regarded as being potentially a secretory unit. Further biochemical and radioautographic studies are needed to delineate the capacity of the axon to participate in hormone and proteincarrier syntheses, transformations, associations and dissociations.

4. Regenerative Capacity of Neurosecretory Systems. The ability of neuro-secretory systems to become functionally operative relatively soon after removal of the neurohemal area, or transection of the tract, has long been recognized. Recent observations on the regeneration of the caudal neurosecretory system in adult teleost *Tilapia* after its *total* removal, indicate the importance of ependymal elements in replacing extirpated neurosecretory elements, at least in lower verte-brates (FRIDBERG et al., 1966). Experiments involving extirpation of neuro-secretory nuclei should consider the potential functional contribution of modified ependymal components, apparently capable of differentiating *de novo* into neuro-secretory cells.

5. Functions of the Dendrite of Neurosecretory Cells. Hypothalamic neuro-secretory neurons, especially in lower vertebrates, often have dendrite-like processes projecting into the III ventricle. Ultrastructural examination of such processes reveals their secretory potential and leaves undecided, but certainly possible, a sensory role in addition (as osmoreceptors or photoreceptors). Caudal neurosecretory neurons also show strong evidence of secretion into the cere-brospinal fluid, especially in regenerating systems (FRIDBERG and NISHIOKA, 1966). The bidirectional secretory capacity of such neurosecretory neurons can be analogized with that of the thyroid cell, which is also capable of secreting apically or basally, depending on the physiological demand. The importance of non-hemal routes of discharge of neurohormone has not yet been properly assessed.

Acknowledgments. I am indebted to FRANCIS KNOWLES for his discussion and accord on the points summarized in this paper, to my colleague RICHARD NISHIOKA for the continuing collaboration basic to attempts to evaluate and develop the concept of neurosecretion, and to the National Science Foundation for its continuing support of our joint research efforts.

References

Specific citations of the literature pertinent to the points summarized above can be found in the following papers

BERN, H. A. (1966): On the production of hormones by neurones and the role of neurosecretion in neuroendocrine mechanisms. Soc. Exper. Biol. Symp. No. 20, "Nervous and Hormonal Mechanisms of Integration".

—, and F. G. W. KNOWLES (1966): Neurosecretion. In: Neuroendocrinology, Vol. 1. (Eds. MARTINI, L., and W. F. GANONG). New York: Academic Press.

FRIDBERG, G., and R. S. NISHIOKA (1966): Secretion into the cerebrospinal fluid by caudal neurosecretory neurons. Science **152**, 90—91.

— — H. A. BERN, and W. R. FLEMING (1966): Regeneration of the caudal neurosecretory system in the cichlid teleost Tilapia mossambica. J. exper. Zool. (in press).

KNOWLES, F. G. W. (1967): The neuronal properties of neurosecretory cells. This Volume.

—, and H. A. BERN (1966): The function of neurosecretion in neuroendocrine regulation. Nature (Lond.) **210**, 271—272.

NISHIOKA, R. S., I. YASUMASU, and H. A. BERN (1966): Photoreceptive features of vesicles associated with the nervous system of cephalopods. Nature (in press).

— — A. PACKARD, H. A. BERN, and J. Z. YOUNG (1966): Nature of vesicles assoscated with the cephalopod nervous system. Z. Zellforsch. (in press).

SCHARRER, E. (1965): The final common pathway in neuroendocrine integration. Arch. d'anat. micr. **54**, 359—370.

SIMPSON, L., H. A. BERN, and R. S. NISHIOKA (1966): Examination of the evidence for neurosecretion in the nervous system of Helisoma tenue (Gastropoda Pulmonata) Gen. Comp. Endocrinol. (in press).

Neuronal Properties of Neurosecretory Cells

F. KNOWLES

Department of Anatomy, Medical School, University of Birmingham, England

Introduction

A most striking and characteristic feature of neurosecretory systems is their ability to synthesize considerable quantities of secretory products, which are hormones in the true sense of the word, (BERN and KNOWLES, 1966). By itself however this feature would hardly command particular attention. It is the fact that these cells lie in the central nervous system and resemble neurons which is especially significant, for it is by reason of their combination of neuronal and endocrine features that they occupy a unique position in neuroendocrinology.

For many years the endocrine activities of neurosecretory cells were of paramount interest. Indeed they have been used as the basis for a definition of neurosecretion. As recently as 1962, at the IIIrd Symposium of Neurosecretion at Bristol, ERNST SCHARRER remarked that 'neurosecretory cells do not form synapses with other neurons or effector organs. Their axons end at blood spaces into which they release the neurosecretory material' (SCHARRER, 1962). Since then however the electron microscope has revealed many instances of direct synaptoid contacts between neurosecretory fibres and other tissues. So, once more, the boundary between neurosecretory cells and other neurons would appear to have become less distinct, and a comparison between the neuronal properties of neurosecretory cells and 'ordinary' neurons («neurones banaux») is therefore of special interest when we attempt to delimit the field of neurosecretion.

Two Categories of Neurosecretion

Before considering the neuronal properties of neurosecretory cells it is necessary to make a clear distinction between two essentially different neurons which have both been termed neurosecretory by various authors. This distinction was first demonstrated at the level of ultrastructure in the pericardial organs of the crustacean *Squilla mantis* (KNOWLES, 1960). It has since been observed in relation to the pituitary of many vertebrates, and it has been shown that the structural differences described are accompanied by biochemical differences also. Two main categories, Type A and Type B, have been postulated (KNOWLES, 1965a); further subdivision may become necessary later. *Type A fibres* generally produce peptide hormones (e.g. ADH, oxytocin) and contain spherical, uniformly electron-dense, elementary vesicles with a diameter greater than 1,000 Å.

Type B fibres appear to contain considerable quantities of monoamines; they contain vesicles which are generally irregular in shape and with electron-dense granules which do not fill the bounding membrane; these vesicles are usually smaller than 1,000 Å in diameter.

Type A fibres are most usually stained with the basic component of the Gomori CAH method.

Type B fibres, in contrast, do not stain blue with the Gomori CAH method though they often stain deeply with the phloxine component of the Gomori CAH-phloxine method.

Recently the fluorescence method of FALCK, 1962 has been used by FUXE, 1964, LICHTENSTEIGER and LANGEMANN, 1965, ENEMAR and FALCK, 1965, and others to trace Type B fibres and we may see as we ascend the vertebrate series that these fibres, as well as Type A fibres, are consistently associated with pituitary control. It is evident that Type A neurosecretion corresponds most closely to the 'classical' neurosecretion postulated by SCHARRER and BARGMANN, and that Type B neurosecretory fibres may represent a special category of 'adrenergic' transmission, possible involving a wide range of dopamine-derivatives. Reasons however for terming both Type A and Type B fibres neurosecretory have been discussed by KNOWLES, 1965b, and KNOWLES and BERN, 1966.

In our present state of knowledge it would be imprudent to delimit the boundaries between Type A and Type B neurosecretion too precisely. It appears that in general neurosecretory fibres containing vesicles of a diameter greater than 1,000 Å seem to be specialised for the production of peptide hormones, while those with vesicles less than 1,000 Å contain monoamines in abundance. Yet the possibility that Type A fibres may also contain monoamines and Type B fibres some peptide hormones must be borne in mind. Moreover the arbitrary dividing line of 1,000 Å (KNOWLES, 1965a) was proposed for convenience, and the discovery of Type A peptide neurosecretion with elementary neurosecretory vesicles less than 1,000 Å in diameter, or Type B neurosecretion with vesicles slightly over the 1,000 Å mark would not invalidate the general postulate that at present at least two categories of neurosecretion, peptide and monamine, seem to be concerned in neuroendocrine regulation. This account of the neuronal properties of neurosecretory cells deals mainly with Type A neurosecretion.

Morphology of Neurosecretory Cells

Morphologically neurosecretory neurons and ordinary neurons have many features in common: Axons and dendrites, extensively developed endoplasmic reticulum equivalent to Nissl bodies, Golgi complexes, a proximodistal transport of axoplasm – these are all characteristic of neurosecretory cells and neurons. Neurofibrillae and synaptic vesicles have also been described in neurosecretory fibres, but there is some reason to doubt that these are exactly equivalent to the structures which they resemble in ordinary neurons.

a) Neurofibrillae. The neurofibrillae of neurosecretory cells show considerable variation in different regions and it may be questioned whether all those fibrillae and tubules which have been described as neurofibrillae or neurotubules are in fact related to one another. In the pericardial organs of *Squilla mantis* for instance neurofibrillae of typical form are found in the more proximal regions of the axon; more distally both these and wider tubules are found: while at the distal end neurotubules, but no typical neurofibrillae, may be seen. The possibility that the fibrillae swell in their distal regions to form the wider neurotubules was studied in *Squilla*, but no evidence for this was found; instead there were indications that the tubules are structurally related to mitochondria which sink from the surface of the axon, and later enlarge to form multilamellate systems (KNOWLES, 1964). Similar multilamellar bodies have been described also in the pituitary pars nervosa of mammals (HOLMES and KIERNAN, 1964; LEDERIS, 1964, 1965; KNOWLES, 1965 b) and appear to represent a distinguishing feature of Type A neurosecretion.

b) Synaptic vesicles. At the terminals of neurosecretory axons many fine vesicles c. 500 Å in diameter have been described and often called synaptic vesicles, because of their size. The possibility that some of these represent neurotubules cut in section cannot be disregarded, for the diameter of some neurotubules also is c. 500 Å. Another interpretation of these vesicles is also possible. KNOWLES, HOLMES, BERN and LEDERIS have all discussed the possibility that these vesicles might arise from the fragmentation of the larger neurosecretory vesicles (see BERN and KNOWLES, 1966). Electrical stimulation of neurosecretory axons of Squilla led to fragmentation of elementary neurosecretory vesicles and the formation of smaller vesicles (KNOWLES, 1963). Such observations would accord also with the experimental work of PALAY, 1957, who showed that ADH release from neurosecretory axon endings led to the disappearance of typical elementary neurosecretory vesicles and a concomitant increase in the number of 'synaptic' vesicles.

Physiology of Neurosecretory Cells

Conduction. The primary business of ordinary neurons is to conduct and transmit impulses. Unfortunately our information about the ability of neurosecretory fibres to conduct impulses is relatively slight. Attempts have been made since the early 1950s to obtain electrophysiological information from neurosecretory systems. It is however not easy to interpret all the data which has been obtained, for, as we have seen, neurosecretory systems may contain more than one structurally and biochemically distinct element; it is therefore not surprising that compound action potentials often result from stimulation. Single unit recordings have however been obtained from several systems, in particular the hypothalamic and caudal neurosecretory systems of fishes (see the review by BERN and YAGI, 1965).

In these experiments there has been one consistent finding which is of particular interest, namely the long *duration* of *action potentials* from neurosecretory fibres – often as much as two to ten times longer than those from adjacent neurons. This difference is most striking in poikilothermous animals; thus far the data obtained from mammals do not indicate such striking differences. Nevertheless it is clear that in many neurosecretory systems the conduction is quantitatively different to that in ordinary neurons.

BENNET and FOX, 1962, have commented on not only the long action potentials but also the very *slow conduction velocities* recorded by them from the terminals of caudal neurosecretory neurons. These findings would be consistent with a view that neurosecretory neurons may differ fundamentally from 'neurones banaux' in their ability to maintain a prolonged and continuous release of neurohormone from their terminals. It is relevant to note at this point that such sustained action may be characteristic not only of neurons which liberate their products into the bloodstream but also those which innervate other endocrine tissues (see KANDEL), 1964 and BERN and YAGI, 1964).

Furthermore the functional hypertrophy of endocrine tissues which follows severance of neurosecretory tracts to them would further indicate that many neurosecretory fibres are normally carrying out a sustained inhibition (see BERN and KNOWLES, 1966).

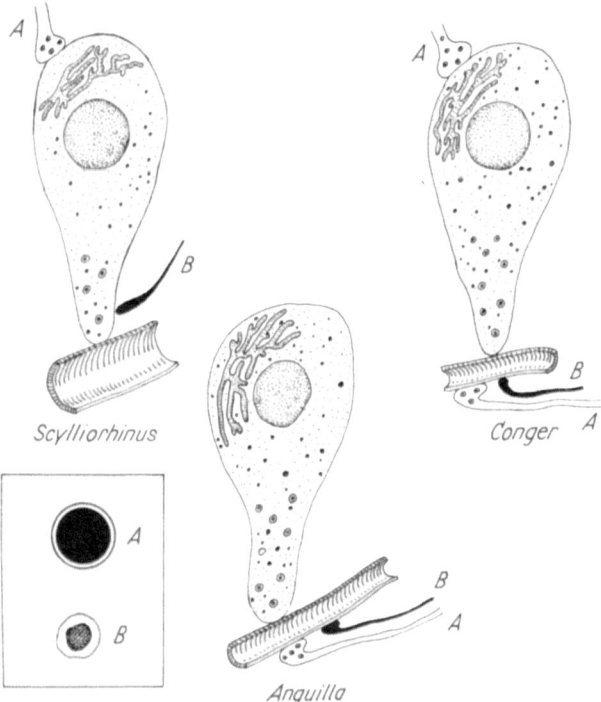

Fig. 1. Three different relationship between Type A and Type B neurosecretory fibres and pars intermedia cells in an Elasmobranch fish (*Scylliorhinus*) and two teleost fishes (*Conger* and *Anguilla*). For an explanation see text. — The distinction in size and appearance between Type A vesicles (c. 1,800 Å in diameter) and Type B vesicles (electron-dense contents c. 750 Å in diameter) is shown inset (see KNOWLES, 1964, and KNOWLES and VOLLRATH, 1966)

Neurosecretory "Innervation" of Endocrine Organs

It has become clear, within recent years, that there are at least two morphologically different relationships between neurosecretory cells and their 'target organs'. The first type, which includes those systems producing the chromactivating hormones of crustaceans and the anti-diuretic hormone of vertebrates, function as endocrine entities, producing and releasing their hormones directly into the bloodstream to affect distant non-endocrine effector organs.

The second type of neurosecretory system however has a more indirect endocrine activity by regulating the action of other endocrine tissues. To this category belong those neurosecretory systems which affect the pituitary. A few selected examples will show that the morphological relationship of this type and its target organ can range in different species from direct synaptoid contact to more distant regulation by blood-born substances.

a) Direct contact. Direct synaptoid contacts between neurosecretory fibres and endocrine cells has been demonstrated in a simple and basic form in the pituitary of the dogfish (KNOWLES, 1965b). Both Type A and Type B fibres terminate on the intrinsic MSH-producing cells.

In the Conger eel a few synaptoid contact between Type A fibres and cells of the pars intermedia have been seen, but other Type A fibres and all Type B fibres discharge into a narrow extravascular channel (KNOWLES and VOLLRATH, 1966). In the freshwater eel also a narrow extravascular blood channel separates the neurosecretory and intrinsic endocrine elements of the pituitary, and neither Type A nor Type B synaptoid contacts were found (Fig. 1).

In *Hippocampus guttulatus* synaptoid contact between Type B fibres and intrinsic secretory cells are common in all parts of the pituitary, but exceedingly few Type A fibre contacts were seen, though Type A fibres are abundant and permeate the whole gland; in *Hippocampus cuda* synaptoid contacts were rare (KNOWLES, VOLLRATH and NISHIOKA, 1966). In *Xenopus* COHEN, 1964, found an extensive system of Type B fibres in the pars intermedia but few if any Type A fibres. This accords with the fluorescence studies of ENEMAR and FALCK, 1965, and the observations by SMOLLER on *Hyla* (SMOLLER, 1965).

A comparison between the neurosecretory innervation of the adenohypophysis in Elasmobranchs, Teleosts and Amphibians suggests that direct contact between A and B fibres and intrinsic endocrine cells may be a primitive feature which later was replaced during phylogeny by an aggregation of fibres to form a kind of neuropil from which substances reach by diffusion the endocrine cells which they affect. It is evident that by this means relatively few neurosecretory fibres could control a larger number of pars distalis cells.

b) Liberation of type A and type B secretion into a portal system. Innervation of the pars distalis in the eel is effected by the discharge of Type A and Type B fibre products into a system of extravascular channels which permeate the pars distalis. This arrangement has been described as a kind of distal median eminence and distal portal system (KNOWLES and VOLLRATH, 1966). In Amphibians also the neurosecretory fibres influencing pars distalis function lie in close conjunction to it (DIERICKX, 1965). In Reptiles and Mammals many neurosecretory fibres generally end at the median eminence, and the space between this region and the pars distalis is usually traversed by an extensive portal system (GORBMANN and BERN, 1952), though even in a primate the pars distalis may be in close opposition to the median eminence (ANAND KUMAR, 1965).

Thus far the finding with the electron microscope show that three main size classes of vesicles are found in the median eminence of higher vertebrates. For instance BERN and NISHIOKA, 1965, found Type A (c. 1,700 Å), Type B (c. 1,000 Å) and a third type (with vesicles c. 300–500 Å in diameter) in the median eminence of some passerine birds.

We have evidence from many sources that both peptides and catecholamines may be involved in neurosecretory control of the pars distalis. Biochemical extraction of peptide releasing-factors has been achieved by GUILLEMIN, SAFFRAN and others: Catecholamines have been demonstrated by the fluorescence method of

FUXE, 1964, and the experiments of MARKEE, EVERETT and SAWYER, 1952, using antiadrenergic drugs reinforce a suggestion that the release of gonadotrophins in rats and rabbits is mediated by catecholamines. At present there is little clear evidence whether an excitatory or inhibitory control is involved.

c) Dual control by neurosecretion of endocrine activity. Our survey of the 'innervation' of endocrine organs by neurosecretory fibres has revealed a considerable diversity in the means whereby the products of the neurosecretory fibres reach the endocrine cells, ranging from direct contact to diffusion through a portal system. One may remark however the consistent occurrence of Type A and Type B fibres in neurosecretory systems concerned in the regulation of other endocrine tissues. This is true not only of the vertebrate pituitary but also has been described in insects (NORMANN, 1965). The significance of such a dual control is not yet clear; it has been suggested that hormone synthesis and hormone release may be independently regulated (KNOWLES, 1965b).

A further possibility is that Type B fibres may innervate Type A fibres and so regulate their function. This is supported by the demonstration of synaptoid contacts between A and B fibres in the insect corpus cardiacum (SCHARRER, 1963; NORMANN, 1965) and the pituitary (BARGMANN, KNOOP and THIEL, 1957).

The Relation between Neurosecretion and Ependymal Elements

Recent studies indicate that the structural and functional relationship between neurosecretory systems and ependyma may be closer than had hitherto been suspected.

Two years ago in Paris ERNST SCHARRER was able to say "The possibility that mechanisms serving the correlation of cerebral and endocrine functions might be provided by secretory ependyma rather than neurons is suggested by the observations of VIGH, AROS, KORITSANZKY, WENGER and CEGLEDI, 1963; LEVEQUE and HOFKIN, 1962; and LEVEQUE and STERN, 1964. However, inasmuch as nothing is known about neural connections of ependymal elements, it would seem premature to discuss their role as mediators in any detail at this time" (SCHARRER, 1965).

Since then many interesting results have been reported from the laboratories of STUTINSKY, LEVEQUE, VIGH and others pointing to the involvement of specialized secretory ependyma (the 'ventricular glands') in neuroendocrine control (see LEVEQUE, STUTINSKY, PORTE and STOECKEL, 1966) and last year apparently functional synaptoid contacts between Type A neurosecretory fibres and secretory ependymal elements were demonstrated in the pituitary of the eel (KNOWLES and VOLLRATH, 1965).

In morphological terms these contacts resembled synapses such as those which have been described elsewhere in the central nervous system, though with some interesting differences. In the first place they were apparently transient. Conditions of illumination and background which led to the colourchange of the eel seemed to promote a greater frequency of these contacts. Secondly, the distribution of osmiophilic material on either side of the synaptic cleft was variable, but usually more osmiophilic material was found on the presynaptic than on the postsynaptic side. It is worthy of note that this absence of post-synaptic darkening is also found in contacts between neurosecretory fibres and pars intermedia cells of *Scylliorhinus* (KNOWLES, 1965b). One may question whether this absence of darkening denotes an absence of post-synaptic events, related to the prolonged release of neurosecretory products.

Recently synaptoid contacts between Type A neurosecretory fibres and ependyma-like elements have been seen in the neural lobe of a prosimian, the

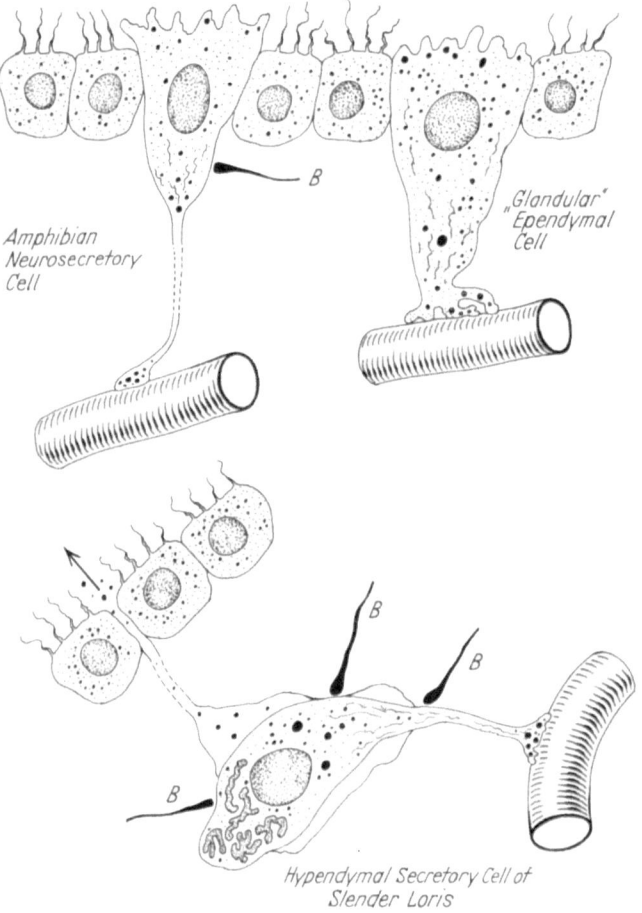

Fig. 2. Some resemblances between a Type *A* neurosecretory cell and modified ependymal elements. The figures, which are semidiagrammatic, show that a bidirectional secretion, both into the cerebrospinal fluid and the blood system, is possible in the types shown, and that Type *B* innervation of neurosecretory cells and modified ependymal elements may be found (see also Fig. 3)

slender loris (KNOWLES and ANAND KUMAR, in preparation) and it seems therefore possible that contacts between neurosecretory fibres and ependyma in the area of the neural lobe may be a consistent feature in Vertebrates.

Moreover contacts between Type B fibres and ependymal elements have been found in a more paraventricular region in the slender loris. The cells thus innervated lie for the most part in a hypendymal layer, but their apical regions are

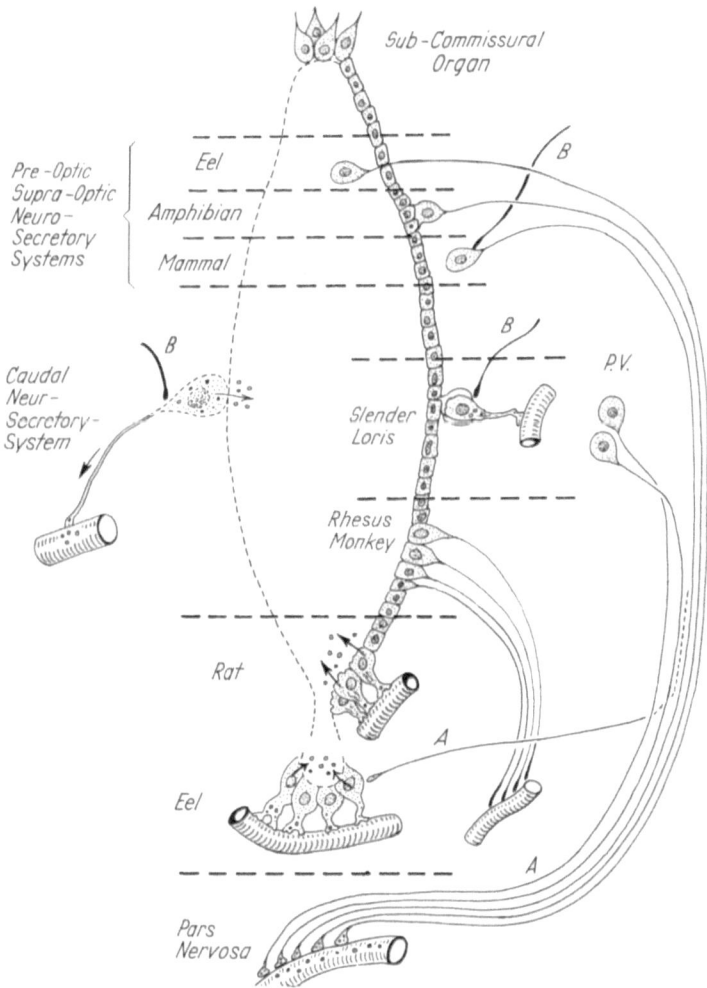

Fig. 3. A schematic drawing to illustrate some comparisons between Type *A* neurosecretory cells and modified ependymal elements of the IIIrd ventricle. — The perikarya of pre-optic, supra-optic, para-ventricular (*P.V.*) and caudal neurosecretory systems exhibit different relationships with the cerebrospinal fluid, ranging from occasional complete immersion in it, as in the eel (BUDTZ, personal communication), through partial contact in *Rana* (DIERICKX, 1962) and in the urophysis (caudal neurosecretory system) of fishes, to no evident contact as in the supraoptic and paraventricular nuclei of mammals. The principal direction of secretion in neurosecretory cells appears to be towards the blood system, through secretion into the cerebrospinal fluid has also been described. — Ventral periventricular glandular ependyma of the rat and eel appears to secrete principally into the ventricle (LEVEQUE, STUTINSKY, PORTE and STOCKEL, 1966; KNOWLES and VOLLRATH, 1966), though some signs of secretion into the blood-stream also have been observed. The main direction of secretion in the specialized lateral periventricular areas of secretory ependyma in the slender loris and Rhesus monkey has not yet been ascertained (KNOWLES and KUMAR, in preparation), though the position of these cells makes secretion either into the ventricle or the blood-system (or both) possible. — It may be seen that most of the cells illustrated form a link between the cerebrospinal fluid and the blood system. — A possible interpretation of this and other resemblances between neurosecretory cells and ependymal elements is discussed in the text

each partially surrounded by a space which appears to be in continuity with the third ventricle of the brain. There are indications that their basal regions are in contact with blood capillaries (Fig. 2).

At present Dr. Anand Kumar and I are studying in our laboratory a periventricular region of modified ependyma in the Rhesus monkey (Fig. 3). These cells which line the ventricle have exceedingly long processes which appear to terminate at blood vessels in or close to the pars tuberalis; these processes are strongly PAS-positive and Gomori-positive but do not stain with silver techniques.

It is interesting to note that various specialized areas of ependyma in the wall of the IIIrd ventricle not only form a cellular bridge between the cerebrospinal fluid and the blood system but apparently may secrete into either. In this respect they resemble the caudal neurosecretory cells of Elasmobranchs which have only short processes and resemble large gland cells with ependymal affinities, set in the spinal cord.

Professor Bern, 1967, has already drawn attention to the bidirectional secretory capacity of these and some other neurosecretory neurons. This and the special form of some neurosecretory cells allows one to raise the issue concerning their cytogenetic relations. For instance the similarity between ependymal cells and neurosecretory cells has been remarked by Olsson, 1963, Clark, 1956, and others, and it has been suggested that superficial cells which originally release from their apical surface secretory material might become secondarily specialised for secretion into body fluids through their basal regions. It is certainly interesting that both secretion and transmission of information are features of the primitive epidermis.

There are indeed reasons to consider whether Type A neurosecretory systems may have closer functional and structural relationships with ependyma than with other elements of the central nervous system, and indeed whether the classical neurosecretory systems and the various secretory ependymal elements in the hypothalamus may represent different modifications of a basic ependymal element with bidirectional secretory capability. A greater specialization of secretion into the cerebrospinal fluid may have given rise to the 'ventricular glands'; conversely greater secretion into the blood-system could have resulted in the evolution of classical neurosecretory neurons (Fig. 2 and 3). This postulate provides some explanation for the position of the perikarya of neurosecretory preoptic neurons in lower vertebrates and receives moreover experimental support in the work of Fridberg, Nisioka, Bern and Fleming, 1966, who have shown that extirpated neurosecretory elements may be replaced by ependymal elements (see also Bern, 1967).

General Discussion

A survey of the neuronal properties of neurosecretory cells, and their relationship to other cellular components of the nervous system emphasises the difficulty, which Bern and I, 1966, have already discussed, of distinguishing between 'neurosecretory' and 'ordinary' neurons, since both Type A (Peptide) and Type B (Monoamine) neurosecretory cells have many typically neuronal qualities, in terms of morphology and function. Of the two, Type A cells can be distinguished from ordinary neurons more easily by their staining reactions, their elementary neurosecretory vesicles and (in some cases) the long duration of action potentials after stimulation; it is also perhaps noteworthy that when synaptoid contacts are made between these Type A fibres and endocrine cells post-synaptic electron density is rare or absent. All these features indicate a 'neuron with glandular activity' (see BARGMANN, 1966, and YAGI and BERN, 1963) distinguished from ordinary neurons by its ability to continue a 'slow and prolonged stimulation of the target organs without fatigue of the activating system' (KNOWLES, 1955).

It is more difficult to make a clear distinction between Type B fibres and adrenergic or other monoamine-containig neurons either on morphological or physiological grounds, and it may be argued that they should not be termed neurosecretory. Yet it is evident that they, no less than Type A fibres, form an integral part of many neuroendocrine control mechanisms. Indeed studies on the pituitary pars distalis and pars intermedia of some vertebrates and the thoracic glands of insects suggests that the activity of these glands may be regulated equally by Type A and Type B fibres. Thus Type A and Type B fibres are both 'engaged directly or in endocrine control and form all or part of an endocrine organ; as such they provide the final common pathway for neuroendocrine regulation' and so may be termed neurosecretory (KNOWLES and BERN, 1966).

If however we make use of this criterion we should at the same time appreciate that some of the elements thus classified may be more 'neuronal' than others. In particular there are some grounds for the postulate that the cytogenetic and phylogenetic relationship between Type A neurosecretory cells and ependyma is closer than that between Type A cells and 'ordinary' neurons, and that Type A neurons may form a special category of neurons distinguished by structural and functional characteristics suggestive of ependyma.

The part played by modified ependyma in neuroendocrine control is as yet a relatively new and unexplored field. A discharge of P.A.S. positive material from certain specialised ependyma into the cerebrospinal fluid has been described by various workers (see LEVEQUE, STUTINSKY, PORTE and STOECKEL, 1966). In the eel the release of P.A.S. positive material into the infundibular recess appeared to be related to activity of the Type A neurosecretory fibres regulating colour-change (KNOWLES and VOLLRATH, 1966), and formed the basis for a suggestion that modified ependyma might form part of a feedback system of information connecting the proximal and distal ends of a neurosecretory system (KNOWLES and VOLLRATH, 1965, 1966). According to this concept the cerebrospinal fluid may link different components of the neuroendocrine system with the involvement of modified regions of ependyma lining the third ventricle. Thus far the evidence for this is morphological and inferential and, as Professor BERN, 1967, has pointed out, the importance of non hemal routes of neurohormones has not yet been properly assessed. Recent studies do however indicate exciting possibilities that the cerebrospinal fluid may play a greater part in neuroendocrine regulation than has hitherto been suspected.

References

ANAND KUMAR, T. C. (1965): Structure and histochemistry of the pituitary gland in the slender loris Loris tardigradus lykekkerianus cabr. (Primates). Suppl. **100**, 158. Acta endocr. (Kbh.).

BARGMANN, W. (1966): Neurosecretion. Int. Rev. Cytol. **19**, 183—201 .

Bargmann, W., A. Knoop, and A. Thiel (1957): Elektronenmikroskopische Studie an
    der Neurohypohyse von Tropidonotus natrix (mit Berücksichtigung der Pars intermedia).
    Z. Zellforsch. 47, 114—126.
Bern, H. A. (1967): The hormonogenic properties of neurosecretory cells (This volume).
—, and F. G. W. Knowles (1966): Neurosecretion. In: Neuroendocrinology, Vol. 1. (Eds.
    Martini, L., and W. F. Ganong). New York: Academic Press.
—, and R. A. Nishioka (1965): Fine structure of the median eminence of some passerine
    birds. Proc. zool. Soc. Calcutta 18, 107—119.
—, and K. Yagi (1965): Electrophysiology of neurosecretory systems. Proc. 2nd. Intern.
    Congr. of Endocrinal. Excerpta Med., Intern. Cong. Ser. 83, 577—583.
Bennett, M. V. L., and S. Fox (1962): Electrophysiology of caudal neurosecretory cells in
    the skate and fluke. Gen. comp. Endocrin. 2, 77—96.
Clarke, R. B. (1956): On the origin of neurosecretory cells. Ann. Sci. Nat. (Zool.) 18, 199—207.
Cohen, A. G. (1964): B. Sc. Thesis. University of Birmingham, England.
Dierickx, K. (1962): The dendrites of the preoptic neurosecretory nucleus of Rana tempo-
    raria and the osmoreceptors. Arch. int. Pharmacodyn. 140, 708—725.
— (1965): The origin of the aldehyde-fuchsin-negative nerve fibres of the median eminence
    of the hypophysis: a gonadotrophic centre. Z. Zellforsch. 66, 504—518.
Enemar, A., and B. Falck (1965): On the presence of adrenergic nerves in the Pars intermedia
    of the frog. Rana temporaria. Gen. comp. Endocrin. 5, 577—583.
Falck, B. (1962): Observations on the possibilities of the cellular localization of monoamines
    by a fluorescence method. Acta physiol. scand. Suppl. 197, 4—25.
Fridberg, C., R. S. Nishioka, H. A. Bern, and W. R. Fleming (1966): Regeneration of the cau-
    dal neurosecretory system in the cichlid teleost Tilapia mossambica. J. exp. Zool. (In press).
Fuxe, K. (1964): Cellular localization of monoamines in the median eminence and the in-
    fundibular stem of some mammals. Z. Zellforsch. 61, 710—274.
Gorbman, A., and H. A. Bern (1952): A textbook of Comparative Endocrinology. New York:
    John Wiley.
Holmes, R. L., and J. A. Kiernan (1964): The fine structure of the infundibular process of
    the hedgehog. Z. Zellforsch. 61, 894—912.
Kandel, E. R. (1964): Electrical properties of hypothalamic neuroendocrine cells. J. Gen.
    Physiol. 47, 691—717.
Knowles, F. G. W. (1955): Crustacean colour change and neurosecretion. Endeavour 54,
    95—104.
— (1960): A highly organised structure within a neurosecretory vesicle. Nature (Lond.) 185,
    710—711.
— (1963): Techniques in the study of neurosecretion. In: Techniques in endocrine research
    (Eds. Eckstein, P., and F. Knowles). pp. 57—65. London-New York: Academic Press.
— (1964): Vesicle formation in the distal part of a neurosecretory system. Proc. Soc. B. 160,
    360—372.
— (1965a): Neuroendocrine correlations at the level of ultrastructure. Arch. Anat. micr. 54,
    433—357.
— (1965b): Evidence for a dual control, by neurosecretion, of hormone synthesis and hormone
    release in the pituitary of the dogfish, Scylloirhinus stellaris. Phil. Trans. B. 249, 435—455.
—, and H. A. Bern (1966): The function of neurosecretion in endocrine regulation. Nature
    (Lond.) 210, 271—272.
—, and A. Kumar: In preparation.
—, and L. Vollrath (1965): A functional relationship between neurosecretory fibres and
    pituicytes in the eel. Nature (Lond.) 208, 1343.
— — (1966): Neurosecretory innervation of the pituitary of the eels Anguilla and Conger.
    Phil. Trans. B. 250, 311—342.
— —, and R. S. Nishioka (1966): In preparation.
Lederis, K. (1964): The fine structure and hormone content of the hypothalamo-neuro-
    hypophysial system of the rainbow trout (Salmo iridens) exposed to sea-water. Gen. Comp.
    Endocrin. 4, 638—661.
— (1965): An electron microscopical study of the human neurohypophysis Z. Zellforsch. 65,
    847—868.

Leveque, T. F., and G. A. Hofkin (1962): A hypothalamic periventricular PAS substance and neuroendocrine mechanisms. Anat. Rec. **142**, 252.

—, and J. I. Stern (1964): A periventricular PAS reactive site in the frog hypothalamus. Anat. Rec. **148**, 306.

— F. Stutinsky, A. Porte, et M. E. Stoeckel (1966): Morphologie fine d'une differentiation glandulaire du recessus infundibulaire chez le rat. Z. Zellforsch. **69**, 381—394.

Lichtensteiger, W., and H. Langemann (1965): Uptake of exogenous catecholamines by monoaminecontaining neurons of the central nervous system; uptake of catecholamines by arcuato-infundibular neurons. J. Pharmac. exp. Ther. **151**, 400—408.

Markee, J. E., J. W. Everett, and C. H. Sawyer (1952): The relationship of the nervous system to the release of gonadotrophin and the regulation of the sex-cycle. Rec. Progr. Hormon. Res. **7**, 139—163.

Normann, T. C. (1965): The neurosecretory system of the adult *Calliphora erythrocephala*. Z. Zellforsch. **67**, 461—501.

Olsson, R. (1963): The evolution of neurosecretory cells and systems. Proceedings. XVI Int. Congr. Zool. (Wash.) **3**, 38—43.

Palay, S. L. (1957): The fine structure of the neurohypophysis. In: Ultrastructure and Cellular Chemistry of Neural Tissue. (Ed. H. Waelsch) 31—49. (Progress in Neurobiology), Vol. 2. (Eds. Korey and Nurnburger). New York: Hoeber.

Scharrer, B. (1963): Neurosecretion XIII. The ultrastructure of the corpus cardiacum of the insect *Leucophaea maderae*. Z. Zellforsch. **60**, 761—796.

Scharrer, E. (1962): Mem. Soc. Endocrin No. **12**, 421—424.

— (1965): The final common path in neuroendocrine integration. Arch. Anat. micr. **54**, 359—370.

Smoller, C. G. (1965): Neurosecretory processes extending into the third ventricle: secretory or sensory? Science **147**, 882—884.

Vigh, B., B. Aros, T. Wenger, S. Koritsansky, and G. Cegledi (1963): Ependymosecretion. (Ependymal Secretion) IV. The gomori-positive secretion of the hypothalamic ependyma of various vertebrates and its relation to the anterior pituitary. Acta. Biol. Hung. **13**, 407—419.

Yagi, K., and H. A. Bern (1963): Electrophysiologic indications of the osmoregulatory role of the teleost urophysis. Science **142**, 491—493.

Mode de libération des produits de neurosécrétion

M. Herlant

Université Libre de Bruxelles, Laboratoire d'Histologie, Laboratoire de Microscopie électronique

Le mode de libération du neuro-sécrétat dans les vaisseaux irriguant le lobe postérieur demeure un problème très controversé. La vasopressine et l'ocytocine sont bien véhiculées par les granulations qui viennent s'accumuler à l'extrémité des fibres neuro-sécrétrices, mais ces hormones qui sont des octopeptides n'existent apparemment pas à l'état libre dans les granulations. Elles sont associées à une molécule protéique beaucoup plus volumineuse (van Dyke et coll., 1942, Hild et Zetler, 1953; Acher, 1958). Acher a désigné cette association protéique sous le terme de «neurophysine». La neurophysine a été isolée et, actuellement, on lui attribue un poids moléculaire de 25.000 (Ginsburg et Ireland, 1963). Au cours de leur libération, les hormones demeurent apparemment associées à leur substrat protéique (van Dyke et coll., 1955; Heller, 1955; Acher, 1958; Ishii et coll., 1962).

Le problème qui se pose donc à nous consiste à envisager si l'excrétion de ce matériel protéique dans les vaisseaux peut être saisi morphologiquement et, dans l'affirmative, à en préciser les modalités.

A l'heure actuelle, la question ne peut être tranchée que par la microscopie électronique qui seule, nous révèle la nature granulaire du neuro-sécrétat.

Les bases morphologiques du problème reposent tout d'abord sur l'étude des barrières que doivent franchir les produits excrétés. Il nous faut donc analyser en premier lieu, la nature des rapports existant entre les extrémités des fibres neuro-sécrétrices et les vaisseaux sanguins.

I. Rapports entre les terminaisons nerveuses et les capillaires

Chez les Mammifères, la nature des contacts entre les terminaisons nerveuses et les vaisseaux a été étudiée chez le Rat (Palay, 1957; Hartmann, 1958), le Lapin (Fujgita et Hartmann, 1961), l'Opossum (Bodian, 1963), l'Homme (Lederis, 1965). Nous avons repris personnellement son analyse chez la Chauve-Souris, Myotis myotis.

Une première constatation importante doit être soulignée: les fibres nerveuses à leur extrémité sont toujours séparées de l'endothelium par un espace périvasculaire important, occupé par une substance amorphe d'apparence homogène, très pauvre en fibrilles collagènes. C'est dans cette substance fondamentale que viennent baigner les terminaisons des fibres neurosécrétrices et les expansions des pituicytes. La limite externe de l'espace périvasculaire est souvent très diffuse car on le voit s'insinuer profondément entre les fibres nerveuses, tantôt sous

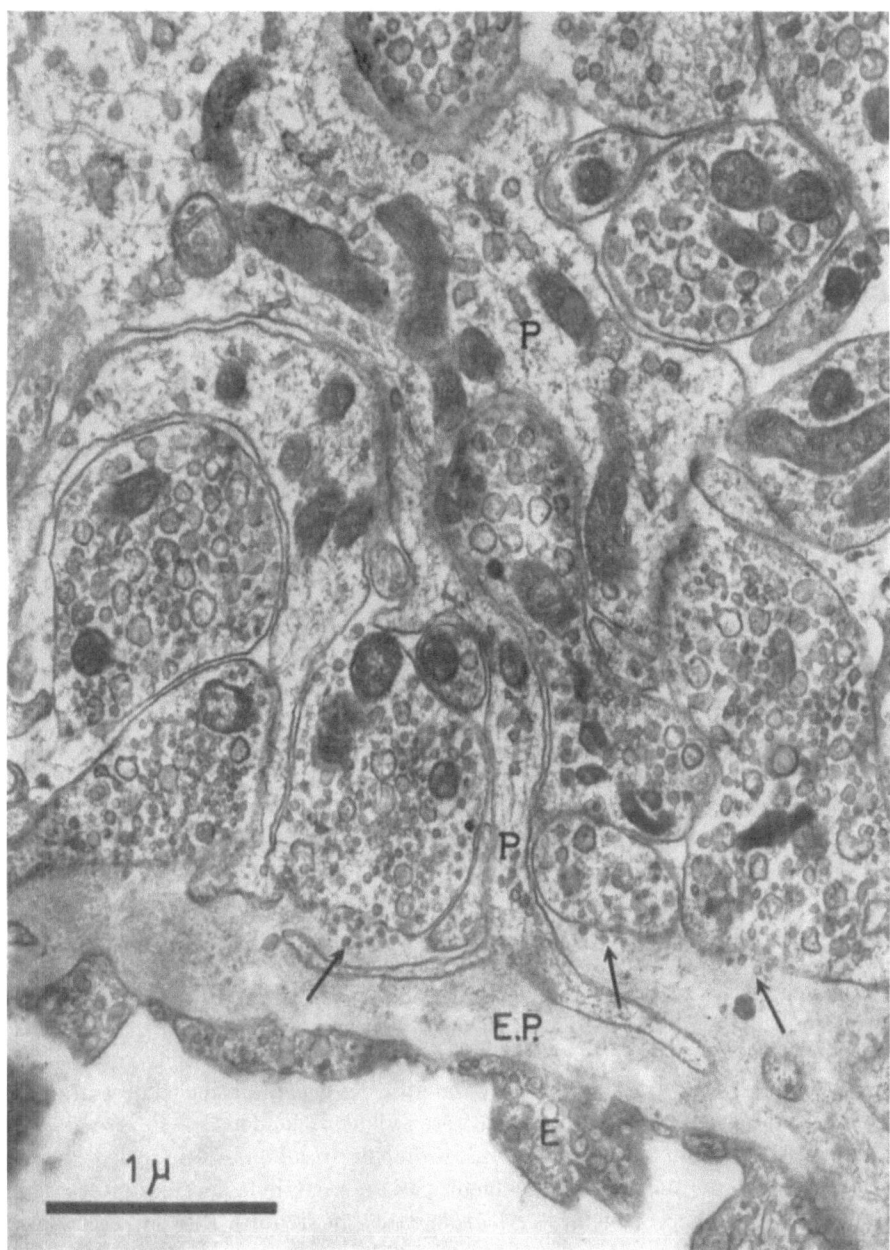

Fig. 1. Chauve-Souris (Myotis myotis) en lactation. Lobe postérieur. Fix: Palade. Incl.: Vestopal. Col.: acétate d'uranyle + Reynolds. X 44.000. Fibres neurosécrétrices au contact d'un capillaire. E: cytoplasme d'une cellule endothéliale contenant des vésicules de pinocytose. E.P.: espace péri-vasculaire renfermant un matériel amorphe. P: prolongement d'un pituicyte venant s'arboriser dans l'espace péri-vasculaire. Les flèches montrent des microvésicules apparemment libérées au niveau de la membrane terminale des fibres neurosécrétrices. Ces dernières contiennent des granules élémentaires en voie de déplétion dont beaucoup présentent des images de bourgeonnement

l'aspect d'interstices étroits, tantôt sous l'aspect de lacunes irrégulières. Par suite de l'existence de ces lacunes, il n'est pas aisé de se faire une idée précise de la morphologie des extrémités nerveuses. Les terminaisons en massue ne sont vraisemblablement qu'apparentes. Fréquemment, comme Bodian l'a observé chez l'Opossum, nous avons constaté la présence de digitations irrégulières de taille variable correspondant apparemment aux ramifications terminales d'une même fibre. Ces digitations demeurent tantôt assemblées, tantôt, elles s'écartent les unes des autres dans les lacunes de l'espace périvasculaire (fig. 1 et fig. 3).

Autour de la lumière du vaisseau, le cytoplasme des cellules endothéliales forme un revêtement continu d'épaisseur variable. Chez la Chauve-Souris, comme chez le Rat, le Lapin et l'Homme, il semble présenter de nombreux pores, mais un examen attentif montre qu'à ce niveau, la lumière vasculaire demeure séparée de l'espace périvasculaire par une membrane mince qui résulte bien, comme l'a décrit Palay, de la coalescence des membranes externe et interne de la cellule endothéliale. Vers la lumière, le cytoplasme des cellules endothéliales ne présente que des expansions peu développées, mais dans l'espace périvasculaire, il peut se prolonger par des languettes irrégulières souvent étendues. En outre, de place en place, l'espace périvasculaire est occupé par des cellules conjonctives qui semblent des histiocytes.

II. Les granules élémentaires

Comme la plupart des cellules glandulaires qui sécrètent des protéines, les cellules neuro-sécrétrices sont le siège d'un phénomène de ségrégation, elles élaborent leur secrétion sous la forme de granulations figurées. Elles ne diffèrent d'éléments glandulaires banaux que par le fait qu'elles sont en outre des neurones et que les granules qu'elles élaborent s'écoulent le long de leurs axones. Ce phéno-mène de ségrégation granulaire se retrouve chez tous les Vertébrés. Depuis les observations de Green et van Bremen, 1955, chez le Rat, le Chat et l'Opossum, de Palay, 1955, 1957, chez le Rat, de Bargmann et Knoop, 1957, chez le Chat et le Chien, de Fugita, 1957, chez le Chien mais aussi celles de Dunkan, 1956, chez le Coq, de Bargmann, 1958, chez la Couleuvre, de Gerschenfeld, Tra-mezzani et de Robertis, 1960, chez le Crapaud, de Bargmann et Knoop, 1960, de Follenius et Porte, 1961, chez les Poissons on sait qu'au microscope élec-tronique, le neuro-sécrétat se présente sous l'aspect de granulations figurées. Les corps de Hering, en particulier, correspondent à des accumulations de ces granules et c'est sous cet aspect que le neuro-sécrétat vient se condenser à l'extrémité des fibres nerveuses. Chez les Mammifères, au niveau du lobe postérieur, le diamètre de ces granules ne montre pratiquement pas de variations spécifiques et oscille entre 1.000 et 3.000 Å, leur taille est cependant plus réduite chez les Poissons et ne dépasse guère 750 à 875 Å (Follenius, 1965).

Comme toutes les granulations élaborées par des cellules glandulaires, les granules élémentaires du neuro-sécrétat sont entourés d'une membrane d'origine golgienne. On peut donc en conclure que le neuro-sécrétat est formé de vésicules arrondies contenant un matériel dense. Ce dernier présente habituellement un aspect homogène. Cependant, chez le Hérisson, par exemple, (Holmes et Kernan, 1964), le contenu des granules offre une structure d'apparence cristalline, il apparait formé de bâtonnets hexagonaux et la membrane d'enveloppe est elle-même striée. Plus suggestifs encore sont les aspects que révèlent à très fort grossissement, les granules élémentaires chez l'Homme (LEDERIS, 1965). On y distingue en effet une accumulation de microvésicules de 50 à 100 Å de diamètre. Or, à un grossissement de x 120.000, nous avons retrouvé les mêmes micro-vésicules dans des granules élémentaires de Myotis myotis (fig. 4).

Le granule élémentaire apparait donc comme la base morphologique de la sécrétion. Ce n'est pas un élément statique, il peut se vider de son contenu. En effet, ces organites se présentent, tantôt comme des corpuscules pleins, tantôt comme des vésicules vides correspondant uniquement à leur membrane d'enve-loppe. On peut de plus, saisir toutes les étapes de leur déplétion depuis le stade où le matériel dense emplit toute la membrane qui l'entoure jusqu'à sa disparition complète en passant par des phases où les granules offrent un aspect ombiliqué et ne contiennent qu'un amas dense central entouré d'un espace clair.

D'autre part, des contrôles biologiques ont démontré que les granules élémen-taires étaient bien les véhicules des activités hormonales. La technique des centri-fugations différentielles a permis leur isolement à partir de neurohypophyses de boeufs, de lapins, de rats (SCHIEBLER, 1952; PARDOE et WEATHERHALL, 1955; WEINSTEIN, MALAMED et SACHS, 1961; HELLER et LEDERIS, 1962; LA BELLA, BEAULIEU et REIFENFSTEIN, 1962). Les suspensions de granules ainsi obtenues se sont révélées beaucoup plus riches en vasopressine et en ocytocine que le liquide surnageant. C'est ainsi par exemple qu'HELLER et LEDERIS, 1962, sont arrivés à récupérer dans la fraction granulaire, respectivement 78,4% et 77,7% de la teneur en vasopressine et en ocytocine contenue dans un homogénat total de lobe posté-rieur. Certaines constatations semblent suggérer que les granules vecteurs de l'ocytocine puissent être distincts de ceux contenant la vasopressine, mais à l'heure actuelle, cette distinction repose essentiellement sur des gradients de densité différents au cours des centrifugations (HELLER et LEDERIS, 1962; LA BELLA, BEAULIEU et REIFFENSTEIN, 1962). Ces résultats ne permettent toutefois pas d'affirmer avec certitude que les deux activités hormonales sont véhiculées par des fibres neuro-sécrétrices distinctes.

III. Les vésicules synaptiques ou soi-disant telles

Dans les terminaisons des fibres neuro-sécrétrices, les granules élémentaires sont toujours associés à des corpuscules de taille beaucoup plus réduite se pré-sentant habituellement sous l'aspect de petites vésicules qu'à la suite de PALAY, 1957, qui fut le premier à les décrire, on considère classiquement comme des vésicules synaptiques.

Leur diamètre oscille entre 200 et 600 Å. Comme les vésicules synaptiques, ces organites sont entourés d'une membrane nettement bilaminée et généralement, leur contenu n'apparait que faiblement plus dense que le cytoplasme avoisinant. Des densités plus élevées sont le plus souvent attribuables à des coupes tangen-tielles, cependant, on peut constater que ces vésicules contiennent parfois un corpuscule plus dense. Leur présence apparait limitée aux terminaisons nerveuses. Leur répartition est très variable, tantôt, elles sont disposées en amas condensés comme dans une terminaison nerveuse banale, tantôt, elles sont éparpillées entre les granules élémentaires, tantôt encore, elles viennent s'accumuler au voisinage de la membrane plasmatique. Certaines fibres semblent ne contenir que des micro-vésicules, cependant, des coupes favorables montrent qu'en d'autres segments de leur trajet, elles renferment également des granules élémentaires.

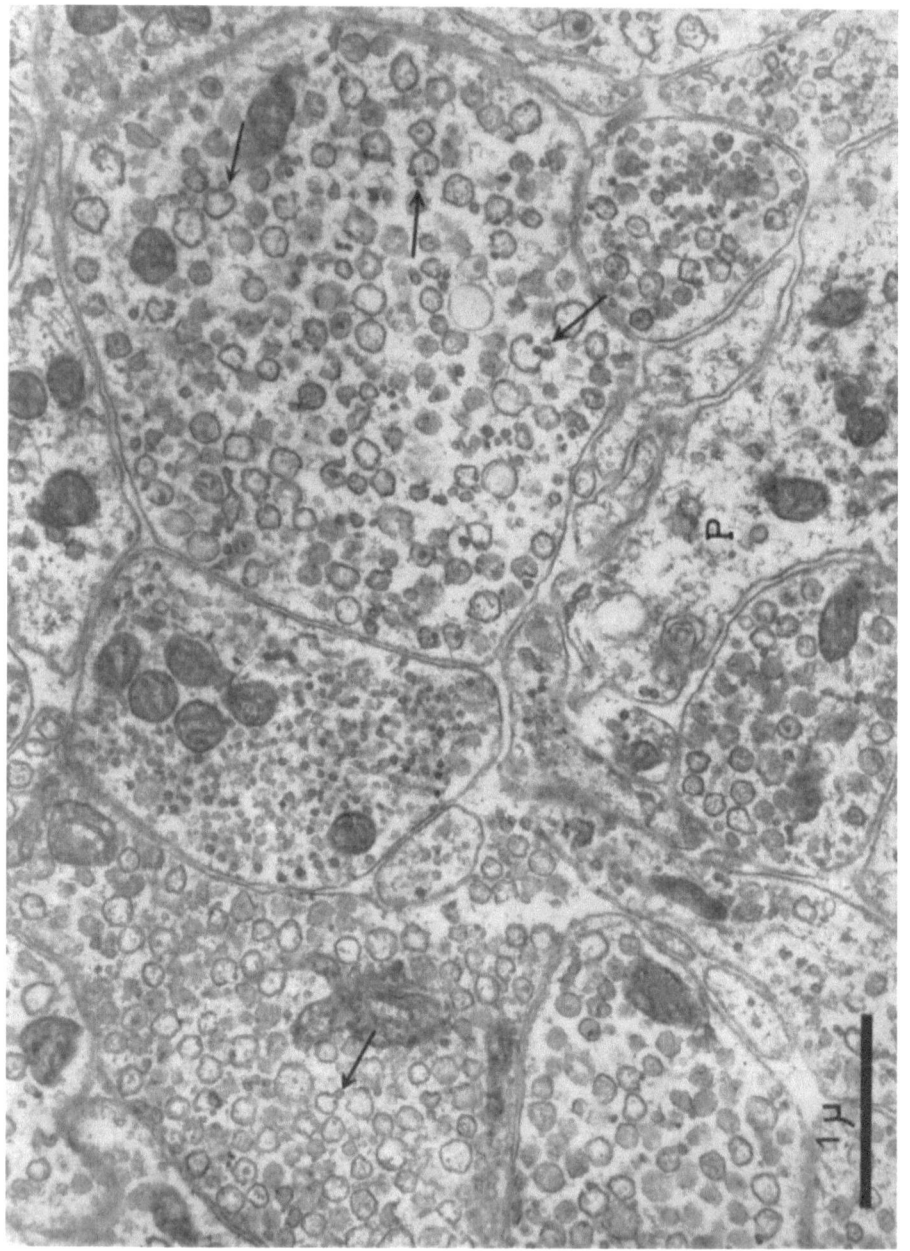

Fig. 2. Même matériel que la figure 1. Fibres neurosécrétrices contenant des granules élémentaires en voie de déplétion. Au niveau de ces granules, les images de bourgeonnement sont particulièrement abondantes. Trois d'entre elles sont désignées par des flèches. Au centre, une fibre semble uniquement contenir des microvésicules dont certaines paraissent contenir un matériel dense. P: Cytoplasme d'un pituicyte

Malgré une convergence d'aspect évidente, il n'existe pas actuellement d'argu-ments décisifs permettant de conclure que toutes ces microvésicules correspondent indistinctement à des vésicules synaptiques. Dans le système nerveux central, on sait que les vésicules synaptiques sont les véhicules de l'acétylcholine et des enzymes participant à sa synthèse, mais cette connaissance est basée sur l'étude neurochimique de vésicules synaptiques isolées par centrifugation différentielle (WHITTAKER, 1959; DE ROBERTIS, 1961, 1964). Or, jusqu'à présent, l'isolement des microvésicules contenues dans les terminaisons nerveuses du lobe postérieur n'a pas été réalisée et l'analyse de la teneur du lobe postérieur en acéthylcholine et en cholinestérases a livré des résultats contradictoires. Une richesse particulière en corps cholinergiques a été mise en évidence chez la Vache (UEMURA et coll., 1963), mais chez les Mammifères du moins, la répartition des activités cholinestérasiques semble très variable. Une réaction faiblement positive a été signalée chez le Chat (KOELLE et GEESEY, 1961), mais HOLMES, 1962, n'a obtenu de résultat positif que chez le Hérisson; chez le Furet, la réaction s'est révélée inconstante et elle était négative chez le Macaque, le Rat, le Lapin. La présence de ces enzymes semble plus généralisée dans le lobe postérieur des Vertébrés non mammaliens; elle a été signalée chez divers Passereaux, chez un Chélonien, chez un Urodèle, chez la Carpe (UEMURA, 1964; KOBAYASHI et FARNER, 1964; KOBAYASHI, 1964).

Dynamique de l'excrétion hormonale. La localisation des hormones associées à un substrat protéique au niveau des granules élémentaires étant démontrée, il nous faut à présent envisager le problème de leur libération à partir de ces granules et leur excrétion dans les vaisseaux sanguins. Il semble certain que ce processus s'effectue d'une manière distincte de celui que l'on observe au niveau de cellules glandulaires élaborant également des protéines sous l'aspect de granulations figurées. Depuis la mise en évidence de ce dernier mode d'excrétion au niveau des cellules acidophiles du lobe antérieur de l'hypophyse (FARQUHAR, 1961) il est actuellement bien connu et il a été observé dans les parenchymes glandulaires les plus divers. Il a en réalité pour effet d'isoler jusqu'à leur excrétion, les produits de sécrétion du cytoplasme. En effet, au cours de l'excrétion, l'enveloppe du grain qui est d'origine golgienne se soude à la membrane plasmatique, celle-ci s'ouvre à l'extérieur, le contenu du grain est libéré dans l'espace périvasculaire, tandis que son enveloppe persiste sous l'aspect d'une vésicule vide. On n'a jamais saisi de manière certaine un phénomène similaire au niveau des terminaisons des fibres neuro-sécrétrices. On n'a jamais signalé jusqu'à présent d'accolement de granules élémentaires à la membrane de la terminaison nerveuse ni de libération d'un matériel figuré dans l'espace périvasculaire.

L'excrétion hormonale semble uniquement se traduire morphologiquement par la disparition *in situ* du contenu des granules élémentaires avec conservation de leur membrane d'enveloppe. En effet, l'apparition massive de vésicules vidées de leur contenu au niveau des terminaisons neurosécrétrices a été observée chez le Crapaud soumis à la deshydratation (GERSCHENFELD et coll., 1960) de même que chez des rats et des lapins traités par des libérateurs des hormones posthypophysaires (HARTMANN, 1958; FUJITA et HARTMANN, 1961). Le stimulus de la tétée a une influence similaire chez la ratte en lactation, il a également pour effet de vider totalement les granules élémentaires de leur contenu dense (MONROE et SCOTT, 1966). Lorsque des femelles sont sacrifiées alors qu'elles allaitent, la plupart des terminaisons nerveuses ne contiennent que des vésicules vides, cependant, le renouvellement des granules élémentaires semble rapide; en effet, si le sacrifice est pratiqué une heure après que les rattes aient été séparées de leur portée, on assiste à une réapparition massive de granules denses.

Chez nos Chauves-Souris en lactation que nous avons sacrifié alors qu'elles allaitaient, nous avons également constaté qu'un grand nombre de terminaisons nerveuses contenaient des vésicules complètement ou presque complètement vidées de leur contenu (fig. 1, 2 et 3). Le phénomène ne semblait toutefois pas aussi

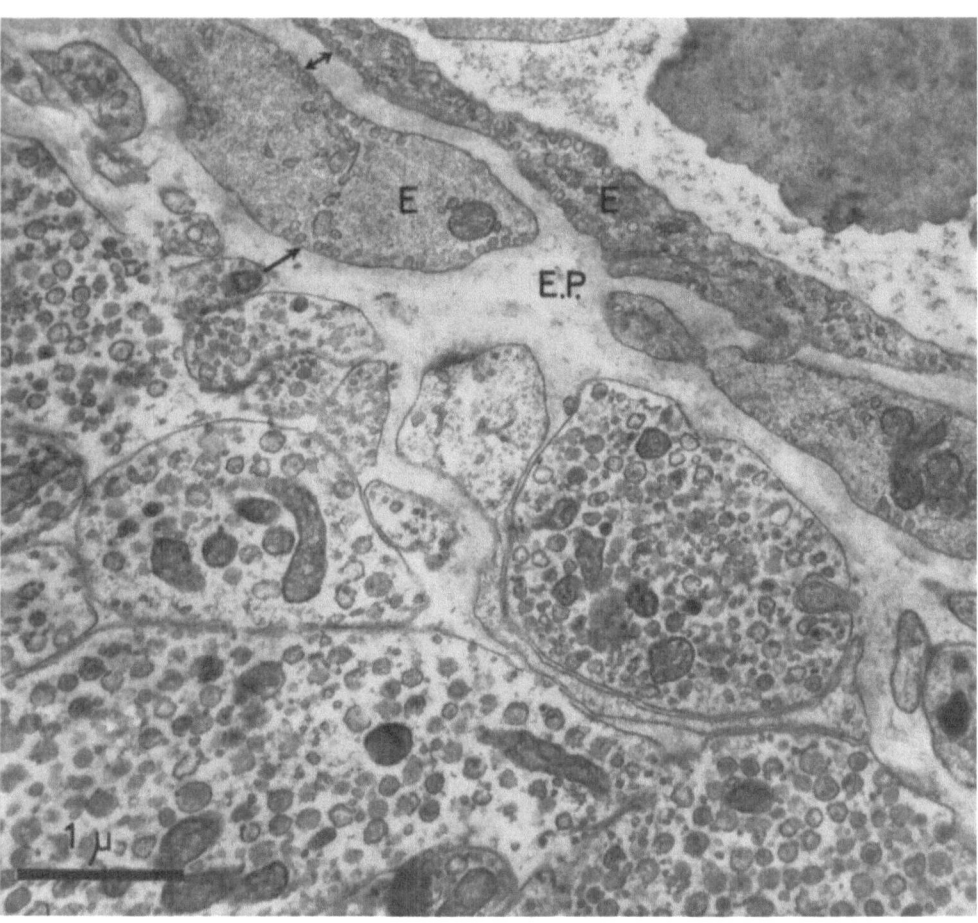

Fig. 3. Même matériel. Même traitement. X 32.000. Rapports des fibres neurosécrétrices avec la paroi du capillaire. E. P.: espace péri-vasculaire séparant les fibres de la paroi endothéliale et s'insinuant entre les terminaisons nerveuses. Abondance massive de vésicules de pinocytose (flèches) au niveau de la membrane plasmatique des cellules endothéliales. Ces vésicules forment par endroits un liseré continu

généralisé que celui décrit par Monroe et Scott chez la ratte en lactation. Sa distribution apparait régionale car chez un même animal, on peut observer autour d'autres capillaires, la présence de terminaisons nerveuses qui toutes, sont bourrées de granules denses. Il est possible d'ailleurs qu'on puisse expliquer de cette manière certaines discordances entre les constatations morphologiques et les dosages. Chez le Lapin comme le Rat par exemple, on peut observer une déplétion massive des granules élémentaires à la suite d'une saignée ou d'une anesthésie prolongée sans qu'elle s'accompagne d'une chute importante de la teneur du lobe postérieur en hormones (LEDERIS, 1964). De même chez l'Homme, LEDERIS, 1965, a observé des variations individuelles considérables au niveau des terminaisons neuro-secrétrices, dans certains lobes postérieurs, celles qui ne contenaient que des vésicules vidées de leur contenu semblaient beaucoup plus abondantes que dans d'autre et cependant, la teneur de ces lobes en vasopressine et en ocytocine n'ét ait nullement abaissée par rapport à la moyenne relevée chez l'Homme. On ne peut toutefois conclure à une déplétion granulaire généralisée qu'à la condition d'examiner un grand nombre de prélèvements exécutés dans toute l'étendue de l'organe. Il est possible comme le suggère LEDERIS que la disparition du matériel dense au niveau des granules élémentaires corresponde à une dissociation entre les hormones et leur substrat protéique et à la redistribution des deux composantes au sein de la fibre nerveuse, mais nous n'en n'avons nullement la preuve.

La disparition du contenu des granules *in situ* au travers d'une membrane encore apparemment intacte n'explique pas encore le mécanisme de l'excrétion hormonale dans les vaisseaux. Ce problème demeure très discuté car deux théories opposées s'affrontent, la théorie du transfert synaptique, la théorie «transformationiste» suivant laquelle les microvésicules résulteraient du morcellement des granules élémentaires.

A. Théorie du transfert synaptique.

Cette théorie a été échafaudée par l'école de DE ROBERTIS (GERSCHENFELD, TRAMEZZANI et DE ROBERTIS, 1960; DE ROBERTIS, 1964), elle est actuellement considérée comme classique. Suivant cette conception, les microvésicules présentes dans les terminaisons des fibres neuro-secrétrices doivent être considérées comme de véritables vésicules synaptiques, c'est à dire comme des réceptacles de substances cholinergiques. Celles-ci sont libérées à la suite de la stimulation des neurones d'origine des fibres et agissent au niveau de la membrane de la terminaison nerveuse pour modifier sa perméabilité et permettre l'excrétion hormonale. Cette théorie est également défendue par l'école de KOBAYASHI. Pour OOTA, 1963, par exemple, au cours d'une excitation des cellules neuro-secrétoires, les stimuli se propagent le long des fibres jusqu' aux vésicules synaptiques présentes à leurs extrémités. Il est exact que la stimulation électrique stéréotaxique des noyaux supraoptiques et para-ventriculaires entraine une excrétion de vasopressine rapide (STUTINSKY et GUERNE, 1965); des influx peuvent donc se propager le long des fibres neurosecrétrices, mais il n'est pas démontré qu'ils y provoquent la libération de substances cholinergiques.

Soulignons aussi que les défenseurs de cette théorie assimilent étroitement le lobe postérieur à l'éminence médiane et à l'urophyse des Poissons. La richesse de ces deux organes en substances cholinergiques et en cholinestérases a été effectivement démontrée. C'est ainsi, par exemple, que l'urophyse des Poissons marins a une teneur en substances cholinergiques 100 fois plus élevée que celle du cerveau (KOBAYASHI et coll., 1963). De même l'éminence médiane du Rat, des Oiseaux, des Reptiles, des Batraciens est également riche en substances cholinergiques et en cholinestérases (KOBAYASHI, 1964; KOBAYASHI et coll., 1966). Cependant, aussi bien l'urophyse des Poissons que l'éminence médiane ont une constitution beaucoup plus complexe que le lobe postérieur, l'une et l'autre contiennent des catégories distinctes de fibres nerveuses. De plus, alors que l'existence des jonctions synaptiques au niveau du lobe postérieur demeure discutée, de véritables synapses

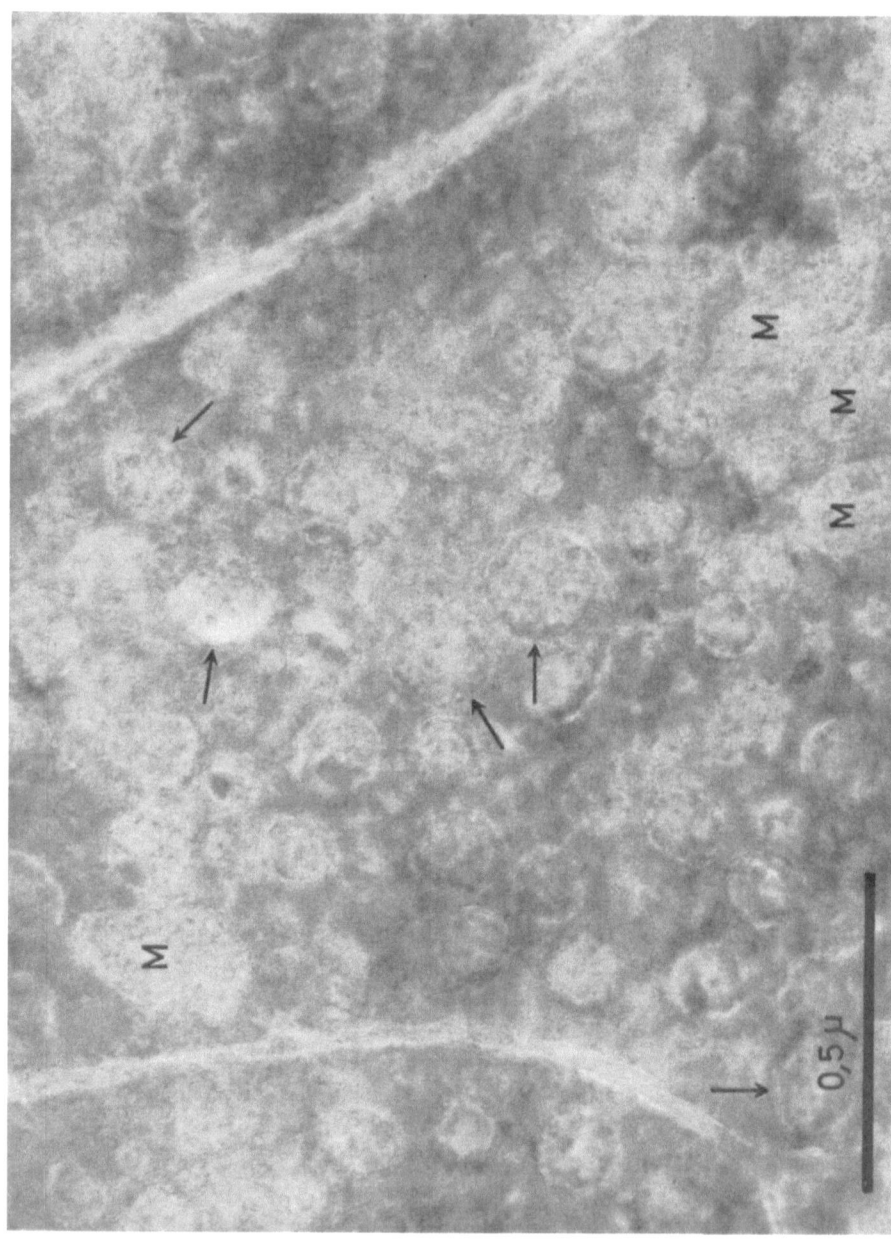

Fig. 4. Image négative à fort grossissement (X 120.000) après dissociation de l'osmium par H₂O₂ de granules élémentaires dans une fibre neurosécrétrice de Chauve-Souris en lactation. Les granules apparaissent formés d'une accumulation de

ont été observés aussi bien dans l'urophyse des Poissons (Bern et coll., 1965) que dans l'éminence médiane où elles semblent abondantes (Kobayashi et Oota, 1964; Kobayashi, Hirano et Oota, 1965). Certes, ces deux organes contiennent aussi des terminaisons nerveuses chargées comme celles du lobe postérieur, de granules élémentaires et de microvésicules mais il n'est nullement exclu que la teneur élevée de l'urophyse des Poissons et de l'éminence médiane en substances cholinergiques et en cholinestérases soit en rapport avec la présence de ces jonctions synaptiques.

Si les microvésicules présentes dans les terminaisons des fibres neuro-secrétrices correspondent bien à des vésicules synaptiques, elles joueraient un rôle distinct de celui qu'elles exercent normalement dans le système nerveux comme le soulignent fort justement PICARD et STAHL, 1966, dans leur rapport; en effet, les substances cholinergiques qu'elles contiendraient n'auraient pas pour action la transmission d'un influx nerveux à un autre neurone ou à un effecteur, mais bien une modification de perméabilité membranaire permettant une libération d'hormone. L'hypothèse demeure en réalité défendable puisque l'on sait que la libération d'acétylcholine au niveau des synapses entraine des modifications de perméabilité membranaire. On peut d'ailleurs invoquer l'exemple de la médullaire surrénalienne, qui n'est pas sans analogies avec les organes neuro-sécrétoires. La libération des catécholamines à partir des cellules de la médullaire à la suite de la stimulation électrique du nerf splanchnique a été suivie au microscope électronique (DE ROBERTIS et VAS FERREIRA, 1957). Sous l'effet de cette stimulation, les vésicules synaptiques contenues dans les terminaisons du nerf splanchnique viennent s'accumuler au voisinage de la zône de contact de la fibre avec la cellule glandulaire, mais à ce niveau, la membrane est épaissie et forme une véritable jonction synaptique, de plus, aux deux côtés de la jonction on observe un accroisse-

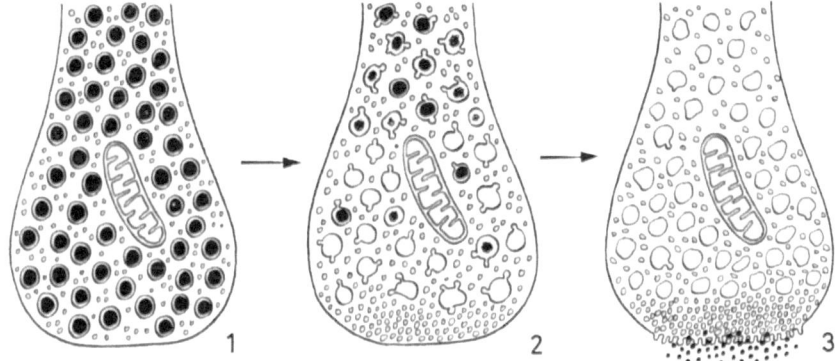

Fig. 5. Schéma possible du mécanisme d'excrétion au niveau des extrémités des fibres neuro-sécrétrices. 1. Accumulation de granules élémentaires pleins à l'extrémité de la fibre. 2. Bourgeonnement des granules aboutissant à la formation de microvésicules qui se libèrent. Ces microvésicules viennent s'accumuler contre la membrane basale. 3. Expulsion du matériel neuro-sécrétoire à partir des microvésicules. L'extrusion aboutit à la libération dans l'espace péri-vasculaire d'un matériel corpusculaire figuré

ment considérable de la densité électronique. D'autre part, au niveau de la cellule glandulaire, la libération des catécholamines s'effectue suivant les mêmes modalités que dans des cellules sécrétant des protéines. En effet, les vésicules contenant les catécholamines viennent s'accoler à la membrane plasmatique et libèrent leur contenu à l'extérieur. A nouveau, le produit de sécrétion n'entre pas en contact

avec le cytoplasme de la cellule glandulaire. Les conditions sont toutefois différentes au niveau des terminaisons neuro-sécrétrices. En effet, si les microvésicules
qui s'y accumulent correspondent à des vésicules synaptiques, il faut tout d'abord
admettre, comme le souligne DE ROBERTIS, 1964, l'intégration de deux mécanismes
neurohumoraux distincts dans une même cellule. En effet, les neurones d'origine
de ces terminaisons sont simultanément responsables de l'élaboration d'un matériel
sécrétoire et du médiateur assurant sa libération. Cette hypothèse peut évidemment
se défendre car les neurones du système hypothalamo-hypophysaire apparaissent
comme des éléments hautement spécialisés.

Le fait que les granules élémentaires semblent se vider de leur contenu dans
le cytoplasme de la terminaison nerveuse étonne davantage. Il implique comme
le suggère BARGMANN, 1966, que le médiateur libéré par les vésicules synaptiques
n'agit pas uniquement au niveau de la membrane plasmatique, mais qu'il modifie
également la paroi des granules.

B. Théorie «Transformationiste» du morcellement des granules en microvésicules

Cette disparition *in situ* du matériel dense contenu dans les granules élémentaires sans qu'on arrive à saisir son excrétion dans les vaisseaux demeure un
phénomène singulier. On a bien signalé la présence dans les capillaires du lobe
postérieur de gouttelettes présentant les mêmes affinités tinctoriales et les mêmes
propriétés histochimiques que le matériel neuro-sécrétoire (HANSTRÖM, 1952;
ROTHBALLER, 1953; SCHARRER et FRANDSON, 1954; HELLER et LEDERIS, 1962).
Mais la libération de ce matériel à partir des terminaisons nerveuses n'a pas été
observée jusqu'ici à l'échelle de la microscopie fine.

La théorie «transformationiste» de BERN (BERN, 1963; BERN, YAGI et NISHIOKA,
1965; FRIDBERG, IWASAKI, YAGI, BERN, WILSON et NISHIOKA, 1966) apparait
susceptible de dissiper cette énigme. Sans exclure la présence de vésicules synaptiques dans les terminaisons nerveuses, BERN et ses collaborateurs sont d'avis que les
granules élémentaires pourraient donner naissance à des microvésicules, comparables
d'aspect aux vésicules synaptiques. Dans l'urophyse des Poissons en particulier,
après stimulation électrique, ils observent l'apparition de microvésicules pleines
au contact de granules élémentaires en voie de déplétion. Cette théorie a été
également défendue par HOLMES et KNOWLES, 1960, et par LEDERIS, 1963, 1964,
1965. Pour LEDERIS, 1965, l'aspect structuré qu'il observe dans les granules
élémentaires pourrait correspondre à des microvésicules susceptibles de se libérer
dans l'axoplasme au moment de la déplétion du granule. Dans la discussion de
leurs observations sur le lobe postérieur de rattes en lactation, MONROE et SCOTT,
1966, envisagent également l'éventualité d'une fragmentation de la membrane
des granules en microvésicules et ils émettent l'hypothèse d'un transfert hormonal
par ces microvésicules.

L'étude du lobe postérieur de Chauve-Souris (Myotis myotis), en lactation que
nous avons personnellement pratiquée, livre également des images qui plaident
en faveur de la théorie «transformationiste». Nous avons déjà signalé que dans les
terminaisons nerveuses au voisinage des vaisseaux, on peut observer toutes les
étapes de la déplétion granulaire. Chez les femelles sacrifiées alors qu'elles allaitaient, les fibres contenant des vésicules vides prédominent mais au sein de ces

terminaisons, on retrouve également des granules contenant du matériel dense à divers stades de sa déplétion. Or, au niveau de très nombreux granules, on observe des images qu'on peut interpréter comme un phénomène de bourgeonnement. Ce phénomène peut affecter deux modalités distinctes : les vésicules vidées deviennent souvent pléomorphes comme l'ont signalé MONROE et SCOTT, 1966, leur paroi apparait rompue et forme un anneau incomplètement fermé dont les deux extrémités s'enroulent et donnent naissance à une microvésicule de même dimension qu'une vésicule synaptique. Cette ouverture du granule peut s'observer alors qu'il contient encore du matériel dense. Mais un examen attentif montre aussi que la paroi de multiples grains en voie de déplétion peut être le siège d'une ou de plusieurs hernies arrondies dans lesquelles s'engage du matériel dense. Ces hernies de la membrane semblent ultérieurement se transformer en microvésicules et se libérer (fig. 1 et fig. 2).

Nous reconnaissons volontiers que ces images doivent être interprétées avec une grande prudence et qu'on ne peut d'emblée leur attribuer une signification fonctionnelle. Soulignons tout d'abord que le bourgeonnement de microvésicules à partir de membranes lipoprotéiques ne constitue pas un phénomène exceptionnel. Il s'observe en particulier de manière constante au niveau de l'appareil de Golgi lorsqu'il est actif. L'apparition de microvésicules aux dépens de membranes disloquées et vidées de leur contenu pourraient simplement correspondre au morcellement de la paroi des granules élémentaires après leur déplétion.

Les images de bourgeonnement que nous avons retrouvé en grande abondance chez des Chauves-Souris en lactation et même chez les Chauves-Souris gravides sont justifiables d'une autre interprétation. On peut en effet admettre que c'est par un tel processus que se réalise la déplétion des granules élémentaires. Leur paroi, en bourgeonnant, donne naissance à des vésicules de taille beaucoup plus réduite dans lequel s'accumule le matériel hormonal. Le transfert de métabolites cellulaires par l'intermédiaire de microvésicules n'est nullement une simple vue de l'esprit. C'est ainsi que pour PALADE, 1960, pour ZEIGEL et DALTON, 1962, les protéines élaborées dans les saccules ergastoplasmiques seraient transportées vers les vacuoles golgiennes par un flux de microvésicules naissant par bourgeonnement à partir des membranes ergastoplasmiques. De même, dans des oeufs d'Invertébrés, PASTEELS, 1965, a observé un éparpillement de microvésicules à partir de corps multivésiculaires.

Cette conception n'exclut nullement la théorie du transfert synaptique. On peut fort bien admettre qu'il existe dans les extrémités neurosécrétrices deux catégories distinctes de micro-vésicules, les unes correspondant à des vésicules synaptiques, les autres naissant par bourgeonnement de la paroi des granules élémentaires. Certaines constatations suggèrent même des distinctions morphologiques entre ces deux classes de microvésicules. La variabilité de leur dimension a été relevée par de nombreux auteurs, elle semble beaucoup plus grande qu'au niveau des vésicules synaptiques classiques chez les Oiseaux par exemple, on a admis l'existence de deux classes de vésicules soi-disant synaptiques, les unes d'un diamètre moyen de 350 Å, les autres, plus grandes atteignant 500 à 600 Å de diamètre (OOTA et KOBAYASHI, 1962; KOBAYASHI et coll., 1961). Cette variabilité dans la taille des microvésicules a été également soulignée dans l'hypophyse des Poissons par FOLLENIUS, 1965, et il conclut également à la possibilité d'un phéno-

mène de bourgeonnement à partir des granules élémentaires et à l'hypothèse
d'une filiation directe entre les granules et une classe de microvésicules.

Chez les Chauves-Souris, les terminaisons neuro-sécrétrices semblent également
contenir deux catégories de microvésicules. Les unes sont assemblées en amas
denses, leur diamètre varie peu et oscille autour de 360 Å, leur contenu apparait
uniformément peu dense. Les autres sont éparpillées, leur diamètre moyen est
de 480 Å (sur 100 mesures) mais il montre des oscillations beaucoup plus grandes
et peut atteindre 600 Å. leur contenu est manifestement plus dense. Apparemment,
ce sont ces dernières vésicules qui résultent du bourgeonnement de la membrane
des grain.

Or, certaines images suggèrent que c'est sous cette forme que s'effectue
l'excrétion du matériel hormonal. Chez les Chauves-Souris en lactation en effet, on
retrouve non seulement la présence fréquente d'un liseré de microvésicules au
niveau de la membrane des terminaisons nerveuses, mais, en outre on peut observer
l'existence de corpuscules dans l'espace périvasculaire. Ces corpuscules sont
comparables à ceux relevés par BERN, YAGI et HISHOIKA, 1964, au niveau de
l'espace périvasculaire de l'urophyse d'Albula. Chez la Chauve-Souris en lactation,
ces apparentes extrusions d'un matériel dense semblent beaucoup plus fréquentes
(fig. 1).

Nous reconnaissons volontiers que de telles images doivent être interprétées
avec grande prudence et qu'une section tangentielle de la membrane peut à tort
donner l'impression que des corpuscules siègent en dehors de l'axoplasme. De
même, on ne peut prendre en considération que les zônes où l'intégrité de la membrane apparait totale. Cependant, nous avons retrouvé ces images d'extrusion
corpusculaire dans un grand nombre de clichés. Tantôt, on ne relève la présence
que de quelques corpuscules dans l'espace périvasculaire, tantôt ils tapissent la
face externe de la membrane d'un liseré plus ou moins continu, tantôt encore, ils
se répandent à quelque distance de la membrane. Leur fréquence, mais aussi le
fait que nous les ayons observé dans des conditions physiologiques bien déter-
minées, semblent exclu re l'hypothèse d'unartefact. En effet, nous n'avons constaté
de telles images que chez des femelles en cours d'allaitement, nous ne les avons
retrouvé ni chez des Chauves-Souris en début de gestation, ni chez des femelles non
gestantes. En d'autres termes, leur apparition coïncide indubitablement avec un
état de grande activité secrétoire du système hypothalamo-hypophysaire.

A fort grossissement, les images demeurent tout aussi troublantes. En effet,
à X 90.000 on observe des images d'accolement de microvésicules à la membrane
de la terminaison nerveuse et on retrouve également de petites encoches de la
membrane en regard de microvésicules comme on l'observe à une échelle différente
dans des cellules glandulaires sécrétant des protéines sous l'aspect de granulations.
Enfin, on constate à nouveau, la présence de corpuscules libres dans les espaces
périvasculaires et on s'aperçoit qu'ils siègent à quelque distance de la membrane
qui, elle même, apparait intacte. Ces corpuscules présentent un centre dense mais
ils ne semblent pas avoir perdu leur membrane d'enveloppe.

Avant d'atteindre la lumière du vaisseau les produits de sécrétion doivent
encore franchir une dernière barrière représentée par la paroi endothéliale. Or,
cette dernière chez la Chauve-Souris en lactation est le siège de modifications qui
semblent correspondre à ce processus. En effet, on observe à son niveau, une

pinocytose particulièrement intense, sa face externe, en particulier, montre fréquemment un liseré continu de vésicules de pinocytose à contenu tantôt clair, tantôt plus ou moins dense. Les mêmes vésicules se retrouvent au niveau des expansions de l'endothelium occupant les espaces périvasculaires.

Conclusions

Le mode d'excrétion des produits de neuro-sécrétion demeure une énigme. Une explication est proposée, elle rallie les deux thèses en présence, celle du transfert synaptique et celle du fractionnement des granules élémentaires. Des observations basées sur le lobe postérieur de Chauves-Souris en lactation semblent en effet démontrer que les microvésicules associées aux granules élémentaires dans les terminaisons des fibres neuro-sécrétrices se partagent en deux classes distinctes. Les unes correspondent effectivement à des vésicules synaptiques comme le défend la théorie classique, mais les autres résultent de la fragmentation des granules élémentaires. C'est par l'intermédiaire de ces dernières que pourrait se faire l'excrétion du matériel hormonal. Le passage de microvésicules dans les espaces péri-vasculaires a été, en effet, constaté.

Bibliographie

ACHER, R.: Etat naturel des principes ocytocique et vasopressique de la neuro-hypophyse. 2è Intern. Symposium über Neurosekretion. (Ed. par W. BARGMANN, B. HANSTRÖM et E. SCHARRER), p. 71—78. Berlin-Göttingen-Heidelberg: Springer 1958.

BARGMANN, W.: Electronenmikroskopische Untersuchungen an der Neurohypophyse. 2e Intern. Symposium über Neurosekretion. (Ed. par W. BARGMANN, B. HANSTRÖM et E. SCHARRER), p. 4—12. Berlin-Göttingen-Heidelberg: Springer 1958.

— Neurosecretion. Int. Rev. Cytol. 19, 183—201 (1966).

—, u. A. KNOOP: Electronenmikroskopische Beobachtungen an der Neurohypophyse. Z. Zellforsch. 46, 242—251 (1957).

— — Über die morphologische Beziehungen des neurosekretorischen Zwischenhirnsystems zum Zwischenlappen der Hypophyse (Licht- und elektronenmikroskopische Beobachtungen). Z. Zellforsch. 52, 256—277 (1960).

BERN, H. W.: The secretory neuron as a doubly specialized cell. in D. MAZIA et A. TYLER: General Physiology of Cell Specialization. pp. 349—366. New York: McGraw-Hill 1963.

— K. YAGI, and R. S. NISHIOKA: Structure and function of the caudal neurosecretory system of fishes. Arch. Anat. micr. Morph. exp. 54, 217—238 (1965).

BODIAN, D.: Nerve endings, neurosecretory substance and lobular organization of the neurohypophysis. Bull. Johns Hopk. Hosp. 89, 354—376 (1951).

DE ROBERTIS, E.: Histophysiologie des synapses et neurosécrétions. Monographie de Physiologie causale. Vol. IV. Paris: Gauthier-Villars 1964.

— A. PELLEGRINO DE IRALDI, G. RODRIGUEZ, and C. J. GOMEZ: On the isolation of nerve endings and synaptic vesicles. J. biophys. biochem. Cytol. 9, 229—235 (1961).

DUNCAN, D.: An electronmicroscope study of the neurohypophysis of a bird. Anat. Rec. 125, 457—472 (1956).

FARQUHAR, M. G.: Origin and fate of secretory granules in cells of the anterior pituitary gland. Trans. N.Y. Acad. Sci. 23, 346—351 (1961).

FOLLENIUS, E.: Bases structurales et ultrastructurales des correlations hypothalamo-hypophysaires chez quelques espèces de Poissons téléostéens. Ann. Sci. Natur. Zoologie 12è série. VII. 1—150 (1965).

—, et A. PORTE: Etude des différents lobes de l'hypophyse de la Perche au microscope électronique. C.R. Soc. Biol. 155, 128—131 (1961).

FRIDBERG, G., S. IWASAKI, K. YAGI, H. A. BERN, D. M. WILSON, and R. S. NISHIOKA: Relation of impulse conduction to electrically induced release of neurosecretory material from the urophysis of the teleost fisch, Tilapia mossambica. J. exp. Zool. 161, 137—150 (1966).

FUJITA, H., and J. F. HARTMANN: Electron microscopy of neurohypophysis in normal adren-
    aline-treated and pilocarpine treated Rabbits. Z. Zellforsch. 54, 734—763 (1961).
GERSCHENFELD, H. M., J. TRAMEZZANI, and E. DE ROBERTIS: Ultrastructure and function
    in neurohypophysis of the toad. Endocrinology 66, 741—762 (1960).
GINSBURG, M., and M. IRELAND: Isolation hormone-binding capacity and subcellular distri-
    bution of neurophysin. J. Physiol. (Lond.) 169, 114—115 (1964).
GREEN, J. D., and V. L. VAN BREEMEN: Electron microscopy of the pituitary and observations
    on neurosecretion. Amer. J. Anat. 97, 177—227 (1955).
HANSTRÖM, B.: Transportation of colloid from the neurosecretory hypothalamic centres of
    the brain into the blood vessels of the neural lobe of the hypophysis. K. fysiogr. Sällsk
    Lund Förh. 22, 18 (1952).
HARTMANN, J. F.: Electron microscopy of the neurohypophysis in normal and histamine
    treated rats. Z. Zellforsch. 48, 291—308 (1958).
HELLER, H.: Active principles of neurohypophysis. J. Pharm. Pharmacol. 7, 225—247 (1955).
--, and K. LEDERIS: Characteristics of isolated neurosecretory Vesicles from Mammalian
    neural Lobes. Pr. 3 Intern. Symposium on Neurosecretion. Memoirs of the Soc. for Endo-
    crinol. (Ed. by H. HELLER et R. B. CLARK). pp. 35—50. New York: Academic Press 1962.
HILD, W., et G. ZETLER: Experimenteller Beweis für die Entstehung der sogenannten Hypo-
    physenhinterlappenwirkstoffe im Hypothalamus. Ark. ges. Physiol. 257, 169—201 (1953).
HOLMES, R. L.: In discussion of E. DE ROBERTIS paper. Mem. Soc. Endocrinol. 12, 18
    (1962).
—, J. A. KIERNAN: The fine structure of the infundibular process of the hedgehog. Z. Zell-
    forsch. 61, 894—912 (1964).
—, and F. G. W. KNOWLES: "Synaptic vesicles" in the neurohypophysis. Nature (Lond.)
    185, 710 (1960).
ISHII, S., I. YASUMASU, H. KOBAYASHI, Y. OOTA, T. HIRANO, and A. TANAKA: Isolation of
    neurosecretory granules and nerve endings from bovine posterior lobe. Annot. Zool. Jap.
    35, 121 (1962).
KOBAYASHI, H.: Histochemical electron microscopic and pharmacologic studies on the median
    eminence. Proc. second intern. Congress Endocrinol. Lond. 1964. Excerpta Medica Found-
    ation. Intern. Congress serie 83.570—576.
— H. A. BERN, R. S. NISHIOKA, and Y. HYODO: The hypothalamo-hypophysial neuro-
    secretory system of the parakeet, Melopsittacus undulatus. Gen. comp. Endocrinol.
    1961 I, 545—564.
—, and Y. OOTA: Functional electron microscopy of the vertebrate neurosecretory storage-
    release organs. Gunma Symposia Endocrinol. 1964 I, 63—79.
— H. UEMURA, Y. OOTA, and S. ISHII: Cholinergic substances in the caudal neurosecretory
    storage organ of fish. Science 141, 714—716 (1963).
—, and D. S. FARNER: Cholinesterase in the hypothalamo-hypophysial neurosecretory
    system of the white crowned sparrow, Zonotricha leucophrys gambelii. Z. Zellforsch. 63,
    935 (1965).
— T. HIRANO, and Y. OOTA: Electron microscopic and pharmacological studies on the median
    eminence and pars nervosa. Arch. Anat. microsc. 54, 277—293 (1965).
— Y. OOTA, H. UEMURA, and T. HIRANO: Electron microscopic and pharmacological Studies
    on the Rat median Eminence. Z. Zellforsch. 71, 387—404 (1966).
KOELLE, G. B., et C. GEESEY: Localization of acetylcholinesterase in the neurohypophysis
    and its functional implications. Proc. Soc. exp. Biol. Med. 106, 625—628 (1961).
LA BELLA, F. S., G. BEAULIEU, and R. J. REIFFENSTEIN: Evidence for the existence of separate
    vasopressin and oxytocin-containing granules in the neurohypophysis. Nature (Lond.)
    193, 173—174 (1962).
LEDERIS, K.: A preliminary report on the ultrastructure of the human neurohypophysis.
    J. Endocrinol. 27, 133—135 (1963).
— Relationship between fine structure and function of the vertebrate hypothalamo-neuro-
    hypophysial system. Proc. Second intern. Congress, Endocrinol. Londres 1964. Excerpta
    Medica fundation. Part. I. 563—569.
— An electron microscopical study of the human neurohypophysis Z. Zellforsch. 65, 847—868
    (1965).

MONROE, B. G., and D. E. SCOTT: Ultrastructural Changes in the Neural Lobe of the Hypophysis of the Rat during lactation and Suckling. J. Ultrastruct. Res. 14, 497—517 (1966).

OOTA, Y.: On the synaptic vesicles in the neurosecretory organs of the carp, bullfrog, pigeon and mouse. Annot. Zool. jap. 36, 167—172 (1963).

—, and H. KOBAYASHI: Fine structure of the median eminence and pars nervosa of the Pigeon. Annot. Zool. Jap. 35, 128—138 (1962).

PALADE, G. E.: Cell electron Microscopy, in: Anatomy (Eds. BOYD, JOHNSON and LEVER). Baltimore: Williams & Wilkins 1961.

PALAY, S. L.: The fine structure of the neurohypophysis, in: Progress in Neurobiology II. Ultrastructure and cellular chemistry of neural tissue. pp. 31—49. (Eds. S. KOREY and J. J. NÜRNBERGER). New York 1957.

— An electron microscope study of the neurohypophysis in normal, hydrated and dehydrated rats. Anat. Rec. 121, 348 (1955).

PARDOE, A. U., and M. WEATHERHALL: The intracellular localization of oxytocic and vasopressor substances in the pituitary glands of rats. J. Physiol. 127, 201—212 (1955).

PASTEELS, J. J.: Aspects structuraux de la fécondation vus au microscope électronique. Arch. Biol. (Liège) 76, 463—509 (1965).

PICARD, D., et A. STAHL: La cellule neurosécrétrice chez les Vertébrés. Bull. Ass. Anat. 130, 1—75 (1966).

ROTHBALLER, A. B.: Changes in the rat neurohypophysis induced with painfull stimuli, with particular reference to neurosecretory material. Anat. Rec. 115, 21—41 (1933).

SCHARRER, E., and R. D. FRANDSON: The mode of release of neurosecretory material in the posterior pituitary of the dog. Anat. Rec. 118, 350—351 (1954).

SCHIEBLER, TH. H.: Cytochemische und elektronenmikroskopische Untersuchungen an granülaren Fraktionen der Neurohypophyse des Rindes. Z. Zellforsch. 36, 563—576 (1952).

STUTINSKY, F., et Y. GUERNE: Effets des stimulations électriques hypothalamiques sur la pression artérielle du Rat. C.R. Soc. Biol. 159, 1420—1422 (1965).

UEMURA, H.: Cholinesterases in the hypothalamo-hyposial neurosecretory system in the bird. Zoosterops palpebrosa japonica. Zool. Mag. (Tokio) 15, 118 (1964).

— H. KOBAYASHI, and S. ISHII: Cholinergic substance in the neurosecretory storage release organ. Zool. Mag. (Tokio) 72, 204—212 (1963).

VAN DYKE, H. B., B. CHOW, O. R. GREEP, and A. ROTHEN: The isolation of a protein from the pars neutralis of the ox pituitary with constant oxytocic, pressor and diuresis hinibiting activities. J. Pharmacol. exp. Ther. 74, 190—204 (1942).

— K. ADAMSON, and S. L. ENGEL: Aspects of the Biochemistry and Physiology of the Neurohypophyseal Hormones. Rec. Progr. Hormone Res. 1955 11, 1—41.

WEINSTEIN, H., A. MALAMED, and H. SACHS: Isolation of vasopressin containing granules from the neurohypophysis of the dog. Biochim. biophys. Acta (Amst.) 50, 386—389 (1961).

WHITTAKER, V. P.: The isolation and characterization of acetylcholin containing particles from the brain. Biochem. J. 72, 694—706 (1959).

ZEIGEL, R. F., and A. J. DALTON: Speculations based on the morphology of the Golgi systems in several types of protein-secreting cells. J. Cell. Biol. 15, 45—54 (1962).

Etude préliminaire au microscope électronique du noyau infundibulaire chez le Cobaye

M. Mazzuca

Laboratoire d'Histologie, Faculté de Médecine et Service de Microscopie électronique, Institut Pasteur, Lille

Cette étude du noyau infundibulaire chez le Cobaye entre dans le cadre de nos recherches sur les relations hypothalamo-hypophysaires. Nous avons été amené à l'entreprendre pour les raisons suivantes:

1. La microscopie électronique de la Zone infundibulaire externe de l'éminence médiane (du Cobaye en particulier) révèle une hétérogénéité de la structure fine des terminaisons nerveuses péricapillaires (6). Cette notion d'hétérogénéité est renforcée par le fait que ces terminaisons nerveuses ne réagissent pas de la même manière à l'action de la réserpine (7).

Or, d'après les résultats obtenus en technique argentique par plusieurs auteurs (1–4–5) ces extrémités présynaptiques péricapillaires sont celles d'axones appartenant au tractus tubéro-hypophysaire. Les fibres qui entrent dans la composition de ce faisceau proviendraient en majeure partie du noyau infundibulaire.

2. D'autre part les travaux de Fuxe (2) utilisant une technique spécifique de mise en évidence des monoamines par la fluorescence révèlent la présence de catécholamines dans les cellules du noyau arqué chez le Cobaye.

3. Enfin les recherches de Hálasz et Szentagothai (3–8) sur le rat les conduisent à penser que cette région du noyau infundibulaire serait la Zone hypophysiotrophe de l'hypothalamus.

Sur ces données nous avons tenté de préciser la structure fine des cellules du noyau infundibulaire, de leurs afférences et des éléments qui transitent dans cette région.

Nos observations portent jusqu' à présent la partie antérieure du noyau infundibulaire de Cobayes mâles adultes. Leurs cerveaux ont été fixés par perfusion intracardiaque de solution tamponnée de glutaraldéhyde (suivie d'une post-fixation osmique) ou de solution tamponnée d'acide osmique; cette dernière méthode donne semble-t-il, de meilleurs résultats.

Après inclusion dans l'Araldite les fragments d'hypothalamus ont été coupés frontalement, la région du noyau infundibulaire étant repérée à l'aide du microscope optique sur des coupes semi-fines colorées par une solution alcaline de bleu de Toluidine.

Les coupes ultrafines ont été contrastées par du citrate de Pb selon Reynolds ou de l'hydroxyde de Pb selon Karnovsky.

Les cellules de la partie antérieure du noyau infundibulaire présentent les caractères suivants: d'une taille de 20 μ en moyenne, elles apparaissent comme des éléments ovalaires lorsque la coupe intéresse une région dépourvue de prolongement (fig. 1).

Leur noyau très volumineux (10 à 11 μ) arrondi dans la plupart des cas présente généralement de nombreuses et profondes incisures. Son nucléole, très gros, est le plus souvent central. Tout au long de la membrane nucléaire on peut observer de nombreux pores annelés.

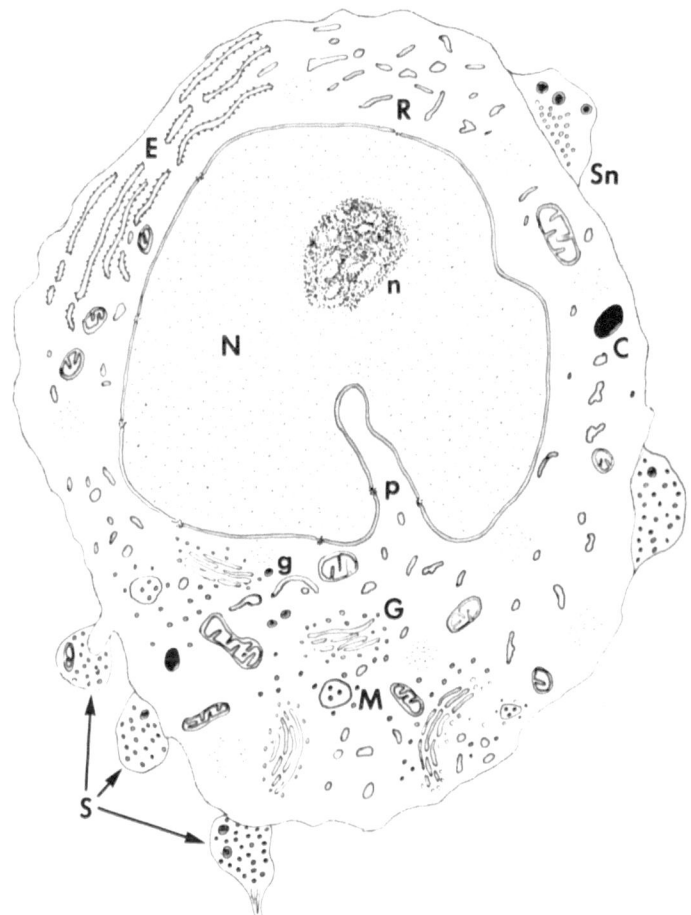

Fig. 1. Schéma d'une coupe de cellule du noyau infundibulaire passant par une région dépourvue de prolongement. *N* Noyau; *n* Nucléole; *p* pores; *E* Ergastoplasme; *R* Réticulum endoplasmique; *G* Appareil de Golgi; *G* Granules denses; *M* Corps multivésiculaires; *C* Corps dense; *S* Synapses; *Sn* Synapse neurosécrétoire

L'ergastoplasme de type classique varie considérablement d'importance d'une cellule à l'autre; il peut se présenter sous plusieurs aspects: lamellaire, généralement groupé et rejeté contre la membrane cellulaire, plus rarement vésiculaire sans localisation précise dans le cytoplasme.

En dehors de l'ergastoplasme, il existe de nombreux polysomes disséminés dans le cytoplasme; on trouve également du réticulum endoplasmique lisse.

L'appareil de Golgi, très dispersé dans le reste du cytone apparaît surtout sous forme vésiculaire. A son voisinage immédiat on rencontre (fig. 2):

Des vésicules dont la taille varie entre 1.000 et 1.500 Å centrées par un granule dense aux électrons d'environ 600 Å de diamètre (fig. 2 b): matériel neurosécrétoire ? Toutefois ces éléments sont en nombre restreint.

Des corps multivésiculaires.

Des corps denses dont la taille est approximativement de 3.000 Å, d'aspect granuleux, entourés le plus souvent par une double membrane.

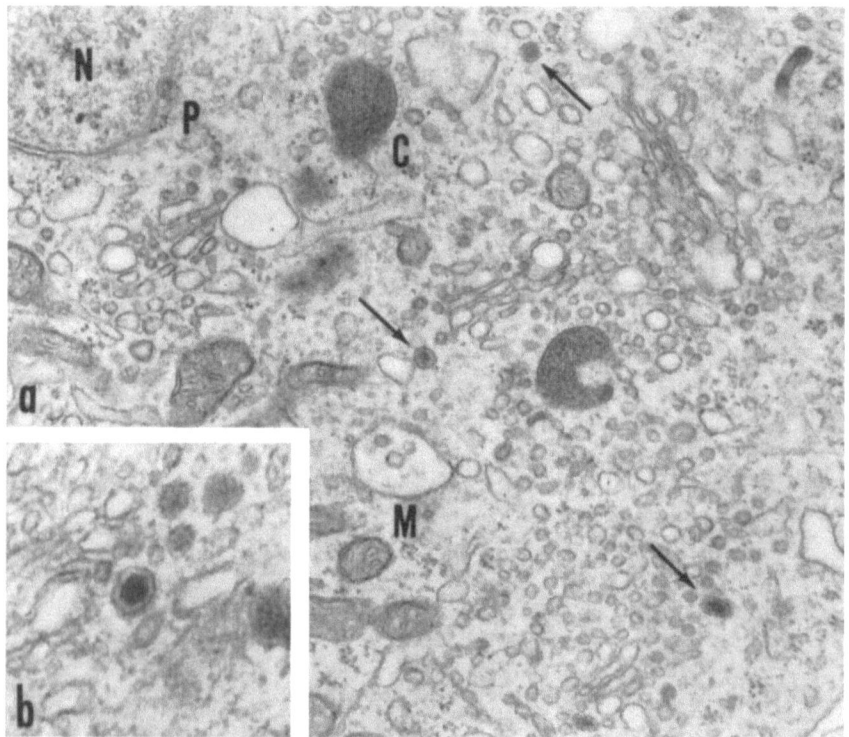

Fig. 2a et b. a) Région de l'appareil de Golgi. *N* Noyau; *C* Corps dense; *M* Corps multi-vésiculaire; *P* Pore — les flèches indiquent les granules denses — $(G = 32.000)$. b) Granules denses à un plus fort grossissement $(G = 64.000)$

Le cytone émet de petites expansions en doigt de gant; chacune d'elles est littéralement coiffée par une extrémité présynaptique.

En coupe frontale, il a été possible de suivre sur un très long trajet les dendrites de ces cellules (60 µ). Ces dendrites possèdent de nombreuses épines de Cajal et des gémules dont la taille peut atteindre 3 à 5 µ (fig. 3).

Des fibres nerveuses se terminent en grand nombre au contact du cytone et des dendrites, soit directement, soit sur les épines de Cajal et les gémules.

Ces extrémités présynaptiques sont de type très différents:

Synapse renfermant des microvésicules synaptiques associées à des vésicules plus grandes (9 à 1.200 Å) centrées par un granule osmiophile, de densité variable; ces synapses sont les plus nombreuses.

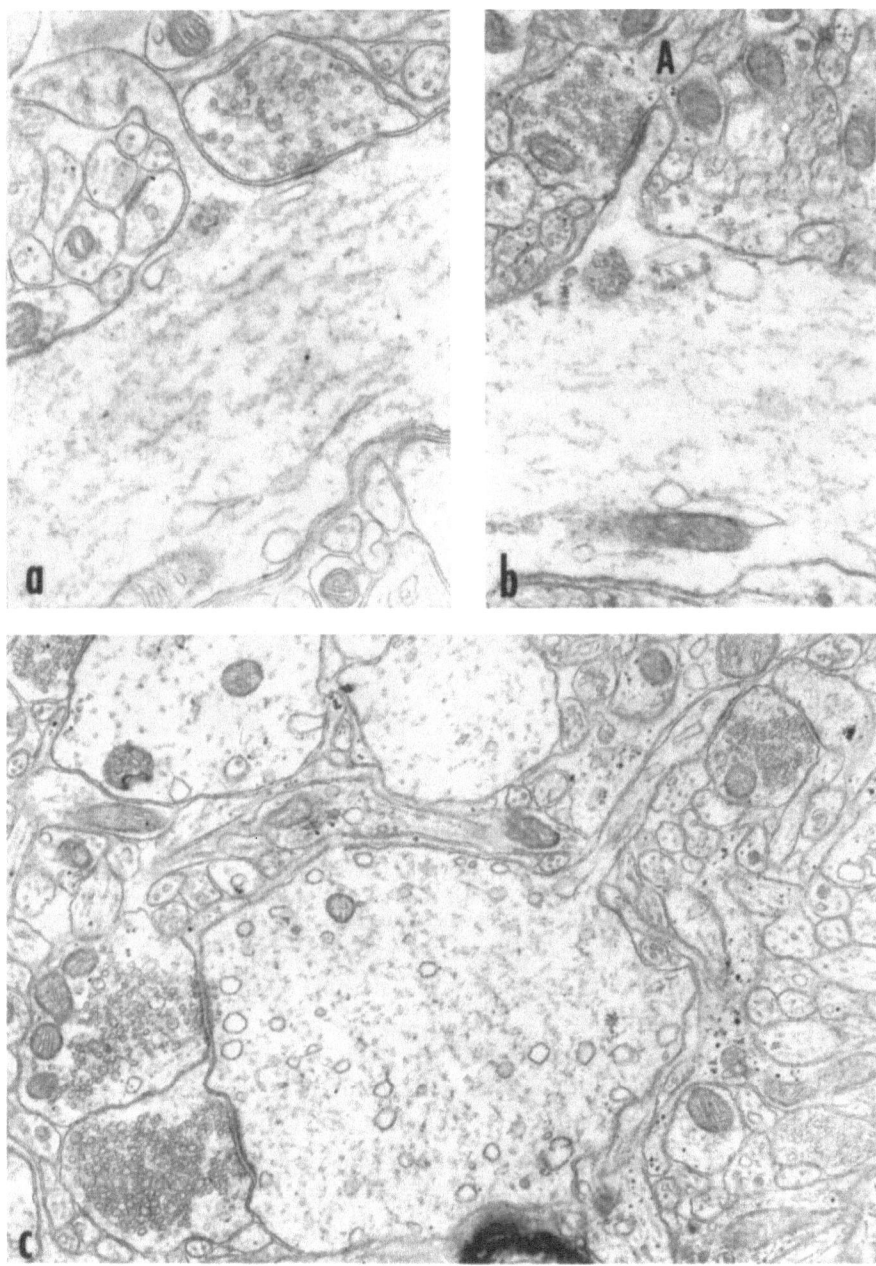

Fig. 3a—c. Dendrites de cellule du noyau infundibulaire. a) Coupe longitudinale = Gémule; noter à son voisinage une synapse axo-dendritique ($G = 24.000$). b) Coupe longitudinale: Epine de Cajal sur laquelle un axone vient faire synapse; A Axone ($G = 24.000$). c) Coupe transversale: Synapses axo-dendritiques et synapse au contact d'une gémule. — Noter la double polarisation de cette extrémité présynaptique ($G = 22.000$)

Synapses neurosécrétoires contenant des microvésicules synaptiques, ainsi que des granulations neurosécrétoires denses; ce genre de synapse, le moins répandu, se rencontre autour du péricaryon et des dendrites.

Synapses constituées par l'association de microvésicules synaptiques et de vésicules de taille très variable à centre clair (fig. 4).

En dehors des cellules et de leurs prolongements dendritiques on observe dans la partie antérieure du noyau infundibulaire de nombreuses fibres myélinisées;

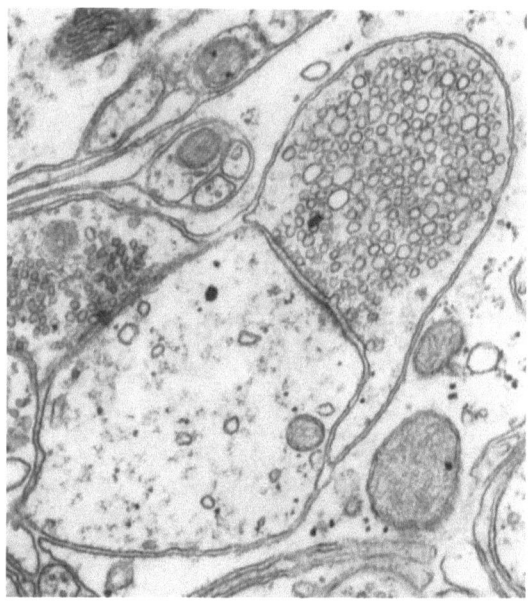

Fig. 4. Synapse axo-dendritique contenant en dehors des microvésicules synaptiques des vésicules claires de taille très variable. Noter la microvésicule synaptique qui semble s'ouvrir dans l'espace intersynaptique ($G = 28.000$)

certaines présentent des images de démyélinisation ce qui laisse supposer qu'elles se terminent dans cette région.

D'autre part il faut noter également la présence de nombreux axones dont l'origine est difficile à préciser. Certains d'entre eux contiennent des vésicules de 1.000 Å de diamètre centrées par un granule osmiophile (fig. 5).

Enfin certaines images laissent supposer que des axones font seulement «synapse en passant» (fig. 5).

En conclusion — de cette étude partielle du noyau infundibulaire on peut retenir que dans sa partie antérieure il semble n'y avoir qu'un seul type de cellule.

Le cytoplasme de ces cellules infundibulaires contient des granules dont la nature neurosécrétoire reste à déterminer.

Si l'on se base sur l'hétérogénéité de structure des pieds terminaux périsomatiques et péridendritiques (puisqu'il existe même des synapses neurosécrétoires) les afférences des cellules du noyau infundibulaire semblent être d'origine différente.

Des axones font «synapse en passant» dans cette région.

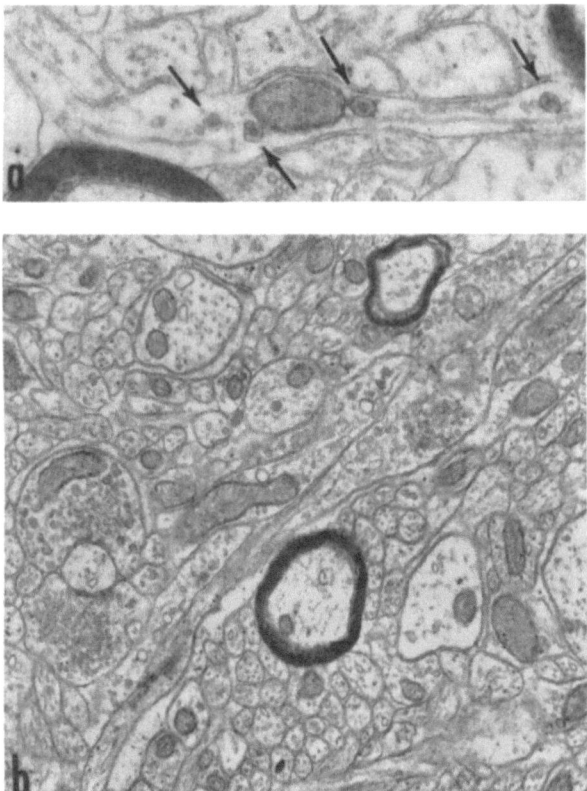

Fig. 5a et b. a) axone dans la région antérieure du noyau infundibulaire qui renferme des microtubules et des granules denses (Flèches) ($G = 27.000$). b) image d'un axone faisant «synapse en passant» (flèche) ($G = 17.000$)

Bibliographie

1. Barry, J. (1960): Recherches sur l'innervation hypothalamique de l'éminence médiane chez le cobaye. Arch. Anat. (Strasbourg) **43**, 187—194.
2. Fuxe, K. (1964): Cellular localization of monoamines in the median eminence and the infundibular stem of some mammals. Z. Zellforsch. **61**, 710—724.
3. Halasz, B., L. Pupp, and S. Uhlarik (1962): Hypophysiotrophic area in the hypothalamus. J. Endocrin. **25**, 147—154.
4. Lefranc, G. (1965): Etude du noyau infundibulaire et de l'éminence médiane du cobaye par la technique de triple imprégnation de Golgi. C.R. Acad. Sci. **260**, 4.087—4.090.
5. Lenys, D. (1962): Etude morphologique des relations neuro-vasculaires hypothalamo-hypophysaires. Thèse Médecine, Nancy p. 195.
6. Mazzuca, M. (1965): Structure fine de l'éminence médiane du cobaye. J. Microscop. **4**, 225—238.
7. — (1966): Action de la réserpine sur les terminaisons nerveuses péricapillaires infundibulaires chez le cobaye. Coll. Ann. S.F.M.E., Bordeaux, Mai.
8. Szentagothai, I. (1964): The parvicellular neurosecretory system. Progr. Brain Research **5**, 135—140.

Cytologie des systèmes neurosécréteurs hypothalamo-hypophysaires des poissons téléostéens

E. Follenius

Laboratoire de Zoologie et Embryologie Experimentale et Département des Applications Biologiques du C.R.N. Strasbourg

I. Introduction

L'analyse des relations hypothalamo-hypophysaires pose plusieurs problèmes cytologiques liés aux différents aspects de l'activité des neurones glandulaires du diencéphale. La production des neurosécrétions, leur transport et leur excrétion considérés dans de nombreux travaux d'histologie et de cytologie classique, ont été abordés d'une façon plus précise grâce au microscope électronique.

Parallèlement on a pu étudier les relations de ces centres glandulaires particuliers avec le système nerveux central d'une part et avec l'hypophyse d'autre part.

Mais à l'heure actuelle, l'exploration des connexions reste encore incomplète. Peu de travaux considèrent à la fois les centres de production des neurosécrétions, les axones et leurs terminaisons. Ces différents niveaux sont en général explorés à part et la reconstitution des voies crinophores est difficile en raison des critères surtout morphologiques qui sont utilisés. Ultérieurement des critères histochimiques devront être trouvés permettant l'identification directe des composés qui forment les différentes catégories de granules. Des essais faits dans cette direction sont inclus dans ce travail consacré à quelques aspects cytologiques des phénomènes neuro-glandulaires et à l'exploration des connexions observées chez plusieurs espèces de Poissons téléostéens.

II. Cytologie des centres de production des neurosécrétions

La cytologie fine des centres neurosécréteurs est connue chez un grand nombre de vertébrés. La première description consacrée à l'un des noyaux hypothalamiques: le noyau préoptique de Carassius (PALAY, 1960) a défini d'emblée les caractères essentiels des cellules neuroglandulaires, ensuite retrouvés chez d'autres espèces: Perche, FOLLENIUS, 1962b; Truite, LEDERIS, 1962 et FOLLENIUS, 1962b; Gadus morrhua et Cottus bubalis (LEDERIS, 1962) et dans d'autres noyaux: N. L. T.: FOLLENIUS, 1962b.

Des divergences apparaissent dans l'interprétation des formations osmiophiles mesurant jusqu'à 1 μ dont PALAY, 1960, décrit l'origine à partir des formations multivésiculaires. LEDERIS, 1962, considère au contraire que ces globules sont constitués par un matériel identique à celui des petits grains de neurosécrétion qui pourraient en dériver. Leur aspect nous (FOLLENIUS, 1962b) avait conduit à admettre qu'il s'agit de lysosomes, distincts des neurosécrétions proprement dites.

L'application de la réaction à l'acide périodique methénamine-argent selon la technique utilisée dans les études sur l'hypophyse (FOLLENIUS et DOERR-SCHOTT, 1966) met en évidence cette différence de la composition chimique. Dans le noyau

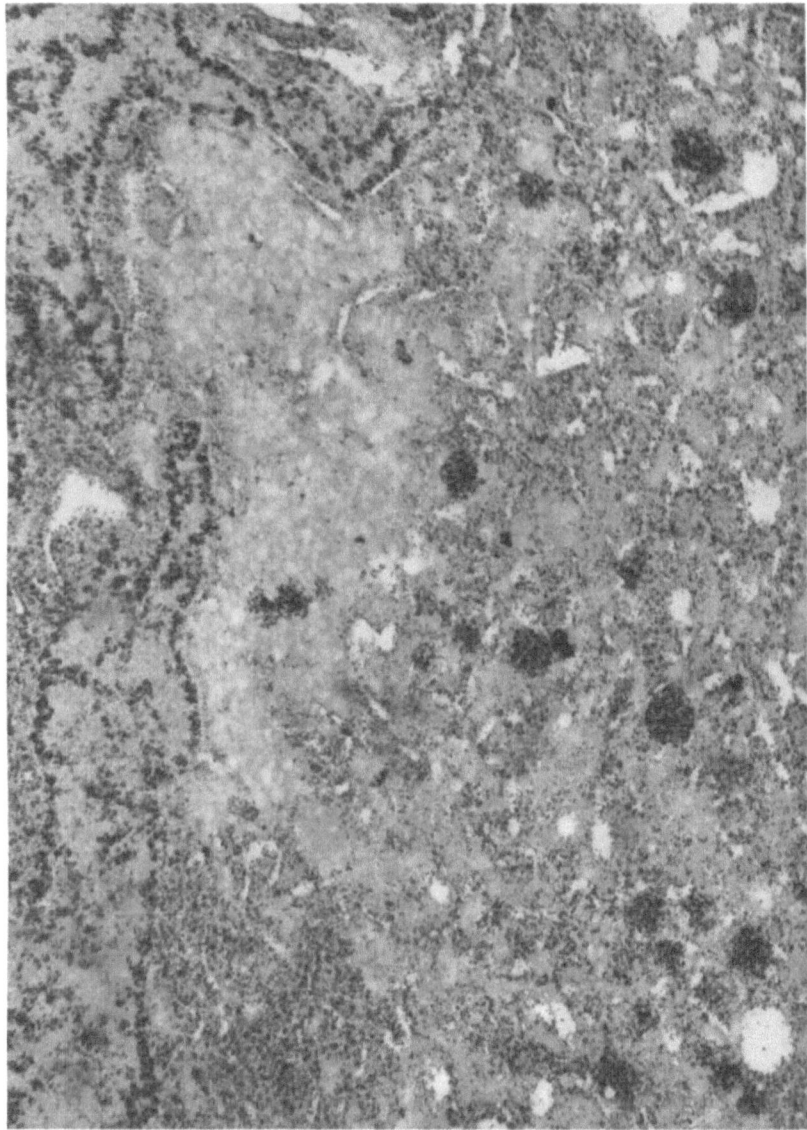

Fig. 1. N.L.T. de la Perche. Réaction à l'acide périodique méthénamine argent. Les neurosécrétions sont négatives. Réaction positive sur les lysosomes. Fix: Glut. Gr 20.000

ventral et latéral du tuber de la Perche les masses osmiophiles réagissent positivement (fig. 1). Leur taille (600 mμ) permet de faire la comparaison avec les coupes semi-fines où elles se colorent nettement à la A.P.S. Cette réaction positive n'est pas vraiment caractéristique des lysosomes comme l'est la mise en évidence de la phosphatase acide dans les formations analogues du noyau supra-optique des mammifères (OSINCHAK, 1963; STUTINSKY et coll., 1963), mais elle présente une valeur signalétique intéressante.

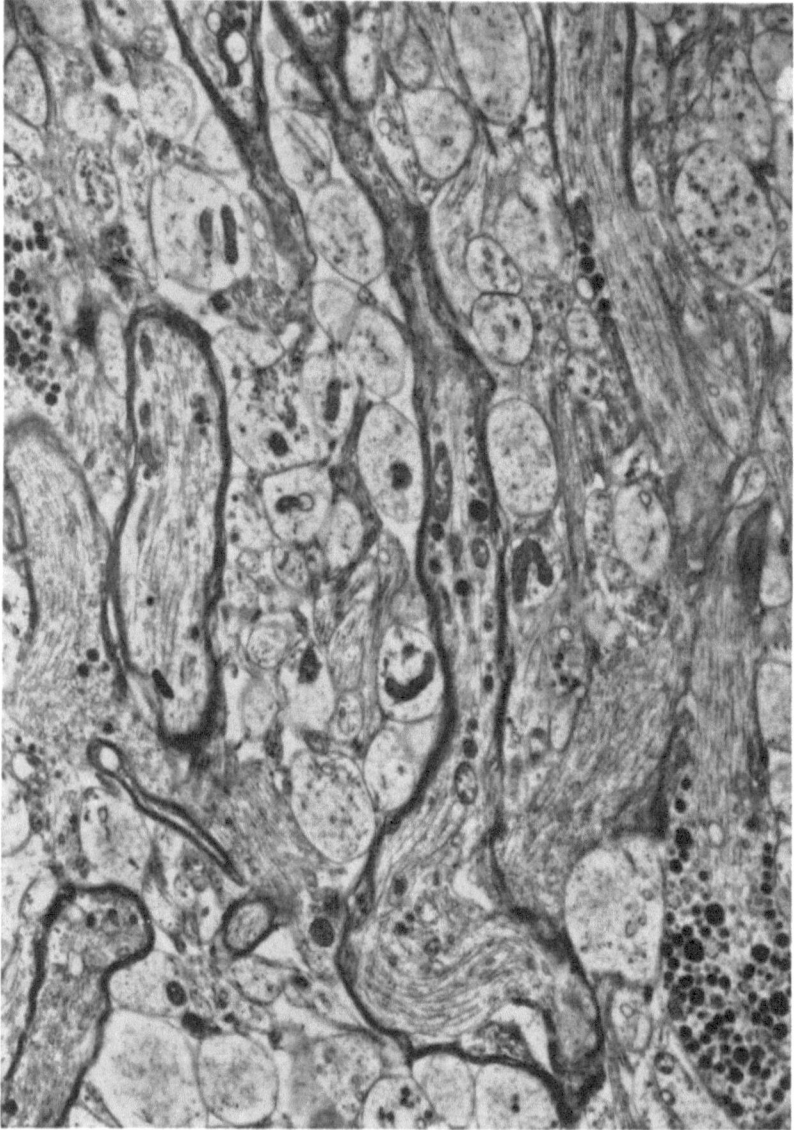

Fig. 2. Coupe frontale dans l'hypothalamus antérieur de la Perche. Morphologie des fibres neurosécrétoires gomori positives myélinisées. Certaines fibres perdent leur gaine à ce niveau. Fix: Pal. Col: A.U. C.Pb. Gr 9.600

La présence de lysosomes dans les cellules neuroglandulaires aurait une signification physiologique précise. Comme dans les cellules hypophysaires, (SMITH, 1966) ils interviendraient dans un processus de résorption intracellulaire des produits de sécrétion bloqués dans la cellule. En fait, nous avons pu observer une variation importante de leur nombre dans les différents neurones pouvant expliquer la colorabilité plus ou moins intense à la A.P.S. signalée en histologie (BREHM, 1958).

L'un des problèmes cytologiques restant en suspens concerne la distinction des granules spécifiques d'origine préoptique de ceux provenant du noyau latéral du tuber. Ces granules réalisent, lors de leur cheminement dans les axones un marquage utilisé, aussi bien en histologie qu'en microscopie électronique, pour la définition des différentes voies. En microscopie électronique les critères distinctifs des deux types de grains ne sont pas satisfaisants chez toutes les espèces. La taille des grains diffère suffisamment chez la Truite: NPO 1460 Å, NLT 1045 Å. Chez les autres espèces la différence est moins évidente ce qui explique les difficultés de l'analyse de l'innervation au microscope électronique. Le diamètre des grains reste constant pendant leur trajet dans l'axone (FOLLENIUS, 1962 b).

Chez la Perche, les fibres préoptico hypophysaires sont faiblement myélinisées et, de ce fait, colorables par la réaction de KLUVER et BARRERA, 1953. Elles contiennent des grains de neurosécrétions caractéristiques qui cheminent entre les neurofibrilles (fig. 2). Au voisinage du noyau latéral du tuber une partie des fibres perdent leur gaine; elles ont à partir de ce niveau l'aspect banal des fibres préoptiques. Quelques fibres conservent leur gaine jusque dans la neurohypophyse où elles se terminent (FOLLENIUS et PORTE, 1962).

Des essais ont été entrepris pour caractériser le contenu des grains grâce à des réactions histochimiques applicables en microscopie électronique. Ces tentatives se heurtent au fait que seule la composition chimique des produits de sécrétion du noyau préoptique est connue (v. SAWYER, 1965). Il s'agit de polypeptides associés à une protéine support. Partant des données fournies par l'histochimie classique (BREHM, 1958) nous avons traité des coupes passant par le noyau latéral du tuber à l'acide périodique méthénamine-argent sans obtenir un résultat positif (fig. 1) au niveau des grains.

Le traitement des coupes par la solution de methénamine argent ou par la solution de Fontana sans oxydation préalable ne donne pas lieu à une réaction argentaffine sur les grains de sécrétion.

Aucune des ces méthodes ne permet de caractériser sélectivement au microscope électronique les neurosécrétions du noyau latéral du tuber par rapport à celles du noyau préoptique. Il semble que les différences de leur constitution chimique soient moins importantes que ne le laissaient prévoir les études histochimiques classiques ou que les méthodes actuellement disponibles ne soient pas encore en mesure de les révéler sur les coupes fines.

III. Contrôle des neurones glandulaires

Les neurones glandulaires, à la fois cellules glandulaires et nerveuses (PALAY, 1960; et BERN, 1962), sont, comme le montrent les études expérimentales, sensibles à un certain nombre de facteurs. Les variations d'activité observées aussi bien dans les noyaux préoptiques supraoptiques et paraventriculaires que dans le noyau latéral du tuber (BILLENSTIEN, 1962) supposent une régulation de l'activité glandulaire et au cours du fonctionnement une régulation de l'excrétion. La microscopie électronique a permis de localiser les jonctions nerveuses pouvant intervenir dans ces processus. Chez la Perche, un certain nombre de synapses sont situées sur les péricaryons du N.P.O. et sur le départ de l'axone. L'examen de la région infundibulaire, au voisinage de la «tige hypophysaire», laisse apparaître d'autres possibilités de connexions entre des fibres banales et les fibres du tractus préoptico-hypophysaire. Des synapses analogues ont également été décrites par KOBAYASHI et coll., 1965, dans l'infundibulum de Rana catesbiana. Leur présence laisse entrevoir le possibilité d'une modulation des processus d'excrétion. Il n'est pas exclu, qu'il existe, en plus, comme l'a suggéré BERN, 1962, un contrôle distal de l'excrétion par l'intermédiaire de jonctions terminales, mais jusqu'à présent, aucune image concernant ce point particulier n'a été observée.

Il n'en reste pas moins qu'à l'ensemble de ces possibilités de contrôle liés à l'existence des jonctions nerveuses s'ajoute celle d'un mécanisme humoral inaccessible aux méthodes d'études morphologiques.

IV. Analyse de la structure du complexe neuro-hypophysaire et des relations avec l'adénohypophyse

Un certain nombre de points concernant les rapports entre la neuro-hypophyse dans son ensemble et l'adénohyophyse apparaissent à la lumière des études de cytologie fine consacrées à plusieurs espèces de Poissons: Salmo irideus et Cyprinus carpio (LEGAIT et LEGAIT, 1958); Cottus bubalis — Gadus morrhua; Anguilla vulgaris (BARGMANN et KNOOP, 1960 et LEDERIS, 1962); Lebistes reticulatus — Phoxinus laevis — Perca fluviatilis et Salmo irideus (FOLLENIUS, 1962a, b); Salmo irideus; (LEDERIS, 1962, 1964 et BODDINGIUS, 1965); Anguilla vulgaris (KNOWLES, 1965). Depuis, nous avons également comparé les relations neuro-adénohypophysaires de l'Epinoche avec celles des espéces précédemment considérées.

Chez tous les poissons téléostéens, la surface de contact entre la neuro-hypophyse et l'adénohypophyse est très développée et, comme le montraient les études histologiques antérieures (v. BARGMANN, 1953; LENYS, 1962), leur intrication donne lieu à des dispositions très variées selon l'espèce et selon l'âge de l'individu.

En dépit de ces différences, l'organisation submicroscopique, bien que complexe, présente des caractères communs.

Bien que la neuro-hypophyse vienne au contact de tous les lobes adéno-hypophysaires, sa partie proximale voisine de la proadénohypophyse et sa partie distale allant au contact de la métaadénohypophyse peuvent, ayant été étudieés chez plusieurs espèces, être décrites d'une façon assez détaillée.

La figure 3 montre la disposition et l'importance des contacts proximaux chez l'Epinoche. Chez toutes les espèces les rapports entre la neuro-hypophyse antérieure et la «bandelette chromophobe», en fait constituée de cellules à petits grains, est identique. Les terminaisons, disposées en palissade, contiennent un grand nombre de vésicules synaptiques et quelques grains à coeur dense. On remarque l'homogénéité très prononcée de cette innervation pratiquement constituée par des fibres à neurosécrétions fines. Les grains de sécrétions ont, quelque soit l'espèce (PERCHE-LEBISTES-EPINOCHE-TRUITE) un diamètre compris entre 600 et 800 Å. Leur coeur dense, décollé de la membrane périphérique ressemble aux grains de neurotransmetteurs décrits dans les fibres sympathiques (GRILLO et PALAY, 1962 et TAXI, 1965). D'après les travaux d'histologie (v. ds. FOLLENIUS, 1962b) les fibres tubériennes contenant du matériel P.A.S. positif aboutiraient dans ce secteur. Mais, d'après nos mesures, la dimension des grains ne correspond pas à celle des grains produits au niveau du péricaryon du noyau latéral du tuber. Trois

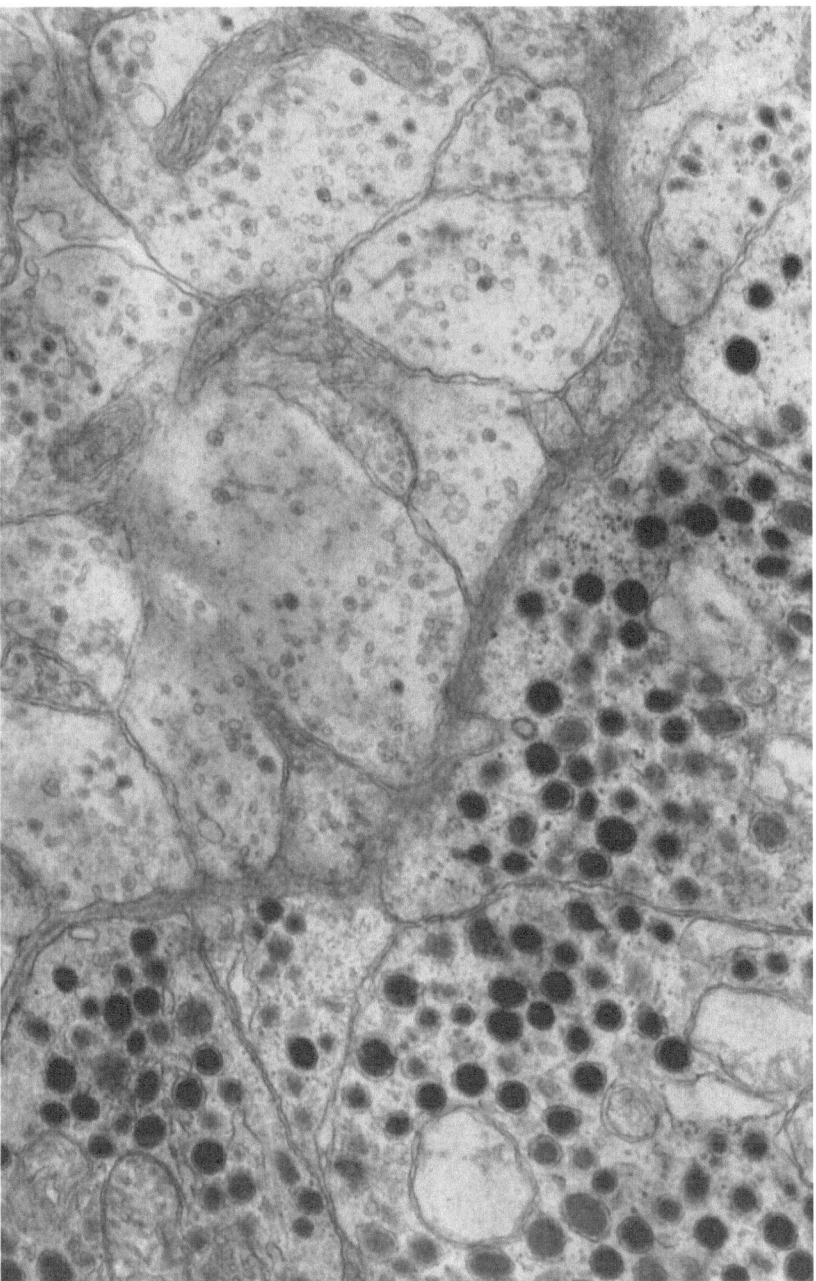

Fig. 3. Contacts neurosécrétoires proximaux chez l'épinoche. Terminaisons nerveuses neurosécrétoires sur la basale entourant la bandelette chromophobe. Gr 30.000

exemples ont pu être étudiés: la pars latéralis du noyau latéral du tuber de la Truite produit des grains de 1045 Å de diamètre alors que ceux des terminaisons du secteur rostral ne mesurent que 700 Å; ceux de la Perche 710 Å (N.L.T. environ 1200 Å) et ceux de l'Epinoche 685 Å (N.L.T. environ 1300 Å).

D'après Knowles, 1965 b, il ne semble pas qu'il y ait chez l'Anguille une différence sensible de taille et d'aspect des grains dans les terminaisons et dans les péricaryons des neurones du noyau latéral du tuber.

Ces fibres contrôlent les cellules corticotrophes (Olivereau et Ball, 1964 et Ball et Olivereau, 1966) formant la «bandelette chromophobe». Des fibres du même type aboutissent également sur les capillaires de ce secteur de la neurohypophyse (Follenius, 1962a, b), où des jonctions neurovasculaires typiques ont été mises en évidence. De par leur position sur le réseau vasculaire elles réalisent un système neurohumoral analogue au système porte des Vertébrés tétrapodes.

Sans insister sur l'innervation de la mésoadénohypophyse (pars proximalis adénohyophysaire), également considérée antérieurement, (Follenius, 1962a, b) nous détaillerons celle très importante, allant à la méta-adénohypophyse (pars intermédia). Les colorations à la chrome-hématoxyline de Gomori, à l'aldéhyde fuchsine ou au Bleu alcian avaient permis de différencier un ensemble de fibres crinophores se colorant très intensément. La répartition de leur terminaisons ne semble pas identique chez toutes les espèces (v. Bargmann, 1953; Bugnon et Lenys, 1960 et Follenius, 1962 b).

A titre d'exemple nous avons plus spécialement comparé les relations entre la neuro et l'adénohypophyse à ce niveau chez deux espèces représentant des types d'organisation.

Chez la Perche, (Kerr, 1942) les fibres bleu alcian positives s'arrêtent sur la basale entourant le lobe nerveux; elles ne franchissent pratiquement pas cette couche. Il est par contre facile de suivre des trajets gomori positifs s'engageant entre les cellules du lobe intermédiaire de l'Epinoche. De tels trajets ont pu être suivis sur des distances assez importantes. Les fibres se détachent du lobe nerveux, passent entre plusieurs cellules claires avant de se renfler en massue terminale contre les cellules A.P.S. positives. Une ou plusieurs massues terminales gomori positives s'appliquent contre la plupart des cellules A.P.S. positives. Chez les deux espèces la répartition des fibres et leur mode de terminaison ont été analysés au microscope électronique. La région de contact entre la neurohyophyse et la métaadénohypophyse de la Perche est très bien délimitée par une basale. Des terminaisons contenant de nombreuses vésicules synaptiques et des grains de neurosécrétions, sont alignées au contact de la basale. D'après la colorabilité de cette zône, sur les coupes histologiques, et d'après la taille des grains élémentaires il s'agit de fibres d'origine préoptique.

Chez l'Epinoche, des fibres venant du lobe nerveux, non délimité par une basale, pénètrent en profondeur. On les voit aboutir au contact des cellules glandulaires. Leurs renflements terminaux sont remplis d'un axoplasme clair contenant des vésicules synaptiques et des granules élémentaires. Sur de nombreuses coupes les granules élémentaires font défaut sans que les vésicules synaptiques soient absentes. Des terminaisons nerveuses ne présentent que très rarement des encroûtements de la membrane où encore des accumulations de vésicules synaptiques centrées sur un point précis. Elles s'appliquent étroitement contre les cellules

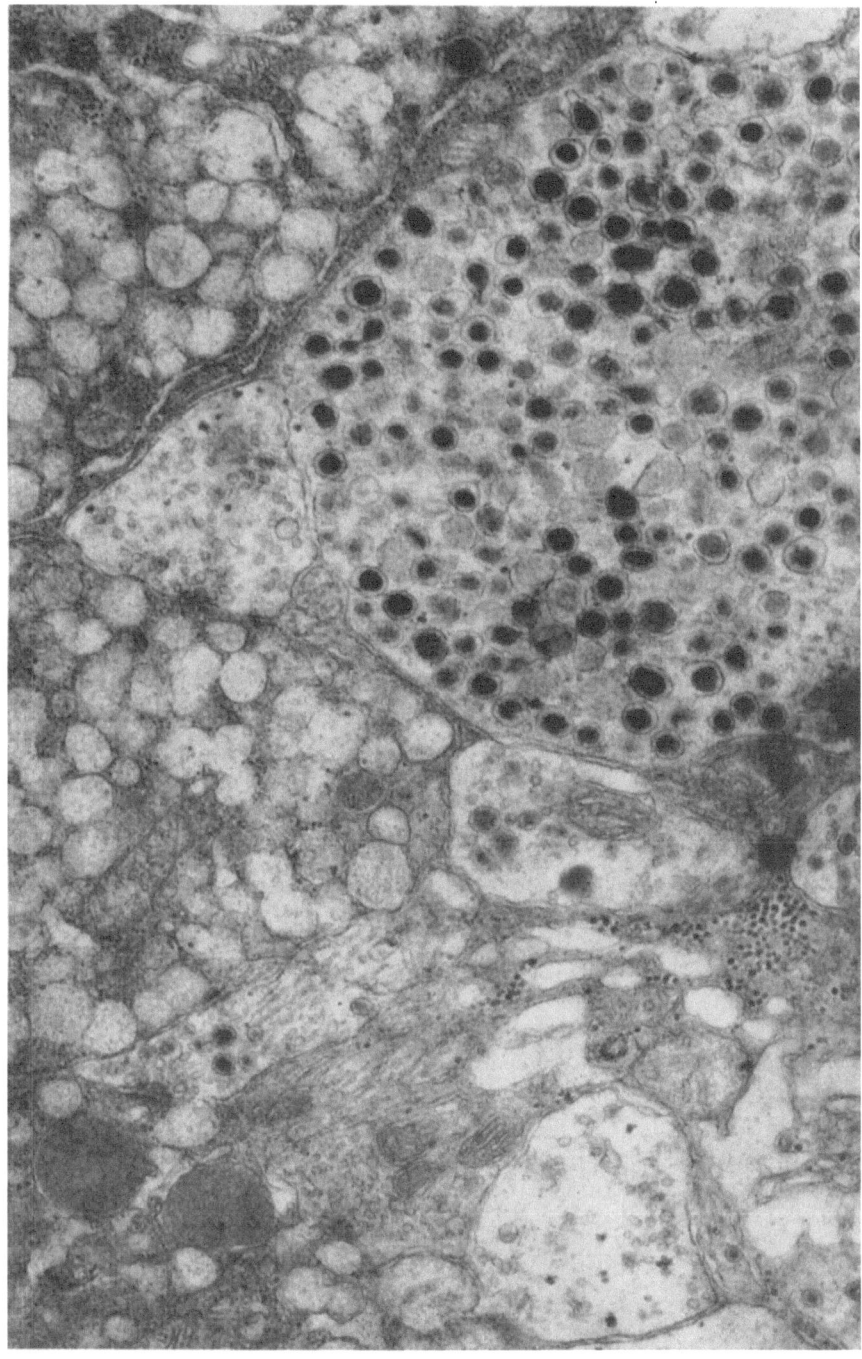

Fig. 4. Aspect des terminaisons nerveuses neurosécrétoires situées entre les cellules de la métaadénohypophyse de l'Epinoche. Gr 30.000

glandulaires dont le cytoplasme ne présente aucune différenciation particulière à leur voisinage.

Dans ces conditions la définition des relations entre les terminaisons et les cellules voisines s'avère délicate. Il est rare que l'on puisse déceler d'une façon indubitable une polarité intéressant particulièrement l'une ou l'autre des cellules voisines. Il est notamment difficile de savoir si les terminaisons agissent sur les cellules glandulaires à une étape particulière de leur cycle sécrétoire. La microscopie électronique confirme l'abondance des terminaisons au niveau des cellules contenant des granulations. Ces jonctions neuro-glandulaires présentent quelques analogies avec les jonctions situées dans les muscles lisses. Dans les deux cas, on note l'absence de sites actifs permettant de définir d'une façon précise l'endroit où se fait l'échange des neurotransmetteurs (Taxi, 1965).

En considérant le contenu et plus précisément la taille et l'aspect des grains denses on distingue deux ou trois types de fibres qui se terminent dans le tissu glandulaire.

Il y a les fibres d'origine pré optique dont les grains denses se reconnaissent par leur diamètre élevé (Epinoche 1580 Å environ) et par l'absence presque complète du liseré périphérique. D'autres par contre, renferment des grains de diamètre plus fin (600–800 Å) dont le contenu moins homogène laisse un liseré périphérique clair plus important sous la membrane. Ces grains présentent des analogies d'aspect avec ceux décrits au niveau des contracts proximaux et dans les fibres sympathiques (Grillo et Palay, 1962; Taxi, 1965). Leur origine et la nature de leur contenu restent à déterminer. En se basant sur les critères de morphologie fine une troisième catégorie, dont l'individualité est discutable, s'impose. Ce sont les terminaisons ne contenant pas des grains denses sur les coupes et pouvant, de ce fait, constituer des terminaisons de fibres nerveuses banales ou de fibres neuro-sécrétoires dépourvues de grains au niveau de la coupe (fig. 4).

Pour des raisons indiquées plus haut il est difficile de déterminer au microscope électronique s'y a, oui ou non, une localisation préférentielle des différents types de terminaisons sur l'une ou l'autre des catégories de cellules, comme il est d'ailleurs difficile de savoir si ces fibres ne forment pas plusieurs renflements successifs ayant des caractères de terminaison. Dans un cas, l'axone neurosécréteur, situé dans le plan de coupe, contourne la cellule glandulaire à grains osmiophiles constituant une partie terminale très allongée.

On peut toutefois considérer que les coupes passant dans la région préterminale d'une fibre diffèrent par leur contenu de celles situées dans la partie terminale. Les segments préterminaux sont, comme l'avait indiqué de Robertis, 1962, chargés en grains de neurosécrétion et pauvres en vésicules synaptiques.

Le problème est posé de savoir quelle est la fonction de chaque type de fibres nerveuses. Quel est le système responsable de l'adaptation chromatique ? Il semble d'après les résultats acquis chez les Sélaciens (Mellinger, 1963 et Knowles, 1965a) et plus récemment chez la Grenouille (Enemar et Falck, 1965) que cette fonction, assurée par l'hormone M.S.H. sécrétée par les cellules du lobe intermédiaire, soit contrôlée à la fois par des fibres gomori positives et par des fibres contenant des catécholamines. L'intervention du système préoptico-hypophysaire dans le contrôle des chromatophores pourrait expliquer le noircissement des Truites observé (Lederis, 1964) après leur transfert de l'eau douce dans l'eau de mer.

Les résultats apportés par la microscopie électronique confirment la pluralité de l'innervation des cellules glandulaires du lobe intermédiaire ce qui laisse prévoir un contrôle complexe des activités secrétices ou excrétrices.

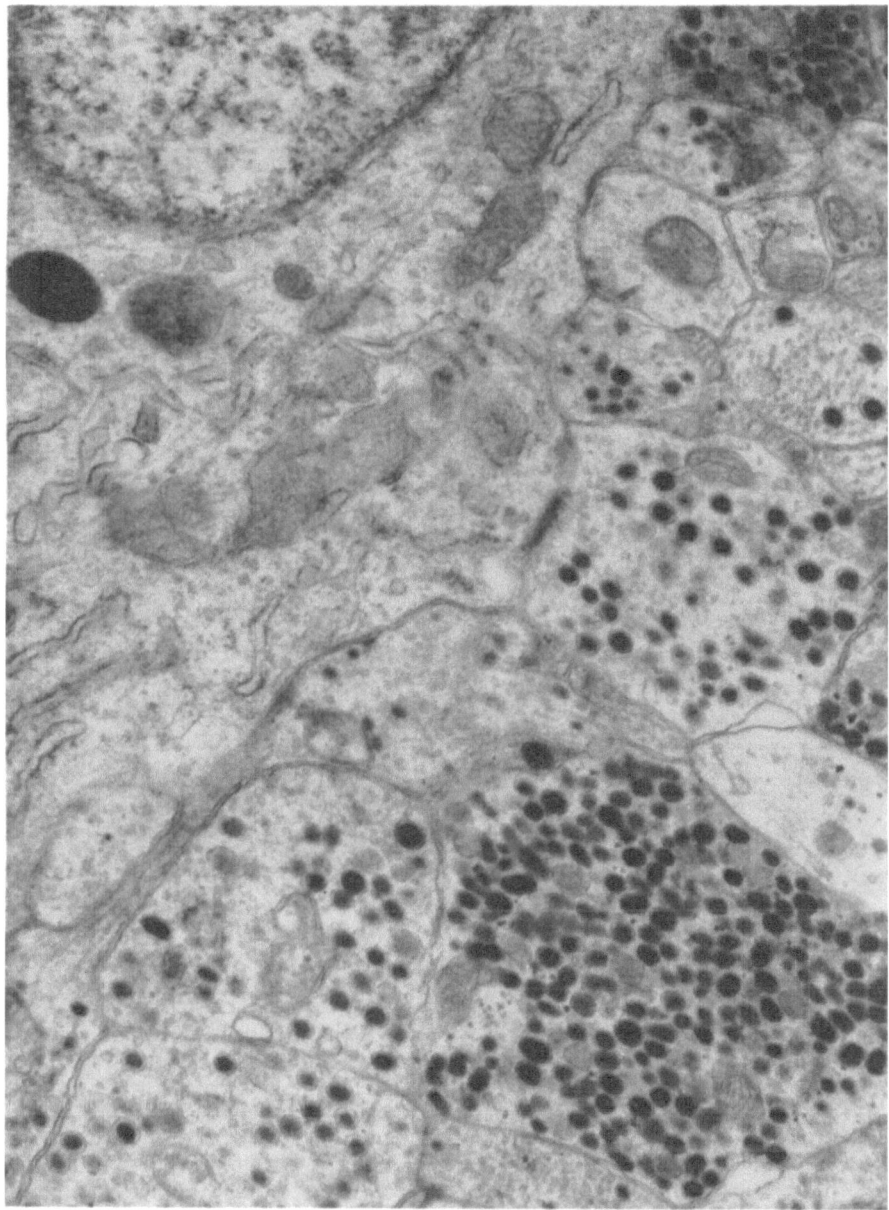

Fig. 5. Contacts synaptiques neurosécrétoires sur les pituicytes du lobe nerveux de l'Epinoche. Fix: Glut. Pal. Gr 21.000

Aussi bien chez la Perche que chez l'Epinoche, de nombreuses fibres gomori positives ne pénètrent pas dans le tissu glandulaire du lobe intermédiaire; elles

4*

s'arrêtent par des terminaisons typiques sur la basale entourant les capillaires du lobe nerveux. La disposition et la structure ces terminaisons, d'abord décrites chez les Mammifères (PALAY, 1957) est identique chez les Poissons (BARGMANN et KNOOP, 1960 et FOLLENIUS, 1962b). Par cette liaison neurovasculaire les hormones hypothalamiques sont susceptibles d'être émises directement dans la circulation sanguine.

Un troisième contingent de fibres neurosécrétrices se termine, non pas sur les capillaires, mais sur des cellules assez peu nombreuses noyées dans le lacis des fibres nerveuses. D'après leur cytologie elles s'apparentent plutôt aux pituicytes qu'aux cellules nerveuses dont la présence dans le lobe nerveux avait été signalé précédemment (STUTINSKY, 1949 et BARGMANN, 1953). Les pituicytes ont chez les différentes espèces de poissons, des aspects assez différents. Ceux de la Perche ont un cytoplasme très clair ne contenant que très peu de structures organisées. Chez l'Epinoche, par contre, ils sont peu nombreux, petits, à noyau encoché et à cytoplasme dense peu abondant contenant quelques citernes ergastoplasmiques et une ou plusieurs inclusions sphériques osmiophiles juxtanucléaires. Quelques fibrilles fines parcourent leur cytoplasme. Leur forme étoilée est plus prononcée que chez la Perche. Il ne semble cependant pas qu'il s'agisse de cellules nerveuses.

Les relations entre fibres nerveuses neurosécrétrices et ces cellules sont tout à fait caractéristiques. Sur les coupes fines, colorées à l'acétate d'uranyle et au citrate de plomb, la membrane synaptique est épaissie et les vésicules synaptiques très nombreuses sont groupées au voisinage immédiat de ces encroûtements (fig. 5). A une certaine distance de la surface synaptique, on distingue des grains de neurosécrétion typiques sur la plupart des coupes. Il s'agit bien de terminaisons synaptiques neurosécrétrices. Chez l'Epinoche, il ne semble pas, en considérant la taille des neurosécrétions que les fibres se terminant sur les pituicytes soient morphologiquement différentes de celles allant sur les capillaires ou sur les cellules adénohypo-physaires. Les pituicytes de l'Epinoche ne sont pas disposés en rosette comme chez l'Anguille (KNOWLES, 1965b, c) où, leur innervation prend un sens particulier en raison des relations qu'ils contractent avec les cavités du troisième ventricule. Ces données nouvelles concernant les relations entre les fibres crinophores et les pituicytes sont à rapprocher des observations de NISHIOKA et coll., 1964, concernant l'innervation neurosécrétoire de l'épendyme chez le moineau. Par cette voie une partie des neurosécrétions est susceptible de passer dans le liquide cérébrospinal. Parmi les observations récentes concernant l'intervention des pituicytes dans les processus neurosécrétoires celles de KUROSUMI et coll., 1964, sur l'accumulation de lipides dans les pituicytes du rat après une vidange des axones neurosécrétoires, sont particulidrement suggestives.

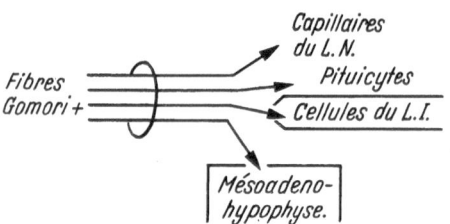

Schéma. Localisation des terminaisons Gomori-positives dans l'adénohypophyse des Poissons téléostéens

D'après l'ensemble des données anatomiques les fibres du tractus hypothalamo-hypophysaire transportant du neurosécrétat gomori-positif ont, en plus de leurs contacts situés dans la mésoadénohypophyse, trois destinations intéressant le lobe nerveux lui même et son voisinage immédiat.

Le schéma page 52 résume ces faits.

V. Discussion

Plusieurs poblèmes sont poés par l'analyse des rapports entre les axones Gomori positifs et les différents récepteurs. Les méthodes d'identification actuelles, basées sur les affinités tinctoriales des neurosécrétions ou sur l'aspect et la taille des granules élémentaires, tendent à faire admettre, malgré une certaine hétérogénéité du contenu de certaines fibres au microscope électronique, qu'elles constituent une classe de fibres particulière. Ces critères morphologiques paraissent insuffisants pour caractériser une diversité fonctionnelle évidente. Chez les Poissons téléostéens, les études à caractère physiologique associent la neurosécrétion gomori-positives à plusieurs fonctions: régulation de l'équilibre hydrominéral (FRIDBERG et OLSSON, 1959; MAETZ ct JULIEN, 1961; MOTAIS, 1961; LEDERIS, 1961); contrôle de l'adaptation chromatique (KNOWLES et VOLLRATH, 1965e).

La multiplicité des lieux de terminaison des fibres gomori positives et celle des fonctions directement ou indirectement contrôlées pourrait s'expliquer soit par une différenciation particulière des fibres échappant encore aux examens morphologiques, soit par une spécificité de réponse des récepteurs innervés. Cette dernière hypothèse pourrait s'appliquer en particulier aux pituicytes ou aux cellules glandulaires de la métaadénohypophyse.

Les deux espèces que nous avons comparées illustrent, du moins en ce qui concerne le lobe intermédiaire, une remarquable organisation tendant à réaliser des relations neuroglandulaires précises. Il appartient aux études expérimentales d'approfondir l'aspect fonctionel que ces dispositions anatomiques laissent entrevoir. Les études ultrastructurales confirment l'importance des terminaisons situées à la périphérie du lobe nerveux et de ses digitations. Leur aspect indique qu'elles prennent, chez les Poissons, part au contrôle des cellules glandulaires adjacentes.

Chez toutes les espèces étudiées jusqu'à présent on distingue un secteur rostral de la neurohypophyse avec des terminaisons nerveuses très nombreuses alignées sur la basale qui le sépare de la bandelette chromophobe.

Les rapports entre le tissus nerveux et le tissu glandulaire de la méso et de la métaadénophypophyse sont différents selon l'espéce. Ils semblent déterminés par l'organisation du tissu glandulaire.

Chez les espèces comme la Perche, où les cellules acidophiles localisées à la périphérie des cordons de cellules glandulaires entourent les cellules basophiles en général situées plus en profondeur, l'innervation reste superficielle. Un grand nombre de terminaisons s'arrête sur la basale qui marque la limite entre le tissue nerveux et le tissu glandulaire.

Dans les hypophyses du type «Epinoche» caractérisées par l'absence d'une localisation précise des différents types de cellules dans la méso et la métaadénohypophyse les fibres nerveuses pénètrent dans le parenchyme glandulaire pour se terminer au contact même des cellules. Il apparaît qu'à la disposition particulière de l'adénohypophyse par rapport au complexe neurohypophysaire correspondent des contacts neuroglandulaires situés dans les différentes parties de l'hypophyse et assurés par plusieurs types de fibres. Comme nous l'avions précédemment souligné une partie du contrôle de l'hypophyse est assurée par un dispositif neurovasculaire situé dans le secteur rostral.

Bibliographie

BAKER, B. I. (1963): Effect of adaptation to black and white backgrounds on the teleost pituitary. Nature (Lond.) **198**, 404.

BALL, J. N., and M. OLIVEREAU (1966): Identification of the A.C.T.H. cells in the pituitary of two teleosts Poecilia latipinna and Anguilla anguilla: correlated changes in the interrenal and in the pars distalis resulting from administration of metopirone (SU 4885). Gen. comp. Endocr. **6**, 5—18.

BARGMANN, W. (1953): Über das Zwischenhirn-Hypophysensystem von Fischen. Z. Zellforsch. **38**, 275—298.

— (1962): Neurosekretorische Nervenfasern und Adenohypophyse. I° Cong. Europ. Anat. Strasbourg 1960 dans Anat. Anz. 109. Ergbd. 260—261.

—, u. A. KNOOP (1960): Über die morphologischen Beziehungen des neurosekretorischen Zwischenhirnsystems zum Zwischenlappen der Hypophyse. (Licht- und elektronenmikroskopische Untersuchungen). Z. Zellforsch. **52**, 256—277.

BERN, H. (1962): The properties of neurosecretory cells. Gen. comp. Endocr. suppl. **1**, 117—132.

BILLENSTIEN, D. C. (1962): The seasonal secretory cycle of the nucleus lateralis tuberis of the hypothalamus and its relation to reproduction in the eastern brook trout Salvelinus fontinalis. Gen. comp. Endocr. **2**, 111—112.

— (1963): Neurosecretory material from the nucleus lateralis tuberis in the hypophysis of the eastern brook trout Salvelinus fontinalis. Z. Zellforsch. **59**, 507—512.

BREHM, H. U. (1958): Über jahreszyklische Veränderungen im Nucleus lateralis tuberis der Schleie (Tinca vulgaris). Z. Zellforsch. **49**, 105—124.

ENEMAR, A., and B. FALCK (1965): On the presence of adrenergic nerves in the pars intermedia of the frog Rana temporaria. Gen. comp. Endocr. **5**, 577—583.

FOLLÉNIUS, E. (1959): Etude histo et cytochimique de l'hypophyse du Cyprinodonte vivipare Lebistes reticulatus R. Ann. endocr. (Paris) **20**, 676—682.

— (1962a): Rapports neurovasculaires et neuroglandulaires dans l'hypophyse de quelques poissons. Etude au microscope électronique. C.R. Acad. Sci. (Paris) **255**, 3474—3476.

— (1962b): Bases structurales et ultrastructurales des correlations hypothalamo-hypophysaires chez quelques espèces de téléostéens. Thèse de Sciences publiée dans. Ann. Sci. Nat. Zool. 18° série tome **7**, 1—150 (1965).

— (1963): Ultrastructure des types cellulaires de l'hypophyse de quelques poissons téléostéens. Arch. Anat. micr. Morph. exp. **52**, 429—468.

— (1965): Bases structurales et ultrastructurales des correlations diencéphalo-hypophysaires chez les sélaciens et les téléostéens. Arch. Anat. micr. Morph. exp. **54**, 195—216.

—, and A. PORTE (1962): Appearance, ultrastructure and distribution of the neurosecretory material in the pituitary gland of two teleost fishes Lebistes reticulatus and Perca fluviatilis. Mem. Soc. Endocr. **12**, 51—69.

—, et DOERR-SCHOTT J. (1966): Mise en évidence sélective au microscope électronique des cellules à sécrétions glycoprotéiques de l'hypophyse par la réaction à l'acide périodique-nitrate d'argent. C.R. Acad. Sci. (Paris) **262**, 912—914.

FRIDBERG, G., and R. OLSSON (1959): The preoptico-hypophysial system, nucleus tuberalis lateralis and subcommissural organ of Gasterosteus aculeatus after changes in osmotic stimuli. Z. Zellforsch. **49**, 531—540.

GRILLO, M. A., and S. L. PALAY (1962): Granules containing vesicles in the autonomic nervous system. 5° Congr. Inter. Micr. Electr. Philadelphia 2. u₁.

KERR, T. (1942): On the pituitary of the perch (Perca fluviatilis). Quart. J. micr. Sci. **83**, 299—316.

KLÜVER, H., and E. BARRERA (1953): A method for the combined staining of the cells and fibres in the nervous system. J. Neuropath. exp. Neurol. **12**, 400—403.

KNOWLES, F. (1965a): Evidence of a dual control by neurosecretion of hormone synthesis and hormone release in the pituitary of the dogfish Scylliorhinus stellaris. Trans. roy. Soc. London B **249**, 435—456.

KNOWLES, F. (1965b): Synaptic contacts between neurosecretory fibres and pituicytes in the pituitary of the eel. Nature (Lond.) **206**, 1168—1169.

— (1965c): A functional relationship between neurosecretory fibres and pituicytes in the eel. Nature (Lond.) **208**, 1343—1344.

— (1965d): Neuroendocrine correlations at the level of ultrastructure. Arch. Anat. micr. Morph. exp. **54**, 343—358.

—, and L. VOLLRATH (1965): Ultrastructure and function in the pituitary of the eel. Gen. comp. Endocr. **5**, 691—692 Abstr.

KOBAYASHI, H., T. HIRANO, and Y. OOTA (1965): Electron microscopic and pharmacological studies on the median eminence and pars nervosa. Arch. Anat. micr. Morph. exp. **54**, 277—294.

KUROSUMI, K., T. MATSUZAWA, Y. KOBAYASHI, and S. SATO (1964): On the relationship between the release of neurosecretory substance and lipid granules of pituicytes in the rat neurohypophysis. Gunma Symp. on Endocrinol. **1**, 87—118.

LEDERIS, K. (1962): Ultrastructure of the hypothalamo-neurohypophysial system in teleost fishes and isolation of hormone containing granules from the neurohypophysis of the cod Gadus morrhua. Z. Zellforsch. **58**, 192—213.

— (1964): Fine structure and hormone content of the hypothalamo-neurohypophysial system of the rainbow trout (Salmo irideus) exposed to sea water. Gen. comp. Endocr. **4**, 638—661.

LEGAIT, E., et H. LEGAIT (1958): Etude de l'hypophyse de quelques téléostéens au microscope électronique. Arch. Anat. (Strasbourg) **41**, 1—45.

LENYS, D. (1962): Etude morphologique des relations neurovasculaires hypothalamo-hypophysaires. Thèse de médecine Université de Nancy n° 57.

MAETZ, J., and M. JULIEN (1961): Action of neurohypophysial hormones on the sodium fluxes of freshwater teleost. Nature (Lond.) **189**, 152—153.

MELLINGER, J. (1963): Etude histophysiologique du système hypothalamo-hypophysaire de Scylliorhinus caniculus (L) en état de mélanodispersion permanente. Gen. comp. Endocr. **3**, 26—45.

MOTAIS, R. (1961): Les échanges du sodium chez un téléostéen euryhalin Platichthys flesus flesus L. Cinétique de ces échanges lors du passage d'eau de mer en eau douce et d'eau douce en eau de mer. C.R. Acad. Sci. **253**, 724—726.

NISHIOKA, R. S., H. A. BERN, and L. R. MEWALDT (1964): Ultrastructural aspects of the neurohypophysis of the white crowned sparrow Zonotrichia leucophrys gambelii with special reference to the relation of neurosecretory axons to ependyma in the nervosa. Gen. comp. Endocr. **4**, 304—313.

OLIVEREAU, M., et J. N. BALL (1964): Contribution à l'histophysiologie de l'hypophyse des téléostéens en particulier de celle de Poecilia species. Gen. comp. Endocr. **4**, 523—532.

OOTA, Y. (1963): Fine structure of the median eminence and the pars nervosa of the turtle Clemmys japonica. J. Fac. Sci. Tokyo Sec. IV. **10**, 169—179.

OSINCHAK, J. (1963): Acid phosphatase activity and the identity of intracellular granules in neurosecretory cells of the rat. J. Cell Biol. **19**, 54A.

PALAY, S. L. (1957): The fine structure of neurohypophysis. Progress in neurology: II. Ultrastructure and cellular chemistry of neural tissue, p. 31—49. S. KOREY et J. I. NURNBERGER édit. New York: Hoeber-Harper.

— (1960) The fine structure of secretory neurons in the preoptic nucleus of the goldfish (Carassius auratus). Anat. Rec. **138**, 417—425.

ROBERTIS, E. DE (1962): Ultrastructure and function in some neurosecretory systems. Mem. Soc. Endocr. **12**, 3—20.

ROBERTSON, O. H. (1951): Factors influencing the state of dispersion of the dermal melanophores in rainbow trout. Phys. Zool. **24**, 309—323.

SAWYER, W. M. (1965): Evolution of neurohypophysial principles. Arch. Anat. micr. Morph. exp. **54**, 295—312.

SMITH, R. E. (1966): Origin and function of lysosomes in protein secreting cells of the adenohypophysis. Electron Micros. and Cytochemistry. Symposium Leiden 1966.

STUTINSKY, F., A. PORTE, J. P. TRANZER et Y. TERMINN (1963): Sur la signification des inclusions colorables par l'aldéhyde fuchsine dans les neurones du système nerveux central du rat. C.R. Soc. Biol. **157**, 2294—2296.

TAXI, J. (1965): Contribution à l'étude des connexions des neurones moteurs du système nerveux autonome. Ann. Sci. Nat. Zool. **12**, série VII, 413—674.

Neurosécrétion hypothalamique Gomori-négative et contrôle gonadotrope chez le Cobaye mâle*

J. Barry

Laboratoire d'Histologie, Faculté de Médecine, Lille

Les observations rapportées dans cet exposé résument les recherches faites au cours des années précédentes par notre groupe de travail sur le contrôle hypothalamique de la fonction gonadotrope préhypophysaire chez le cobaye mâle, ainsi que certains résultats que nous avons obtenus tout récemment en ce domaine. Le point de départ de nos recherches a été la découverte chez le cobaye (1) et chez la taupe (2) de cellules de morphologie neuroglandulaire à grains de sécrétion gomorinégatifs, dispersées au sein de la région hypothalamique latérodorsale et constituant un véritable noyau que nous avons proposé de désigner par l'expression de «noyau hypothalamique latéro-dorsal interstitiel» ou N.H.L.D.I.

Le fait que les cellules de ce noyau semblent particulièrement actives chez la taupe lors de la phase d'activité sexuelle printanière (3) nous a conduit à orienter nos recherches vers l'examen d'une intervention éventuelle des ces éléments dans le contrôle de la fonction gonadotrope préhypophysaire.

L'étude de l'évolution post-natale de ces cellules (4) nous a permis d'établir qu'elles se différencient dès le milieu de la 1ére semaine après les cellules des NSO et NPV mais nettement avant les cellules gonadotropes préhypophysaires; qu'elles présentent une série de phases de mise en charge et des variations individuelles considérables suggérant une activité de type cyclique; enfin qu'elles semblent particulièrement actives à partir de la période qui précède immédiatement la puberté.

L'étude histologique de ces cellules permet de préciser les principaux stades fonctionnels (une douzaine environ) de leur cycle sécrétoire dans diverses conditions physiologiques et expérimentales, les formes dépourvues de grains de sécrétion (type 0) demeurant reconnaissables par leur topographie, leur morphologie générale et, surtout, la présence d'un noyau à deux nucléoles dont l'un au moins en position marginale. L'étude microélectronique de ces cellules (5) a permis de suivre les différents stades d'élaboration des grains dont l'évolution semble se faire principalement à l'intérieur des cavités ergastoplasmiques. La castration bilatérale provoque à partir de la 12 iéme heure environ, une réaction de mise en charge (d'amplitude physiologique) suivie d'une excrétion notable vers la 18 iéme heure (6). La castration unilatérale entraîne une réaction semblable mais d'amplitude beaucoup plus faible (7), cette dernière étant supprimée par l'administration préalable de testostérone (8).

---

* Avec la collaboration technique de Mademoiselle G. Gilibert

La comparaison de séries d'animaux castrés bilatéralement depuis 24, 30, 36, 42, 48, 54 et 72 heures, 10 jours, 1 mois, 5 mois, 6 mois et 7 mois (9, 10) nous a permis de constater l'existence d'une *réaction biphasique* des cellules du N.H.L.D.I. Celle-ci comporte une «réaction hypothalamique précoce» (avec prédominance de phénomènes de synthèse et de mise en charge, d'amplitudes supra physiologiques) suivie, au bout de quelques jours, d'une très longue phase de «réaction hypothalamique tardive» (avec phénomènes de cession l'emportant sur ceux de stockage et déplétion croissante de la charge glandulaire, le nombre de coupes de cellules en état de charge pouvant se réduire de plus de 90 % par rapport aux castrés recents).

L'étude des variations annuelles de la charge glandulaire moyenne au cours de l'année suggère l'existence d'une «phase d'activation printanière» (maximum en Mars environ) (11). L'association de la castration à cette phase d'activation printanière (animaux castrés en Septembre-Octobre et sacrifiés en Mars-Avril permet d'observer une délétion considérable de la charge glandulaire, réduite de plus de 98 %, avec apparition d'images de multinucléolation nucléaire et de margination nucléolaire, qui suggèrent une intensification de la synthèse (12) des ARN impliqués dans l'élaboration de la substance des grains.

Ces diverses observations conduisent à penser que *les cellules du N.H.L.D.I. sont le lieu d'élaboration du facteur hypothalamique* (ISCH-RF) *contrôlant la fonction gonadostimulante B* (ICSH) *préhypophysaire et sont électivement sensibles à la rétroaction négative des androgénes d'origine gonadique (testostérone).*

L'étude caryométrique des cellules du noyau infundibulaire chez des témoins et des mâles castrés depuis 24 heures jusqu'á 35 jours montre l'absence de variations significatives des diamètres (avec une plus grande fréquence à 10 microns dans toutes les séries) et suggère que, chez le cobaye, le noyau infundibulaire (même s'il intervient dans le contrôle de l'axe préhypophyso-testiculaire) n'est pas l'un des sites hypothalamiques spécifiques de rétroaction aux androgènes (13).

L'étude histoenzymologique de l'hypothalamus de cobayes normaux, castrés ou ayant reçu des injections de testostérone, montre que la castration s'accompagne d'une augmentation de l'activité acétylcholinestérasique des cellules du N.H.L.D.I. et met en évidence le fait, très intéressant, que l'activité acétylcholinestérasique paraît localisée électivement à la surface des grains de sécrétion. Il semble donc possible que l'acétylcholine (excitant physiologique probable des cellules du N.H.L.D.I.) intervienne dans l'évolution des grains au niveau des péricaryons, peut-être en déclenchant certaines transformations préalables à leur migration distale (14).

Nous avons tenté de mettre en évidence et de caractériser, dans les extraits du N.H.L.D.I.; la substance active élaborée par les cellules gomorinégatives qui le constituent. Nos observations ont porté sur un total de 1.354 cobayes mâles et de 730 rattes préparées pour le test de déplétion de l'acide ascorbique (15) ou du cholestérol (16) ovariens. Tous les extraits hypothalamiques utilisés ont été préparés à partir de *prélévements dépourvus d'éminence médiane.* Nous avons par ailleurs éliminé toutes les rattes ayant réagi insuffisamment à la préparation par les gonadotrophines sérique et chorionique (ovaires de moins de 60 mg) (17, 18, 19). Nous avons constaté: 1°. que les extraits frais acides totaux d'hypothalamus (EM exclues), à la doses de 5 hypothalamus ratte, entraînent une chute de l'acide ascorbique et du cholestérol ovariens; 2°. que les extraits frais acides de N.H.L.D.I.

(mais non d'hypothalamus «restants») entraînent des chutes significatives de l'acide ascorbique ($P < 0,05$) et du cholestérol ($P < 0,01$) ovariens (fig. 1), ces chutes étant plus accusées avec les extraits préparés en Février et Mars (périodes de mise en charge saisonnière du N.H.L.D.I.) et alors comparables à celles obtenues avec des extraits frais de préhypophyse; 3°. que les extraits frais de N.H.L.D.I. entraînent également une déplétion du cholestérol ovarien chez des rattes préparées pour le test de BELL et al. mais hypophysectomisées depuis peu, donc renferment une substance de type LH.

Le fractionnement, sur Sephadex G 50 perlé, d'extraits acides lyophilisés de N.H.L.D.I. (M. Moschetto sous la direction de M. Biserte)[1] nous a permis de séparer deux fractions actives (A et C) séparées par plusieurs fractions inactives (notamment B et BC) la fraction A possédant une activité de type LH tandis que la fraction C active chez les rattes test normales (déplétions de 22 et 37 % dans 2 séries de 10 et 7 animaux) mais, inactive chez l'animal hypophysectomisé, possède une activité de type LRF.

Ces observations nous conduisent à penser que *les cellules du N.H.L.D.I. élaborent vraisemblablement une substance active de type LRF (ou ICSH-RF), de PM compris entre 1.000 et 2.000 environ et sont en même temps le site hypothalamique électif d'une rétroaction courte, préhypophyso-hypothalamique de LH (ou ICSH).*

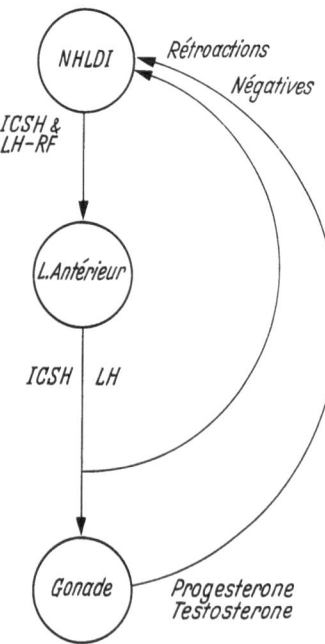

Fig. 1. *Histophysiologie des cellules du N.H.L.D.I.* — Schéma des circuits à rétroactions négatives courtes (LH ou ICSH) et longues (testostérone et progestérone) s'exerçant au niveau du N.H.L.D.I.

Bibliographie

1. BARRY, J.: Sur l'existence de cellules acidophiles de type neurosécrétoire au niveau de l'hypothalamus antérieur chez le cobaye. C.R. Soc. Biol. **148**, 133 (1954).
2. — Recherches sur la neurosécrétion diencéphalique chez Talpa europea. Bull. Soc. Sci. **15**, 49 (1956).
3. — Recherches sur la glande diencéphalique. 1) Recherches sur les cellules du noyau hypothalamique latérodorsal interstitiel de Talpa europaea. C.R. Soc. Biol. **154**, 1.250 (1960).
4. — CL. BUGNON, CHR. GIROD, J. LÉONARDELLI, S. SLIMANE-TALEB et J. F. TORRE: Etude morphologique du noyau hypothalamique latérodorsal interstitiel du cobaye de la naissance à la puberté. C.R. Soc. Biol. **155**, 735 (1961).
5. MAZZUCA, M.: Etude au microscope électronique des cellules neurosécrétoires du noyau hypothalamique latérodorsal interstitiel. C.R. Acad. Sci. (Paris) **258**, 1.898 (1964).
6. BARRY, J., et G. LEFRANC: Recherches sur les variations morphologiques des cellules du noyau hypothalamique latérodorsal interstitiel du cobaye au cours de la période précédant le déclenchement de la «réaction hypothalamique précoce à la castration» C.R. Soc. Biol. **156**, 1.838 (1962).
7. — — Etude des modifications du noyau hypothalamique latérodorsal interstitiel chez le cobaye mâle castré unilatéralement. C.R. Soc. Biol. **157**, 126 (1963).

[1] Laboratoire de Biochimie de la Faculté de Médecine

8 LEFRANC, G., et J. BARRY: Action inhibitrice du stérandryl sur la « réaction hypothalamique précoce à la castration». C.R. Soc. Biol. **156**, 1.827 (1962).

9. BARRY, J., et J. F. TORRE: Etude des modifications morphologiques du Noyau hypothalamique latérodorsal interstitiel (N.H.L.D.I.) chez le cobaye mâle castré. C.R. Soc. Biol. **155**, 2.309 (1961).

10. —, et J. LÉONARDELLI: Etude comparée de la charge glandulaire des cellules du noyau hypothalamique latérodorsal interstitiel chez le cobaye mâle et le cobaye femelle normaux. C.R. Soc. Biol. **158**, 554 (1964).

11. — — Recherches sur les variations de la charge glandulaire des cellules du noyau hypothalamique latérodorsal interstitiel du cobaye au cours de l'année. C.R. Soc. Biol. **158**, 1.618 (1964).

12. — — Effets à long terme de la castration bilatérale chez le cabaye mâle sur la réaction de mise en charge printanière des cellules du noyau hypothalamique latérodorsal interstitiel. C.R. Soc. Biol. **159**, 2.371 (1965).

13. — Etude caryométrique du noyau infundibulaire chez le cobaye mâle normal et castré. C.R. Soc. Biol. **160**, 755 (1960).

14. —, et J. LÉONARDELLI: Variations de l'activité acétylcholinestérasique de l'hypothalamus chez le cobaye mâle castré ou soumis à l'action d'androgènes. C.R. Soc. Biol. **160**, 1.608 (1966).

15. PARLOW, A.: A rapid bioassay method for LH and factors stimulating LH secretion. Fed. Proc. **17**, 402 (1958).

16. BELL, E. T., S. MUKERJI, and J. A. LORAINE: A new bioassay method for luteinizing hormone depending on the depletion of rat ovarian cholesterol. J. Endocr. **28**, 321 (1964).

17. BARRY, J., M. DAUTREVAUX, G. LEFRANC et J. C. FOURLINNIE: Recherches préliminaires sur la topographie du facteur hypothalamique contrôlant la fonction gonadostimulante B préhypophysaire chez le cobaye. C.R. Acad. Sci. **257**, 4.217 (1963).

18. — G. LEFRANC, J. LÉONARDELLI et J. C. FOURLINNIE: Effets de l'injection d'extraits frais de noyau hypothalamique latérodorsal interstitiel de cobaye sur le taux de cholestérol ovarien de rattes préparées pour le test de BELL, MUKERJI et LORAINE. C.R. Soc. Biol. **159**, 1.152 (1965).

19. — G. BISERTE, G. LEFRANC, J. LÉONARDELLI et M. MOSCHETTO: Recherches sur le site hypothalamique d'élaboration du facteur préhypophysiotrope contrôlant le sécrétion de LH-ICSH chez le cobaye. C.R. Acad. Sci. **263**, 536 (1966).

Contribution à l'étude de la neurosécrétion chez le rat par la méthode autoradiographique

J. FLAMENT-DURAND*

Laboratoire d'anatomie pathologique. Faculté de Médecine de l'Université Libre de Bruxelles et Fondation Médicale Reine Elisabeth. (Directeur: Professeur L. DESCLIN)

Lors du deuxième Symposium international sur la neurosécrétion de 1958, J. C. SLOPER apportait les premiers résultats qu'il avait obtenus dans l'étude de la neurosécrétion par autoradiographie à l'aide de cystéine S^{35} (1958). Poursuivant à l'aide de cette technique son étude de la neurosécrétion chez le rat normal, il put montrer qu'un captage intense et sélectif se fait précocément au niveau des neurones magnocellulaires de l'hypothalamus, précédant d'environ 9 heures l'arrivée de matériel radioactif dans le lobe postérieur (1960). Il objectivait ainsi grâce à l'autoradiographie la notion d'un cheminement le long du tractus supra-opticohypophysaire d'un matériel élaboré au niveau des neurones magnocellulaires de l'hypothalamus.

Nous avons repris cette méthode d'investigation chez l'animal normal, chez l'animal hypophysectomisé et chez des animaux placés dans des conditions mettant en jeu les hormones dites posthypophysaires, comme la déshydratation et la lactation (1961, 1962, 1963). Nous avons également étudié des animaux en oestrus permanent à la suite d'une illumination continue (1965). Nous désirions comparer les résultats obtenus par la technique autoradiographique à ceux obtenus par la méthode histologique utilisant la coloration à l'hématoxyline à l'alun de chrome de GOMORI, qui offrait elle, un moyen d'étudier la répartition du neurosécrétat et d'apprécier par caryométrie l'activité métabolique des différents noyaux hypothalamiques. Pour les autoradiographies, tout notre matériel a été traité de la même façon. Après fixation dans du formol 10 % et enrobage à la paraffine, les cerveaux sont coupés en série à 7 μ et les hypophyses à 5 μ. Les coupes sont ensuite couvertes par de l'émulsion Ilford de type K5. Elles sont développées après un temps d'exposition de 10 jours.

Rats normaux

Nos résultats confirment entièrement ceux de SLOPER. Nous avons constaté, chez des rats sacrifiés $^1/_2$ heure après l'injection de 50 microcuries de cystéine S^{35}, un captage intense et sélectif du radioisotope injecté, au niveau des noyaux supraoptiques (NSO) et de la portion magnocellulaire des noyaux paraventriculaires (NPV). A ce moment, aucune radioactivité n'est décelable au niveau du lobe postérieur de l'hypophyse. Il faut attendre un délai de 10 heures pour voir apparaître

* Travail effectué avec l'aide d'une subvention du Fonds National de la Recherche Scientifique Belge.

du matériel radioactif au niveau du lobe postérieur, qui devient encore plus abondant chez les animaux sacrifiés après 24 heures. Avec cet acide aminé, aucun marquage n'apparaît dans le lobe antérieur, ni le lobe intermédiaire.

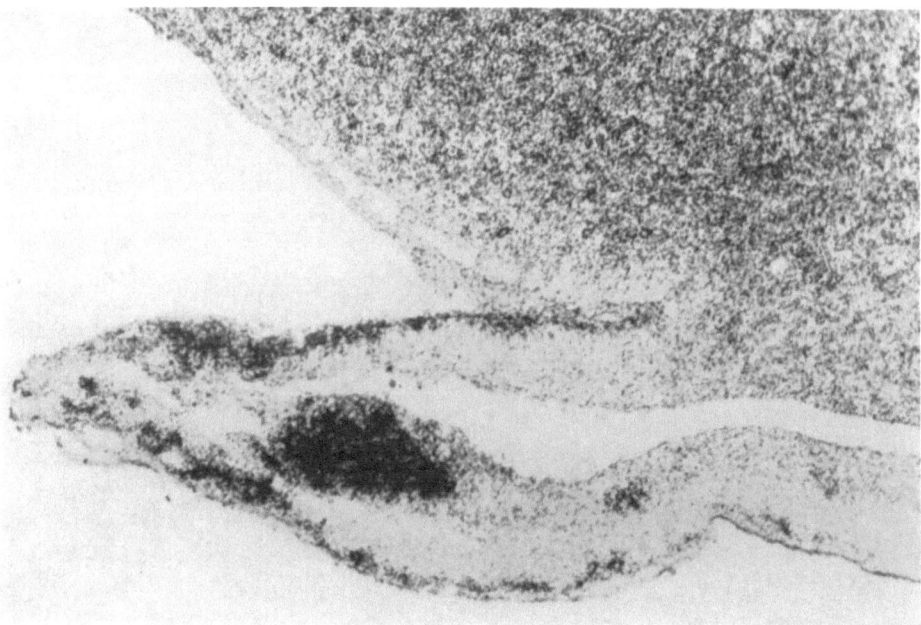

Fig. 1. Coupe sagittale passant par le moignon de tige hypophysaire d'un rat hypophysectomisé depuis 1 mois, sacrifié 24 heures après l'administration de cystéine S^{35}

Rats hypophysectomisés depuis 1 mois

On sait que chez de tels rats, il apparaît une accumulation de substances colorables par l'hématoxyline à l'alun de chrome de GOMORI au niveau du moignon de la tige hypophysaire (STUTINSKY, 1952–1955; BILLENSTEIN et LEVEQUE, 1955).

Les détracteurs de la notion de transport du neurosécrétat considèrent que ce matériel nait sur place à la suite de la dégénérescence des neurites sectionnés, les partisans de la théorie du «transport» estiment au contraire qu'il représente une accumulation des produits de neurosécrétion.

Nous avons étudié par la technique autoradiographique 5 rats hypophysec-tomisés depuis 1 mois. Deux rats sacrifiés $^1/_2$ heure après l'administration du radioisotope montrent un captage intense au niveau des neurones qui forment le NSO. Ce NSO est d'ailleurs fortement réduit de taille chez ces animaux, comme cela a été montré antérieurement (RASMUSSEN, 1937–1940). Après ce délai de $^1/_2$ heure, aucune radioactivité n'est présente dans le moignon de tige. Il faut attendre 10 heures pour voir apparaître de la radioactivité dans le moignon de la tige et ce matériel est encore visible chez les animaux sacrifiés 24 heures après l'injection du radioisitope (fig. 1). Ce délai correspond au temps de cheminement normal de la neurosécrétion et réfute la notion de l'apparition sur place du matériel Gomori positif à la suite de la dégénérescence des neurites sectionnés.

Rats soumis à une déshydratation pendant une période de 1 mois

De nombreux travaux ont étudié *la répartition du neurosécrétat* le long de l'axe hypothalamo-hypophysaire chez des animaux soumis à une déshydratation. Ces travaux ont montré un appauvrissement de l'axe neurosécrétoire en son matériel colorable, surtout important au niveau du lobe postérieur.

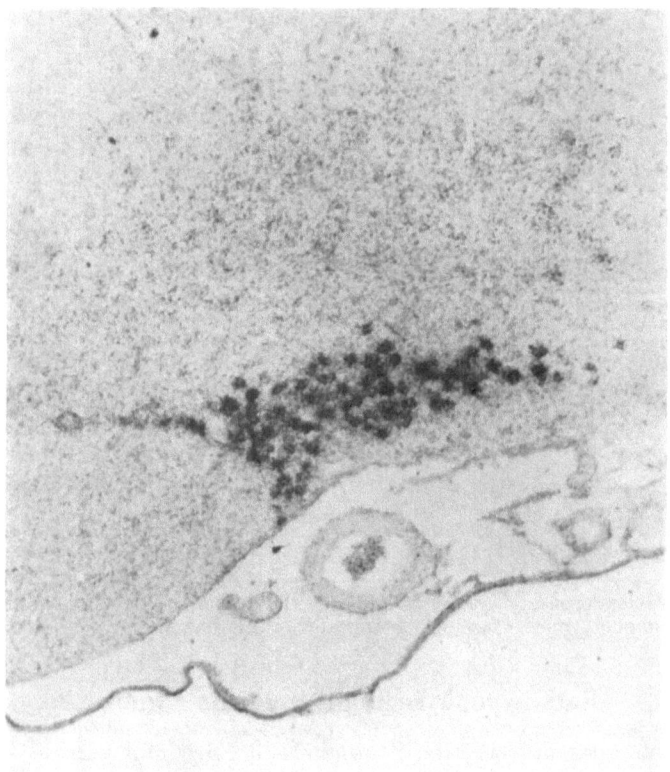

Fig. 2. Coupe frontale au niveau d'un noyau supraoptique d'un rat témoin sacrifié 1/2 heure après l'injection de cystéine S[35]

Par *des méthodes caryométriques*, Hillarp, 1949; Leveque, 1953; Wolter, 1956; Rinne, 1960; Ifft, 1962, ont montré qu'il existe après déshydratation une augmentation significative de la taille des noyaux et des nucléoles des neurones formant les NSO.

Nous avons étudié de tels animaux par la méthode autoradiographique à l'aide de cystéine S[35]. Nous avons comparé des animaux normaux à des animaux soumis à une période de déshydratation de 1 mois. Un premier groupe de 12 rats a reçu pendant 1 mois comme unique boisson de l'eau salée à 2 %. Il est comparé à 12 témoins de même âge, soumis à régime hydrique normal. Chaque animal reçoit une injection sous-arachnoïdienne de 1/10ème de cc. de sérum physiologique contenant en solution 50 microcuries de DL cystéine marquée par le S[35]. Nos animaux sont répartis en 6 groupes (4 animaux par groupe) et sacrifiés $1/_2$, 10 et 24 heures après l'injection du radioisotope.

Resultats

I. *Rats sacrifiés* $^1/_2$ *heure après l'injection du radioisotope:* (fig. 2 et 3). Chez ces animaux, nous avons constaté au niveau des neurones formant les NSO un captage très net, plus intense chez les animaux déshydratés que chez les témoins. Le captage au niveau de la partie magnocellulaire des NPV était moins intense et d'intensité comparable dans les deux groupes. Dans la posthypophyse après ce délai d'une demi-heure, il n'y a aucune radioactivité décelable.

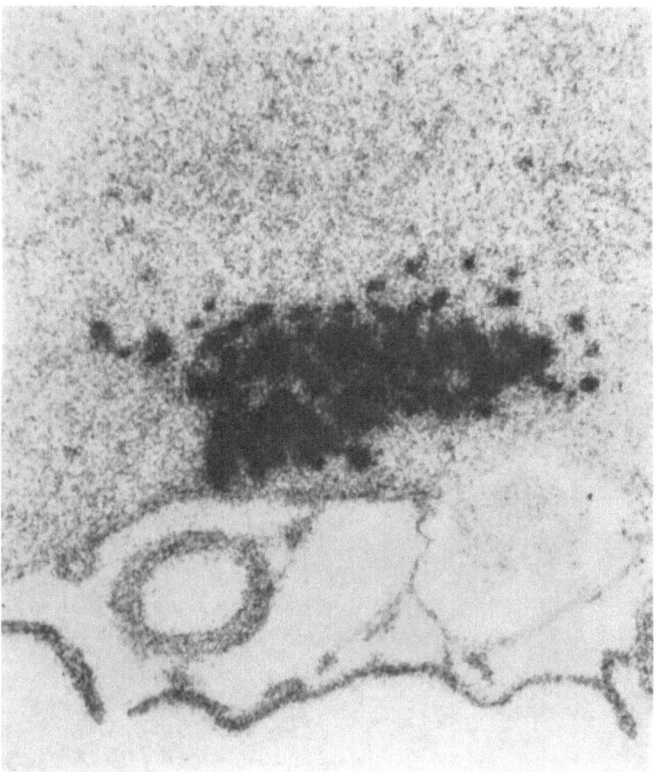

Fig. 3. Coupe frontale au niveau d'un noyau supraoptique d'un tat soumis à une déshydratation depuis un mois et sacrifié 1/2 heure après l'injection de cystéine S[35]

II. *Rats sacrifiés 10 heures après l'injection du radioisotope:* La radioactivité reste présente au niveau des NSO dans les deux groups de rats. Après ce délai de 10 heures il apparaît de la radioactivité dans le lobe postérieur de l'hypophyse, aussi bien chez les témoins que chez les animaux soumis à une déshydratation, mais chez ces derniers l'intensité du noircissement est nettement plus importante que chez les témoins (fig. 4).

III. *Rats sacrifiés après 24 heures.* La radioactivité observée au niveau du lobe postérieur est maintenant nettement moindre chez les animaux déshydratés que chez les témoins (fig. 5).

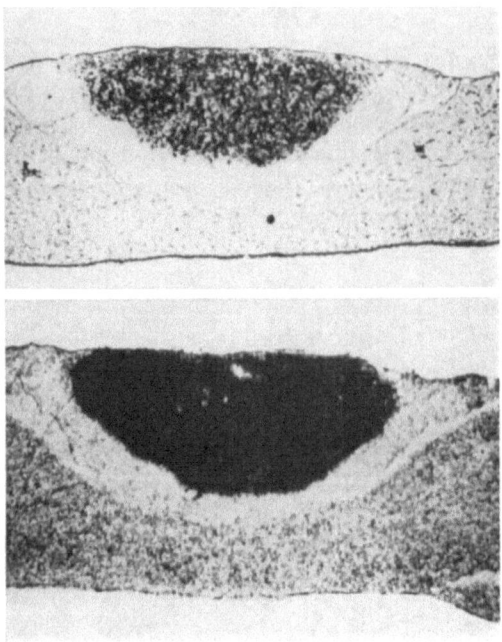

Fig. 4. Hypophyses d'animaux sacrifiés dix heures après l'injection de cystéine S³⁵. *En haut:* animal témoin. *En bas:* animal soumis à une déshydratation depuis 1 mois

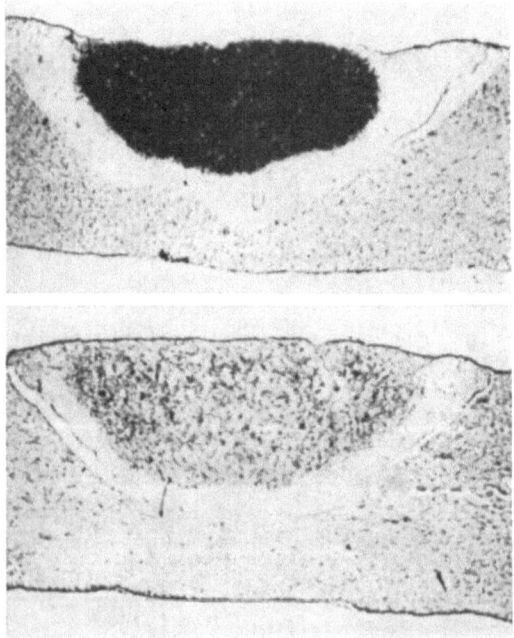

Fig. 5. Hypophyses d'animaux sacrifiés 24 heures après l'injection de cystéine S³⁵. *En haut:* animal témoin. *En bas:* animal soumis à une déshydratation depuis un mois

Conclusion

Il ne nous paraît pas douteux que le captage plus intense des acides aminés marqués par le S^{35} au niveau des NSO traduise de façon beaucoup plus directe le phénomène d'activation métabolique de ces cellules déduit de l'augmentation de taille de leurs noyaux et nucléoles chez les animaux déshydratés, par HILLARP, LEVEQUE, WOLTER, RINNE et IFFT.

L'intérêt de nos observations concerne surtout les renseignements qu'elles fournissent sur la chronologie du cheminement du «neurosécrétat» depuis les noyaux supraoptiques jusqu'au lobe postérieur de l'hypophyse. C'est ainsi qu'elles montrent qu'une radioactivité importante apparaît 10 heures après l'administration du radioisotope dans le lobe postérieur, précédant la déplétion accélérée de ce lobe postérieur en ses produits radioactifs chez les animaux soumis à une déshydratation. La disparition accélérée de la radioactivité au niveau du lobe postérieur chez les animaux déshydratés correspond sans doute à la déplétion en «neurosécrétat» Gomori + constatée au niveau du lobe postérieur par divers auteurs dans ces mêmes circonstances. Par contre, nos résultats révèlent une dissociation entre le comportement du matériel colorable au Gomori et la substance que nous avons marquée. En effet, par nos autoradiographies, nous détectons une radioactivité importante dans le lobe postérieur de l'hypophyse apparaissant 10 heures après l'administration de l'isotope, dans des conditions expérimentales où cette même hypophyse colorée au Gomori aurait montré une déplétion en son contenu en «neurosécrétat» Gomori +.

Nos résultats traduisent l'arrivée accélérée de produits élaborés en quantité plus grande par les noyaux supraoptiques activés et leur utilisation plus rapide.

HILD avait déjà montré une accélération du flux axoplasmique au niveau des NSO dans des cultures de tissu soumises à un milieu hypertonique (1954).

Animaux en lactation

On sait que la succion des mamelons par les jeunes entraine un réflexe neuro-hormonal qui provoque l'éjection du lait, mettant en jeu une libération d'ocytocine. Ce réflexe met-il en jeu les NPV ou les NSO ou ces deux formations ? L'accord n'est pas encore établi à ce sujet. Des explorations de l'axe hypothalamohypophysaire par la technique de GOMORI ont montré une baisse du contenu du lobe postérieur en son matériel neurosécrétoire (STUTINSKY, 1953–1957; MALANDRA, 1956; RENNELS, 1958; RINNE, 1960; chez le rat; RACADOT chez la chatte, 1957; COLLIN et RACADOT chez le cobaye, 1953; BRIGHTMAN chez la souris, 1955). Par contre, aucune donnée de la littérature n'apporte de renseignements caryométriques réflétant l'activité métabolique des neurones magnocellulaires au cours de la lactation, à l'exception des observations de RINNE, 1960, qui ne décèle aucune modification.

Par ailleurs, les tentatives d'établir une corrélation entre contenu en matériel neurosécrétoire colorable par le Gomori et teneur en hormone du lobe postérieur au cours de la lactation n'ont pas toujours abouti à des résultats concordants (STUTINSKY, 1957; RENNELS, 1958; DENAMUR, 1965).

Nous avons étudié des animaux en lactation par la méthode de GOMORI et par la technique autoradiographique et nous les avons comparés à des animaux ayant mis bas à la même date, mais séparés de leurs jeunes dès la mise-bas.

a) *Mesures caryométriques sur du matériel coloré par la méthode de Gomori et étude de la répartition du «neurosécrétat».* 8 rates lactantes ont été comparées à 6 rates ayant été séparées de leurs jeunes dès la naissance. Toutes les bêtes ont été sacrifiés 8 jours après la mise bas. Au moment du sacrifice, le cerveau et l'hypophyse ont été prélevés, fixés au Stieve, puis coupés en série à 7 μ pour les cerveaux et à 5 μ pour les hypophyses. Les coupes ont été colorées par l'hématoxyline à l'alun de chrome de Gomori. Chez les rates lactantes, nous avons constaté une augmentation très nette de la taille des neurones formant les noyaux supraoptiques et paraventriculaires particulièrement marquée au niveau de la portion magnocellulaire de ces derniers. Ces neurones sont augmentés de taille, leur cytoplasme est clair et on ne voit plus que de rares granulations Gomori + à la périphérie du corps cellulaire. Par contre, il existe de nombreux renflements le long des fibres nerveuses émanant de ces neurones ce qui leur donne un aspect moniliforme. Le lobe postérieur des hypophyses des bêtes lactantes contient moins de matériel Gomori + que les lobes postérieurs des animaux séparés de leurs jeunes dès la mise-bas.

Nous avons voulu préciser notre impression par des déterminations caryométriques. Nous avons à cet effet dessiné à la chambre claire 50 neurones du NPV et 100 neurones du NSO chez les animaux des deux groupes à un grossissement constant de 225 X. Les noyaux et les nucléoles ont été mesurés par planimétrie et nous exprimerons nos résultats en unités planimétriques. Ces unités sont arbitraires mais strictement constantes dans les deux groupes d'animaux, elles fournissent donc une mesure quantitative permettant de les comparer.

Les valeurs rapportées dans le tableau 1 indiquent une augmentation significative de la taille des noyaux et des nucléoles des neurones supraoptiques et paraventriculaires, traduisant un accroissement de l'activité métabolique de ces neurones neurosécrétoires au cours de la lactation.

Tableau 1. Expérience lactation

Mesures planimétriques de 50 neurones (par animal) dessinés à la chambre claire à un grossissement constant de 225 X au niveau de la partie magnocellulaire des noyaux paraventriculaires
M ± SEM

	Noyaux		Nucléoles	
Animaux en lactation	Animaux séparés de leurs jeunes dès la mise-bas		Animaux en lactation	Animaux séparés de leurs jeunes dès la mise-bas
$500,9 \pm 7,90$	$419,3 \pm 6,45$		$34,6 \pm 1,53$	$24,2 \pm 1,26$
	P < 0,001			P < 0,001

Mesures planimétriques de 100 neurones (par animal) dessinés à la chambre claire au niveau des noyaux supraoptiques
M ± SEM

Animaux en lactation	Animaux séparés de leurs jeunes dès la mise-bas		Animaux en lactation	Animaux séparés de leurs jeunes dès la mise-bas
$1.047 \pm 22,82$	$921,5 \pm 5,27$		$68,7 \pm 4,57$	$52,7 \pm 0,92$
	P < 0,001			P < 0,001

M: valeur moyenne ± erreur type de la moyenne.
P: représente le degré de signification de la différence des moyennes.

b) Autoradiographies à l'aide de cystéine S^{35}: Afin de préciser cet accroissement de l'activité métabolique des neurones magnocellulaires au cours de la lactation et de voir s'il s'accompagne d'une accélération de la vitesse de cheminement des neurohormones élaborées, le long de l'axe hypothalamo-hypophysaire vers le lobe postérieur, nous avons appliqué la méthode autoradiographique à l'aide de S^{35} L-cystéine chez des animaux en lactation et nous les avons comparés à des contrôles.

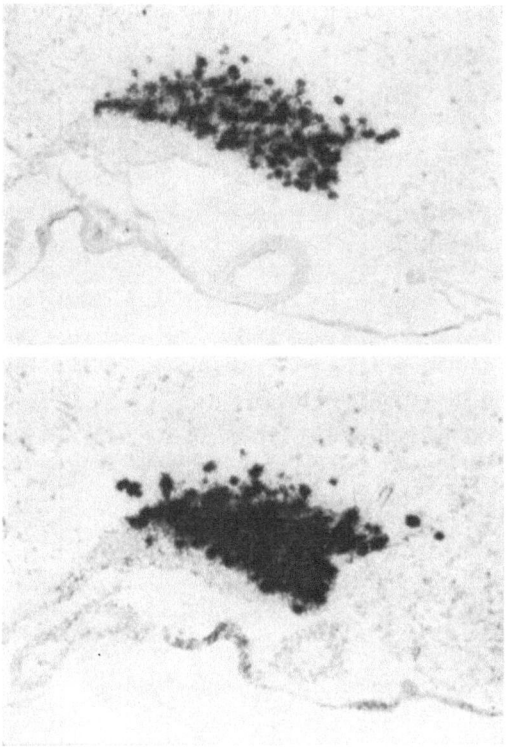

Fig. 6. Coupe frontale au niveau du noyau supraoptique de rats sacrifiés une heure après l'injection de cystéine S^{35}. *En haut:* animal témoin. *En bas:* animal en lactation depuis huit jours

Nous avons comparé 25 femelles allaitant leurs jeunes depuis 8 à 10 jours à 23 femelles de même âge ayant été séparées de leurs jeunes dès la mise bas et que nous utilisons comme groupe contrôle. Nous avons pris soin de laisser à chaque mère en expérience un nombre constant de 6 jeunes. Chacun des animaux a reçu une injection sous-arachnoïdienne de 1/10ème de ml. de sérum physiologique contenant 50 microcuries de L-cystéine S^{35}. Ils sont répartis en différents groupes selon le moment du sacrifice qui prend place 1 heure, 10 heures, 24 heures et 30 heures après l'administration du radioisotope.

Localisations hypothalamiques: Nous avons comparé 5 bêtes lactantes à 5 bêtes séparées de leurs jeunes dès la mise-bas, sacrifiées *1 heure après l'injection du radioisotope.* Nous avons constaté un captage très intense et très sélectif au niveau des noyaux supraoptiques et de la portion magnocellulaire des NPV (fig. 6 et 7).

5*

Le noircissement était nettement plus intense chez les bêtes en lactation que chez les contrôles. Cette impression sujective a pu être confirmée par des mesures histophotométriques permettant d'apprécier la radioactivité par une mesure de densité optique. A ce moment, aucune radioactivité n'est décelable au niveau de l'hypophyse.

Localisations hypophysaires: Nous avons étudié ces localisations chez des animaux sacrifiés 10, 24 et 30 heures après l'administration du radioisotope. Chacun des animaux a reçu une injection sous-arachnoïdienne de 50 microcuries de

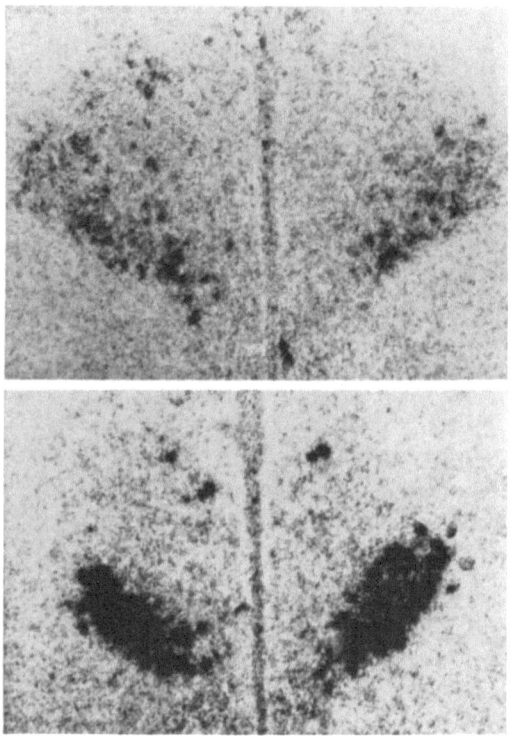

Fig. 7. Coupe frontale au niveau des noyaux paraventriculaires de rats sacrifiés une heure après l'injection de cystéine S^{35}. *En haut:* animal témoin. *En bas:* animal en lactation depuis huit jours

S^{35} cystéine. Nous avons ainsi comparé 8 rats en lactation à 8 rats séparés de leurs jeunes dès la mise bas et *sacrifiés 10 heures après l'injection de S^{35} cystéine.* Dans les deux cas, nous avons observé l'apparition de matériel radioactif sélectivement localisé dans le lobe postérieur de l'hypophyse. Le matériel apparaissant chez les animaux en lactation est nettement plus intense que chez les animaux témoins (fig. 8).

Chez les 6 bêtes sacrifiées *24 heures après l'administration du radioisotope* et que nous avons comparées à 5 bêtes contrôles, la radioactivité augmente au niveau du lobe postérieur chez les animaux contrôles et diminue chez les bêtes en lactation.

Chez les 6 animaux sacrifiés *30 heures après l'injection* et que nous avons comparés à 5 témoins, le degré de noircissement est moindre chez les animaux en lactation que chez les témoins sacrifiés après le même délai.

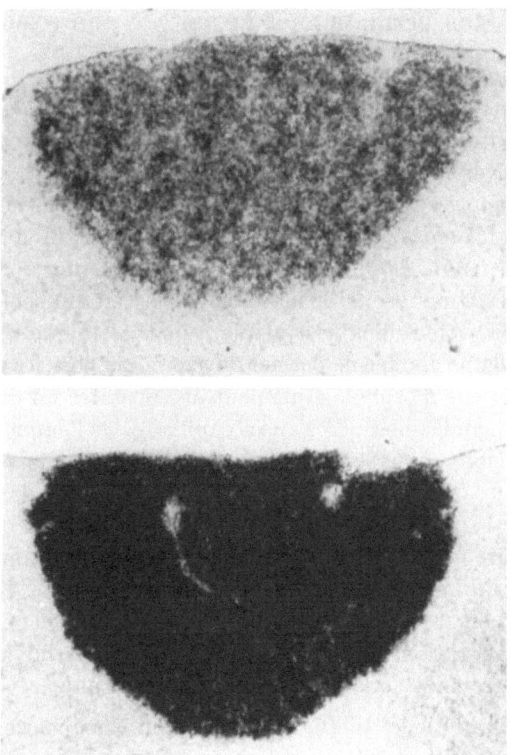

Fig. 8. Lobe postérieur de l'hypophyse d'animaux sacrifiés 10 heures après l'injection de cystéine S³⁵. *En haut:* animal témoin. *En bas:* animal en lactation depuis huit jours

En conclusion

Nos expériences montrent qu'au cours de la lactation il existe une activation métabolique au niveau des neurones formant les noyaux supraoptiques et la partie magnocellulaire des noyaux paraventriculaires, qui se traduit par une augmentation significative de la taille de leurs noyaux et de leurs nucléoles et également par un captage plus intense à leur niveau du radioisotope (L-cystéine S³⁵) que nous administrons. Parallèlement à cette activation métabolique, du matériel radioactif apparait plus précocement et en plus grande quantité dans le lobe postérieur des animaux en lactation que dans celui des témoins. Ce matériel radioactif s'y accumule transitoirement et disparait plus rapidement chez les animaux en lactation que chez les témoins. Il nous parait intéressant de souligner à nouveau que, chez des animaux en lactation où la coloration de Gomori ne révélerait qu'une déplétion en matériel colorable dans le lobe postérieur, nos images histoauroradiographiques permettent de saisir une migration accélérée d'une quantité importante

de substances radioactives 10 heures après le captage au niveau des neurones
magnocellulaires de l'hypothalamus qui est suivie d'une déplétion plus rapide du
lobe postérieur en son matériel radioactif.

Animaux en oestrus permanent à la suite d'une exposition continue à la lumière

A un moment où de nombreuses recherches établissent l'existence de médiateurs
probablement hypothalamiques contrôlant les diverses activités hypophysaires
aucun substrat morphologique ne permet de les visualiser.

Du matériel Gomori négatif et PAS + a été décrit à l'entour des flocules vas-
culaires de l'éminence médiane et dans les sinusoïdes du lobe antérieur chez
l'homme (HERLANT, 1951, 1954). Toutefois, le principal intermédiaire visible entre
l'hypothalamus et l'hypophyse est le matériel neurosécrétoire colorable au Gomori.
Quelle est sa participation dans le contrôle hypothalamique des fonctions anté-
hypophysaires ? Aucune donnée ne permet de le préciser chez les mammifères. Tout
au plus du point de vue morphologique peut-on constater un contact étroit entre
le matériel colorable au Gomori et les anses capillaires de l'éminence qui, on le sait,
vont irriguer l'adénohypophyse. La seule condition où une modification de la
neurosécrétion a pu être observée chez des mammifères, dans des conditions
expérimentales mettant en jeu le lobe antérieur, est l'état d'oestrus permanent
résultant d'un éclairement continu. On sait que l'exposition continue à la lumière
entraine chez le rat un état d'oestrus permanent (BROWMAN, 1937; FISKE, 1941;
EVERETT, 1842; DESCLIN, 1954). FISKE et GREEP, 1959, ont observé chez de tels
animaux une augmentation de la taille des neurones des noyaux supraoptiques
(NSO) et un accroissement de leur activité neurosécrétoire.

Dans un travail antérieur (1960), nous avons pu par une étude caryométrique
apporter un élément quantitatif à cette observation en démontrant une augmentation significative de la taille des neurones des NSO chez le rat maintenu dans des
conditions d'éclairage continu.

Nous nous sommes demandé ce que la technique autoradiographique à l'aide
de cystéine S35 pouvait fournir comme information dans l'étude du retentissement
sur les gonades de l'éclairement continu, condition qui stimule la fonction gonadotrope du lobe antérieur de l'hypophyse. En outre, afin de préciser l'importance de
l'intégrité de la rétine et des voies optiques sur cette action stimulante de la
lumière sur les gonades, nous avons comparé des animaux intacts à des animaux
dont les voies optiques étaient interrompues uni- et bilatéralement.

60 rats femelles âgés de 3 semaines sont répartis en 6 groupes de 10. Trois
groupes comprenant 10 rats intacts, 10 rats énucléés de l'oeil droit et 10 rats
énucléés des deux yeux, soumis à un éclairage continu depuis l'âge de 3 semaines
sont comparés à 3 groupes de 10 rats opérés de la même manière et maintenus dans
les conditions normales d'alternance diurne-nocturne. Dès l'ouverture de l'orifice
vaginal qui a pris place au cours de la 6ème semaine, les frottis ont été étudiés
quotidiennement pendant une période de 6 mois. Au moment du sacrifice, les
ovaires et le tractus génital ont été prélevés et fixés dans du Bouin-Hollande-
sublimé. Les hypophyses coupées en série à 5 μ et les cerveaux coupés en série à 7 μ

ont été colorés par l'hématoxyline à l'alun de chrome de Gomori-phloxine. Les ovaires et le vagin ont été colorés par le trichrome de MASSON.

Résultats

1. *Effets sur le cycle et sur le tractus génital:* Les animaux intacts et borgnes soumis à un éclairage permanent ont rapidement montré des phases d'allongement de leurs périodes oestrales et après 1 mois s'est installé un état d'oestrus permanent qui a persisté pendant toute la durée de l'expérience. Au moment du sacrifice, leurs ovaires contenaient de nombreux follicules et pas de corps jaunes; leur vagin était kératinisé. Les rats énucléés des 2 yeux et soumis à un éclairage continu ont présenté des cycles réguliers de 5 jours. Leurs ovaires contenaient de très nombreux corps jaunes.

2. *Etude caryométrique des noyaux supraoptiques et paraventriculaires:* Nous avons dessiné à la chambre claire à un grossissement constant de 225 X, 100 noyaux et 100 ncléoles des neurones formant le NSO. Nous en avons déterminé la surface à l'aide d'un planimètre. Les unités planimétriques sont arbitraires mais strictement constantes dans les différents groupes d'animaux.

Tableau 2. *Experience oestrus permanent à la suite d'une illumination continue*

Mesures planimètriques de 100 neurones dessinés à la chambre claire à un grossissement constant de 225 X au niveau des noyaux supraoptiques (NSO)
(M ± SEM)

Rats avec voies optiques intactes				Rats énucléés des deux yeux			
Noyaux		Nucléoles		Noyaux		Nucléoles	
Animaux témoins	Animaux exposés à la lumière	Animaux témoins	Animaux exposés à la lumière	Animaux témoins	Animaux exposés à la lumière	Animaux témoins	Animaux exposés à la lumière
868,2 ± 13,54	996,8 ± 14,76	55,8 ± 1,88	68,2 ± 0,98	803,3 ± 23,77	898,0 ± 17,40	52,2 ± 1,56	60,1 ± 1,07

Analyse statistique des valeurs des noyaux

Source de variations	Sommes des carrés	DL	Carrés moyens	F
Enucléation bilatérale/Témoins	66.994	1	66.994	21,14*
Eclairement/Témoins	124.657	1	124.657	39,33*
Interaction	2.873	1	2.873	< 1
Erreur	114.108	36	3.169	

Analyse statistique des valeurs des nucléoles

Enucléation bilatérale/Témoins	342	1	342	16,8*
Eclairement/Témoins	1.030	1	1.030	50,5*
Interaction	51	1	51	2,5
Erreur	734	36	20,4	

* $P < 10^{-3}$

Tableau 3. *Rats énucléés de l'oeil droit*

Mesures planimétriques de 100 neurones dessinés à la chambre claire à un grossissement constant de 225 X au niveau des noyaux supraoptiques (NSO)

(M ± SEM)

Noyaux				Nucléoles			
Animaux témoins		Animaux exposés à la lumière		Animaux témoins		Animaux exposés à la lumière	
NSO G.	NSO D.	NSO G.	NSO D.	NSO G.	NSO D.	NSO G.	NSO D.
799,6	778,5	921,7	915,5	51,0	50,5	61,6	67,2
± 9,83	± 7,68	± 20,25	± 16,42	± 1,11	± 0,84	± 1,51	± 2,19

Analyse statistique des valeurs des noyaux

Source de variations	Sommes des carrés	DL	Carrés moyens	F
Enucléation OD/Témoins	1.863	1	1.863	< 1
Eclairement/Témoins	167.832	1	167.832	80,4*
Interaction	555	1	555	< 1
Erreur	75.116	36	2.086,5	

Analyse statistique des valeurs des nucléoles

Source de variations	Sommes des carrés	DL	Carrés moyens	F
Enucléation OD/Témoins	5	1	5	< 1
Eclairement/Témoins	1.863	1	1.863	82,29*
Interaction	153	1	153	6,76**
Erreur	815	36	22,64	

* $P < 10^{-3}$ ** $P < 0,05$

Nous constatons que, sous l'effet de la lumière, les noyaux et les nucléoles des neurones formant les NSO augmentent de façon significative chez tous les animaux, indépendamment de l'intégrité des voies optiques (tableaux 2 et 3). L'analyse de la variance pour les noyaux donne une valeur de F = 39,33, ce qui aboutit à une probabilité de P < 0,001. D'autre part, la résection bilatérale des voies optiques entraine une réduction de taille significative des NSO (F = 21,14, P < 0,00). Enfin, les effets opposés des 3 facteurs se compensent presque complètement, au point que, chez les animaux aveugles, la stimulation lumineuse permanente a pour effet de ramener les NSO à une valeur comparable à celle d'animaux intacts soumis à l'alternance diurne-nocturne. La différence n'est pas significative (t = 1,3). Comme l'indique le tableau 2, l'analyse de la variance pour les nucléoles chez ces animaux donne également des résultats hautement significatifs. En outre, chez les rats borgnes, nous avons comparé le côté gauche au côté droit chez les animaux placés dans des conditions habituelles et chez des animaux soumis à une illumination continue. L'analyse statistique des valeurs est rapportée dans le tableau 3. Nous avons également mesuré par caryométrie 50 neurones des noyaux paraventriculaires chez 10 animaux normaux comparés à 10 animaux soumis à un éclairement continu. Les valeurs planimétriques obtenues pour ces différents groupes d'animaux ne montrent pas de différences statistiquement significatives.

3. *Etude autoradiographique de l'incorporation de cystéine S^{35} au niveau des noyaux magnocellulaires de l'hypothalamus.* 30 animaux âgés de 2 mois au début de

l'expérience ont été répartis en 2 groupes: le premier groupe a été soumis à un éclairement continu pendant une période de 3 mois, le second groupe a été maintenu dans les conditions habituelles d'alternance diurne-nocturne pendant la même période. Les frottis vaginaux ont été observés pendant 3 mois; à la fin du premier mois d'exposition continue à la lumière, un oestrus permanent s'est installé tandis que les contrôles présentaient des cycles réguliers de 4 à 6 jours. Ces 30 animaux ont alors reçu 50 microcuries de L-cystéine S^{35} par injection sous-arachnoïdienne. Ils ont été sacrifiés 1 h., 10 h. et 24 h. après l'injection du radioisotope.

Chez les animaux en oestrus permanent résultant d'une illumination continue, nous avons observé un accroissement important par rapport aux témoins du captage de la cystéine S^{35} par les neurones des noyaux supraoptiques, 1 heure après l'injection. Ce captage accru s'est accompagné chez les animaux éclairés d'une apparition plus intense de produits radioactifs au niveaux du lobe postérieur de l'hypophyse 10 heures après l'administration du radioisotope, qui a été suivie d'une déplétion accélérée du lobe postérieur en son matériel radioactif chez les animaux sacrifiés après 24 heures.

En conclusion

Il existe chez les animaux en oestrus permanent par la lumière une augmentation de l'activité métabolique des NSO qui se traduit par une augmentation de taille des noyaux et nucléoles des NOS et par une incorporation plus importante de l'acide aminé marqué qui s'accompagne d'une migration accélérée de matériel radioactif le long de l'axe hypothalamo-hypophysaire.

Notre étude autoradiographique nous permet donc de conclure que cette activation des NSO semble liée à un phénomène mettant en jeu les hormones du lobe postérieur évoluant parallèment à l'illumination continue et non lié au contrôle de la fonction gonadotrope de l'antéhypophyse. Rappelons à ce sujet que Rodeck a signalé des troubles de la fonction antidiurétique chez des enfants aveugles dès la naissance.

La méthode autoradiographique nous a permis de récolter des renseignements qu'il était impossible d'obtenir par la technique de GOMORI seule, sur la dynamique et la chronologie des phénomènes de neurosécrétion.

Nous avons pu confirmer la notion du cheminement le long du tractus supra-opticohypophysaire d'une substance élaborée dans l'hypothalamus chez l'animal normal et hypophysectomisé. Chez des animaux placés dans des conditions expérimentales mettant en jeu la participation des hormones dites posthypo-physaires, comme la déshydratation et la lactation, nous avons pu observer une activation du métabolisme des neurones magnocellulaires qui se traduit par un captage accru du radioisotope. Cette augmentation de l'activité métabolique est présente au niveau des NSO au cours de la déshydratation et au niveau des NSO et NPV au cours de la lactation. Cette augmentation de leur activité métabolique s'accompagne d'une accélération du cheminement du matériel qu'ils élaborent le ong de l'axe hypothalamo-hypophysaire et de leur utilisation accélérée.

Signalons que s'il existe une bonne concordance entre les renseignements fournis par la méthode de GOMORI et la technique autoradiographique, cette dernière nous a permis de déceler des variations dans le temps du contenu du lobe postérieur en matériel radioactif, là où la technique de Gomori ne montrait qu'une déplétion en «neurosécrétat».

Nous pensons que la cystéine S^{35} que nous injectons à nos rats est utilisé par les neurones magnocellulaires qui élaborent des neurohormones étiquetées par le S^{35}.

Notre interprétation trouve une confirmation dans les travaux récents de Sachs et Takabatake, 1964, qui démontrent que la perfusion de cystéine S^{35} dans le 3ème ventricule chez le chien aboutit à l'élaboration de vasopressine marquée par le S^{35}. Nous pensons donc que nous suivons le cheminement des hormones elles-mêmes particulièrement riches en cystéine, tandis que le matériel élaboré colorable par le Gomori serait leur vecteur protéique. Nos résultats sont en accord avec les conclusions récentes de divers auteurs qui insistent sur l'absence de corrélation entre le contenu hormonal de la posthypophyse et sa teneur en matériel Gomori + (Moses, Leveque, Giambattista et Lloyd, 1963; Lederis, 1965).

Nous avons essayé de préciser l'éventuelle participation de la neurosécrétion Gomori + dans le contrôle de la fonction antéhyophysaire. En effet, chez des animaux en oestrus permanent à la suite d'une illumination continue, nous avions constaté, à la suite de Fiske et de Greep une augmentation de taille significative des noyaux et des nucléoles formant les NSO. Nous retrouvions cette augmentation de taille mais à un degré moindre chez des animaux énucléés bilatéralement. Notre étude autoradiographique montre un accroissement du captage du radioisotope au niveau des NSO qui s'accompagne d'une migration accélérée de produit radioactif vers le lobe postérieur de l'hypophyse.

Nous pouvions donc conclure que cette activation semblait liée à un phénomène mettant en jeu les hormones du lobe postérieur, évoluant parallèlement à l'illumination continue et non lié au contrôle de la fonction gonadotrope de l'antéhypophyse.

Nous avons le projet d'essayer de préciser que la substance dont nous suivons la migration représente bien les octapeptides hormonaux en essayant de démontrer que c'est bien dans la fraction hormonale active que se retrouve le pic de radioactivité. Ces travaux sont actuellement en cours.

Disons pour conclure que la technique autoradiographique proposée par Sloper en 1958 fournit un moyen d'investigation intéressant de l'axe neurosécrétoire et de la cinétique des phénomènes de neurosécrétion.

Bibliographie

Bargmann, W., W. Hild, R. Ortmann u. Th. Schiebler: Morphologische und experimentelle Untersuchungen über das hypothalamisch-hypophysäre System. Acta neuroveg. (Wien) 1, 233—245 (1950).

Billenstein, D. C., and T. F. Leveque: The reorganization of the neurohypophysealstalk following hypophysectomy in the rat. Endocrinology 56, 704—717 (1955).

Brightman, M. W.: Neurosecretion and milk ejection in the mouse. Anat. Rec. 121, 268—269 (1955).

Collin, R., et J. Racadot: La chute du taux de la substance Gomori + neurohypophysaire dans le postpartum chez le cobaye. Ann Endocrin. (Paris) 14, 546—549 (1953).

Denamur, R.: The hypothalamo-hypophyseal system and the milk-ejection reflex. Dairy Sci. Abstr. 27, 193—224 and 263—280 (1965).

Ficq, A., and J. Flament-Durant: Autoradiography in endocrine research, p. 73—85. (Ed. P. Eckstein and F. Knowles). London: Academic Press 1963.

FISKE, V. M., and R. O. GREEP: Neurosecretory activity in rats under conditions of continuous light and darkness. Endocrinology **64**, 175—185 (1959).

FLAMENT-DURAND, J.: Etude des relations hypothalamo-hypophysaires à l'aide de radio-isotopes marqués au Soufre 35. C.R. Acad. Sci. (Paris) **252**, 3487—3500 (1961).

— Etude du système hypothalamo-hypophysaire chez des rats déshydrates et chez des rats hypophysectomisés; dans Livre Jubilaire du Dr. LUDO VAN BOGAERT, p. 286—295. Bruxelles: Acta Medica Belgica 1962.

— Action de la lumière sur les noyaux hypothalamiques chez le rat. Ann. Endocr. **26**, (Paris) 609 —613 (1965).

— Contribution à l'étude des relations hypothalamo-hypophysaires. Ann. Soc. roy. Sci. méd. nat. Brux. **19**, 1—119 (1966).

—, et L. DESCLIN: Action d'un éclairage permanent sur les neurones et le neurosécrétat des noyaux hypothalamiques du rat. C.R. Soc. Biol. (Paris) **154**, 513—1515 (1960).

HERLANT, M.: Une forme de neurosécrétion transportée vers le lobe antérieur de l'hypophyse. C.R. Acad. Sci. (Paris) **238**, 1739—1742 (1954).

HILD, W.: Das morphologische kinetische und endokrinologische Verhalten von hypothala-mischen und neurohypophysärem Gewebe in vitro. Z. Zellforsch. **40**, 257—312 (1954).

HILLARP, N. A.: Cell reactions in the hypothalamus following overloading of the antidiuretic function. Acta Endocrin. **2**, 33—43 (1949).

IFFT, J. D.: Evidence of gonadotrophic activity of the hypothalamic arcuate nucleus in the female rat. Anat. Rec. **142**, 1—8 (1962).

LEDERIS, K.: Relationship between fine structure and function of the vertebrate hypothalamo-neurohypophysial system. In: Proceedings of the Second International Congress of Endo-crinology. p. 563—569. London 1964,

—, and H. HELLER: Intracellular storage of vasopressin and oxytocin in the posterior pituitary lobe. In: First Internation Congress of Endocrinology Copenhagen 1960.

LEVEQUE, T. F.: Changes in the neurosecretory cells of the rat hypothalamus following ingestion of sodium chloride. Anat. Rec. **117**, 741—758 (1953).

MALANDRA, B.: Beobachtungen am neurosekretorischen Zwischenhirnsystem der normalen, trächtigen und laktierenden Ratte. Z. Zellforsch. **43**, 594—610 (1956).

MOSES, A. M., T. F. LEVEQUE, M. GIAMBATTISTA, and C. W. LLOYD: Dissociation between the content of vasopressin and neurosecretory material in the rat neurohypophysis. J. Endocrin. **26**, 273—278 (1963).

ORTMANN, R.: Morphologisch experimentelle Untersuchungen über das diencephal hypo-physäre System im Verhältnis zum Wasserhaushalt. Klin. Wschr. **28**, 449 (1950).

— Über experimentelle Veränderungen der Morphologie des hypophysen Zwischen-Hirn-system und die Beziehung der sog. „Gomorisubstanz" zur Adiuretni. Z. Zellforsch. **36**, 92—140 (1951).

RACADOT, J.: Neurosécrétion et activité thyroïdienne chez la chatte au cours de la gestation et de l'allaitement. Ann. Endocr. (Paris) **18**, 628—634 (1957).

— La neurohypophyse de la chatte au cours de la gestation et de l'allaitement. C.R. Soc. Biol. (Paris) **151**, 764—766 (1957).

RASMUSSEN, A. T.: Reaction of the supraoptic nucleus to hypophysectomy. Proc. Soc. exp. Biol. **36**, 729—731 (1937).

— Effects of hypophysectomy and hypophysial stalk resection on the hypothalamic nuclei of animals and man. Res. Publ. Ass. nerv. ment. Dis. **20**, 245—269 (1940).

RENNELS, E. G.: Effects of lactation on the neurohypophysis of the rat. Tex. Rep. Biol. Med. **16**, 219—231 (1958).

RINNE, V. K.: Neurosecretory material around the hypophysial portal vessels in the median eminence of the rat. Studies on its histological properties and functional significance. Acta endocr. (suppl.) **57**, 9—108 (1960).

SACHS, H., and Y. TAKABATAKE: Evidence for a precursor in vasopressin biosynthesis. Endo-crinology **75**, 943—948 (1964).

SLOPER, J. C.: The application of newer histochemical and isotope techniques for the locali-sation of protein-bound cystine or cysteine to the study of hypothalamic neurosecretion in normal and pathological conditions. Internationales Symposium über Neurosekretion 1955, 2. 20.

Sloper, J. C., D. J. Arnott, and B. C. King: Sulphur metabolism in the pituitary and hypothalamus of the rat: a study of radioisotope uptake after injection of S³⁵ DL-cystéine, methionin and sodium sulphate. J. Endocrin. 20, 9—23 (1960).

Stutinsky, F.: Sur l'origine diencéphalique des hormones dites posthypophysaires. C.R. Soc. Biol. 146, 1691 (1952).

— Sur la substance Gomori-positive du complexe hypothalamo-hypophysaire du rat. C.R. Ass. Anat. 70, 942—949 (1952).

— La neurosécrétion de l'anguille normale et hypophysectomisée. Z. Zellforsch. 39, 276—297 (1953).

— La neurosécrétion au cours de la gestation et le post-partum chez la rate. Ann. Endocr. (Paris) 14, 722—731 (1953).

— Effets de l'hypophysectomie totale ou partielle sur la neurosécrétion hypothalamique du rat. C.R. Ass. Anat. 92, 1256—1266 (1955).

— Recherches expérimentales sur le complexe hypothalamo-neurohypophysaire. Arch. Anat. micr. Morph. exp. (suppl.) 46, 93—158 (1957).

Wolter, R.: Mesure de l'activité sécrétoire des cellules du noyau supra-optique dans diverses conditions expérimentales. Arch. Biol. (Liège) 67, 555—569 (1956).

Eine licht- und elektronenmikroskopische Analyse des neuroendokrinen Zwischenhirn-Vorderlappen-Komplexes der Vögel*

A. Oksche, Gießen

Anatomisches Institut der Justus Liebig-Universität Gießen

Einleitung

Auf dem 3. Internationalen Symposium über Neurosekretion (Bristol 1961) haben wir in zwei Vorträgen (Oksche; Farner, Oksche und Lorenzen) über das neurosekretorische System von *Zonotrichia leucophrys gambelii* (Aves, Passeriformes, Fringillidae) berichtet. Aus den damaligen neurohistologischen Befunden wurde geschlossen, daß die *Eminentia mediana (infundibuli)* dieses Vogels sowohl mit dem supraopticoparaventriculären neurosekretorischen System als auch mit den Tuberkernen nervös verknüpft ist (Abb. 1). Die mit Neurosekretmethoden sehr intensiv färbbare Palisadenschicht ihres rostralen Abschnittes wurde als ein *zweites*, vom Hypophysenhinterlappen unabhängiges *Neurosekretdepot* gedeutet. Eine Arbeitshypothese hatte zum Ziel, lichtabhängige Gonadenreaktionen (Benoit u. Assenmacher, 1953, 1959) mit Neurosekretschwankungen in der Eminentia mediana in Einklang zu bringen.

In den vergangenen fünf Jahren konnte vom Arbeitskreis Farners ein im einzelnen wesentlich präziseres Bild der Eminentia mediana entworfen werden. Diese Befunde betreffen vor allem die regionalen Unterschiede in der Enzymverteilung (histochemische Studien von Kobayashi, 1964/65) und den anatomischen Aufbau des portalen Hypophysenkreislaufs (Modellrekonstruktionen nach Gefäßinjektion von Vitums u. a., 1964, 1966). Sowohl der rostrale als auch der caudale Wulst der Eminentia mediana sind als *neurohämale Regionen* aufzufassen, die voneinander unabhängig auf dem *Gefäßweg* mit dem Hypophysenvorderlappen verbunden sind.

Von den *histochemischen* Befunden verdient die Tatsache Beobachtung, daß — ungeachtet der unterschiedlichen Neurosekretdichte — der Nachweis von Acetylcholinesterase und Monoaminoxydase sowohl im rostralen als auch im caudalen Abschnitt der Eminentia mediana positiv ausfällt (Kobayashi, 1964/65).

Weiterhin zeigten die *stereotaktischen Operationen* von F. E. Wilson, 1965, daß bei *Zonotrichia leucophrys gambelii* die lichtabhängigen Hodenreaktionen (Gewichts- und Größenzunahme) im wesentlichen wohl über die Tuberkerne vermittelt werden. Eine proximal von der Eminentia mediana durchgeführte vollständige Durchtrennung der neurosekretorischen Bahn war ohne Einfluß auf die von der Photoperiode abhängige Hodenaktivierung.

Schließlich haben Bern u. a., 1966, mit dem *Elektronenmikroskop* nachgewiesen, daß die Nervenendigungen der Eminentia mediana von *Zonotrichia leucophrys gambelii* einen kleinen (um 400 Å), scheinbar leeren Granulatyp, der nicht den Hinterlappeneinschlüssen entspricht, enthalten. Eine Unterscheidung der beiden, neurohistologisch doch so verschiedenen Abschnitte der Eminentia mediana ist auf Grund des Ultrastrukturbildes nicht möglich.

* Mit Unterstützung durch die Deutsche Forschungsgemeinschaft. Einen Teil des Tiermaterials verdanke ich Herrn Prof. Dr. D. S. Farner, Seattle, Wash., USA (Grant from the National Institutes of Health NB 01353).

Fragestellung

Da die Spezifität der Paraldehydfuchsin-Färbung nach neueren Erfahrungen nicht sehr groß ist (vgl. Bern, 1966/67), muß gefragt werden, ob das elektiv tingierte Material in der Palisadenschicht der Eminentia mediana tatsächlich dem *Tractus supraoptico-paraventriculo-hypophyseus* entstammt und nicht etwa in den Endigungen des *Tractus tubero-infundibularis* entsteht.

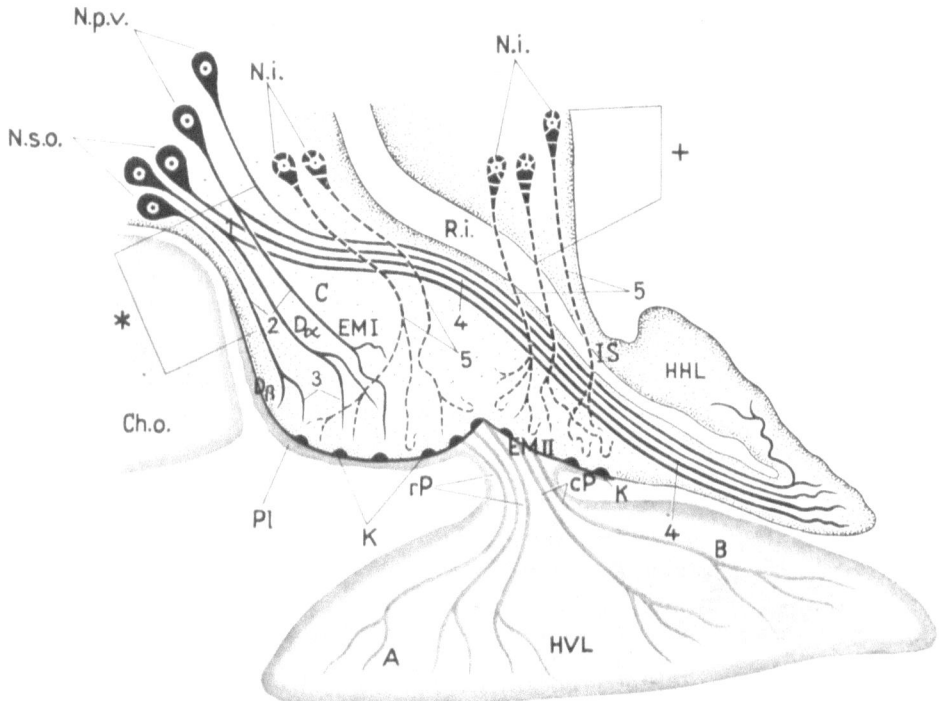

Abb. 1. *Zwischenhirn-Hypophysensystem* eines *Spatzenvogels*, dargestellt nach Befunden bei *Zonotrichia leucophrys gambelii* (Schematischer Sagittalschnitt, gez. I. Völker). — *Ch. o.-* Chiasma opticum, *R. i.-*Recessus infundibuli. *HHL-*Hypophysenhinterlappen; *HVL-*Hypophysenvorderlappen mit seinem Lobus cephalicus (*A*) und Lobus caudalis (*B*); *PI-*Pars infundibularis (tuberalis); *EM I-*rostraler Wulst; *EMII-*caudaler Wulst der *Eminentia mediana*; *IS-*Infundibularstamm. *N. s. o.-Nucl. supraopticus*; *N. p. v.-Nucl. paraventricularis*; *1* und *4-Tr. supraoptico-paraventriculo-hypophyseus*; *2-*gebündelte elektiv färbbare Fasern, die in die *Palisadenschicht* (*3*) der Eminentia mediana eindringen. Die Frage, ob diese als Axone besonderer neurosekretorischer Zellen oder als Kollateralen des Tr. supraoptico-paraventriculo-hypophyseus aufzufassen sind, ist ungeklärt. *N. i.-Nucl. infundibularis, 5-Tr. tubero-infundibularis* (caudal verdichtet). *Portales Gefäßsystem* mit dem primären Capillarnetz (*K*), einem rostralen (*rP*) und einem caudalen (*cP*) portalen Gefäßbündel. (Zur Erläuterung der Abb. 4 und 5. Besondere Stellen der Materialentnahme für elektronenmikroskopische Untersuchungen bei *Passer domesticus*: *C*, D_α, D_β — drei verschieden tiefe Zonen der Zona externa; + s. Abb. 5 A—D; * s. Abb. 5 E, F)

Zur Klärung dieses Problems sind die folgenden Fragen zu beantworten: 1. Ist die mit Paraldehydfuchsin färbbare Substanz der Palisadenschicht — ähnlich wie das Neurosekret des Hinterlappensystems — ein an SH- bzw. SS-Gruppen reicher Stoff? 2. Kommt ein solches Material auch in den Perikaryen des Nucleus infundibularis oder im Verlauf des Tractus tuberoinfundibularis vor? 3. Ist in Neurosekretfärbungen und silberimprägnierten Nervenfaserpräparaten wirklich ein direktet anatomischer Zusammenhang des Tr. supraoptico-paraventriculohypophyseus mir der Palisadenschicht vorhanden? 4. Welche Typen von Elementargranula finden sich a) in den Perikaryen des Nucleus infundibularis, b) im proximalen, noch vor der Eminentia mediana gelegenen Teil der neurosekretorischen Bahn und c) in den Perikaryen des Nucleus supraopticus.

Befunde

I. Lichtmikroskopischer Teil (Abb. 2 und 3)

1. Die *Palisadenstrukturen* der Eminentia mediana lassen sich bei *Zonotrichia leucophrys gambelii* nicht nur mit Paraldehydfuchsin und Chromalaunhämatoxylin, sondern auch mit den für das cystinreiche Neurosekret spezifischeren Alcianblau- und Viktoriablau-Verfahren darstellen (Methodik s. SLOPER u. a., 1956). Alle diese Färbungen gelingen erst nach vorheriger Oxydation. Die Palisadenschicht zeigt außerdem (nach Oxydation) eine *positive Pseudoisocyanin-Reaktion*, die besonders gut fluorescenzmikroskopisch (Verfahren von STERBA) zu beobachten ist (Abb.2C). Mit dieser sehr empfindlichen Methode wird das Trägerprotein (Neurophysin) der Oxytocine erfaßt (STERBA u. WELLNER, 1963; STERBA, 1965). Eine weitere Stütze dieser Ergebnisse ist der bei der gleichen Vogelart von TAGUCHI u. a., 1966, erhobene Befund, daß nach intraventriculärer Injektion von ^{35}S DL-Cystein radioaktives Material nicht nur im Hinterlappensystem, sondern auch in den Palisaden der Eminentia mediana auftritt.

2. Die Perikaryen des Nucleus infundibularis und ihre im Tractus tuberoinfundibularis zusammengefaßten Nervenfortsätze enthalten *keine* mit den obengenannten Neurosekretfärbungen nachweisbaren Substanzen.

3. Mit allen Neurosekretfärbungen – auch mit Pseudoisocyanin – kann man in Schnittserien ein *elektiv tingiertes Faserbündel* darstellen, das sich am rostralen Rand der *Eminentia mediana* von der neurosekretorischen Hinterlappenbahn trennt und nach basal wendet. Die Körnchenketten dieses Faserzuges werden palisadenwärts immer deutlicher, um schließlich in diesem depotartigen Saum zu verdämmern.

Ein besonders plastisches Bild dieses Fasersystems und seiner räumlichen Beziehungen vermitteln aufgehellte *Totalpräparate* (Abb. 2A, B, D, E), die man sowohl mit Viktoriablau (BRAAK, 1962) als auch mit Paraldehydfuchsin (OKSCHE, MAUTNER u. FARNER, 1964) herstellen kann.

4. Schließlich sind die vom rostralen Teil des Hypothalamus kommenden *Eminentia-Fasern* auch mit *Silberimprägnationstechniken* einwandfrei darstellbar (Abb. 3A). Diese Fasern, die zum Teil auch noch nach Versilberung mit Paraldehydfuchsin tingierbar sind, erscheinen viel zarter als die grobimprägnierten Züge der Hinterlappenverbindung. Im Verband der neurosekretorischen Bahn findet man sie, von den Hinterlappenfasern überlagert, am weitesten basal, unmittelbar auf der Konvexität des Chiasma opticum. Die Ursprungszellen dieser Fasern konnten leider noch nicht ermittelt werden und so wissen wir nicht, ob diese Perikaryen diffus verteilt oder in einem besonderen Kernareal des neurosekretorischen Systems lokalisiert sind. Sollte es sich aber erweisen, daß diese

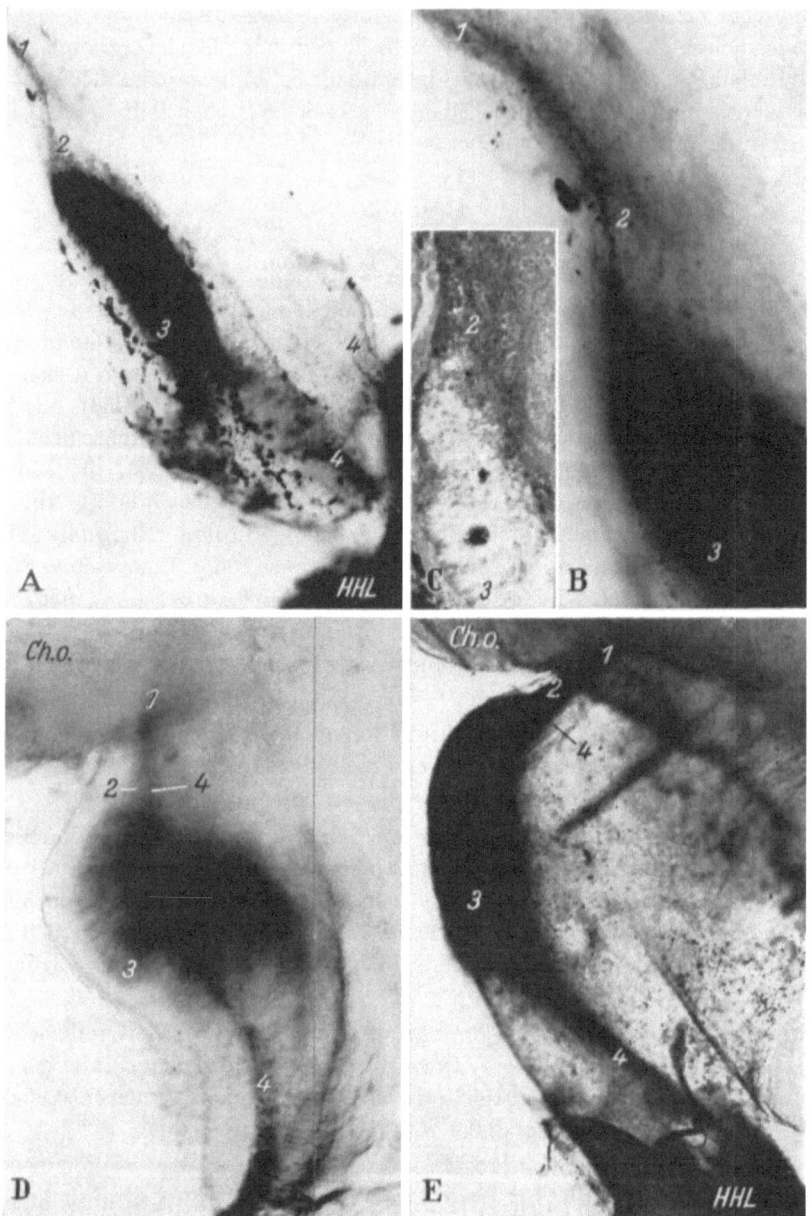

Abb. 2 A—E. Aufgehellte *Totalpräparate* (A, B, D, E) des *neurosekretorischen* Systems (Bouin fix). — *Ch. o.*-Chiasma opticum. *1.* hypothalamischer Teil der neurosekretorischen Bahn, *2.* elektiv gefärbtes Bündel zu den Palisadenzügen der Eminentia mediana (*3*). *4.* neurosekretorische Bahn zum Hypophysenhinterlappen (HHL). A, B: *Zonotrichia leucophrys gambelii*. Paraldehydfuchsin. Sehnervenkreuzung und Tr. opticus durch Präparation entfernt. Vergr. 90 und 225fach. (Das eingefügte Schnittpräparat C zeigt die Sekundärfluorescenz der mit *2* und *3* gekennzeichneten Strukturen. Bouin. *Pseudoisocyanin-Reaktion* n. STERBA; Filter BG 12 und K 530. Vergr. 200fach). D *Passer domesticus*. Viktoriablau. Vergr. 200fach. E *Ente*. Paraldehydfuchsin. Vergr. 30fach

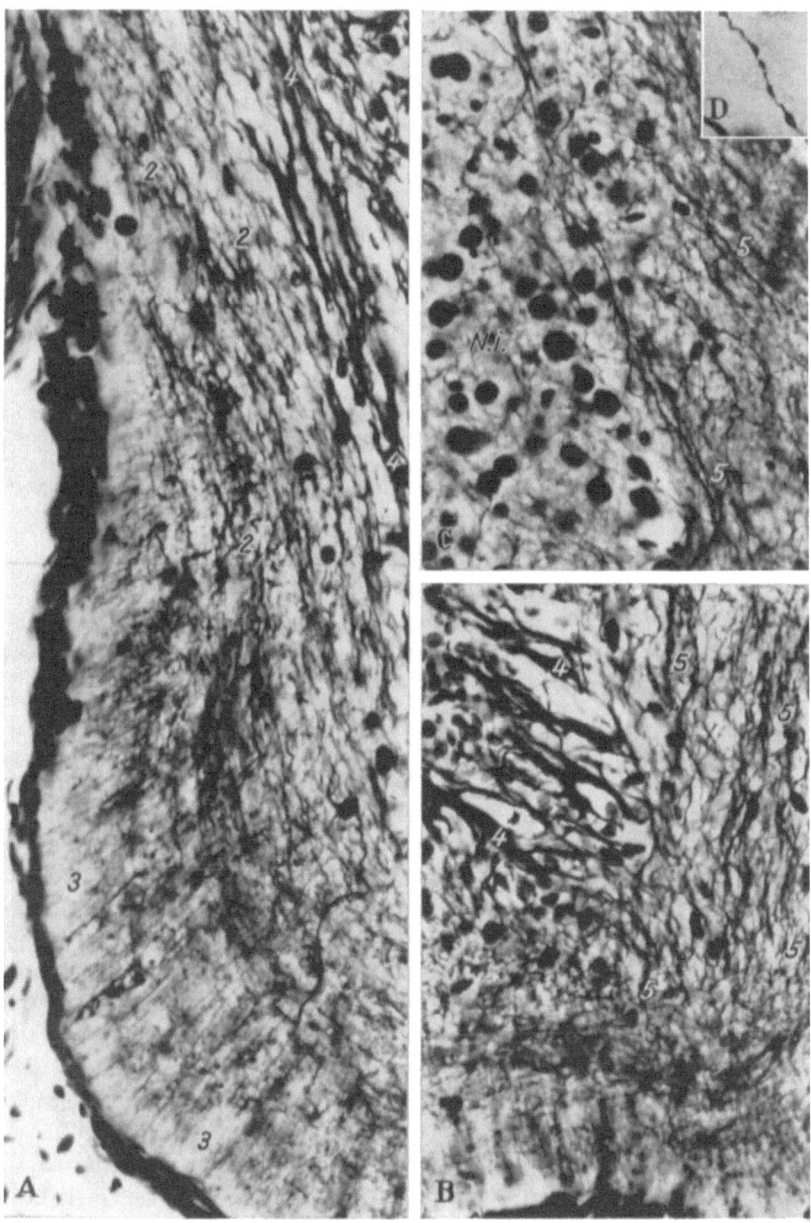

Abb. 3 A—D. *Neurohistologisches* Bild der *Fasersysteme* im *Zwischenhirn-Hypophysensystem* (Sagittalschnitt) von *Zonotrichia leucophrys gambelii* (vgl. Abb. 1). — Formalin. A—C: Bodian-Ziesmer; D: Golgi-Bubenaite. Vergr. 600 mal. A: *rostrale* Randpartie der *Eminentia mediana*. *2.* feine Faserzüge zur Eminentia mediana mit Beziehungen zur Palisadenformation *(3)*. *4*—grobfaserige neurosekretorische Bahn zum Hypophysenhinterlappen; B: *caudale* Randpartie der *Eminentia mediana* mit einstrahlenden Fasern des Tr. tubero-infundibularis *(5)*; C: *Nucl. infundibularis (N. i.)* mit dem Anfangsteil des Tr. tuberoinfundibularis *(5)*; D: Varicöse Faserelemente im Bereich des Nucl. infundibularis

Fasern nicht aus den bekannten neurosekretorischen Kerngebieten hervorgehen, dann muß die Existenz eines Tractus hypophyseus anterior (Wingstrand, 1951) erneut diskutiert werden.

Diskussion

Die Silberpräparate, die in diesem Fall eine besonders subtile Technik erfordern, zeigen deutlich, daß die beschriebenen *neurosekretorischen* Eminentia-Fasern *nicht* als ein Teil des Tr. tubero-infundibularis aufzufassen sind. Die Faserzüge des letzteren sind noch viel zarter und anders strukturiert (Abb. 3 B−D). Am deutlichsten sind sie am caudalen Rand des Hypothalamus zu erkennen. Die Eminentia mediana wird in rostrocaudaler Richtung immer stärker von Fasern des Tubersystems durchsetzt; dieses System ist aber grundsätzlich auch im rostralen Eminentia-Wulst vertreten.

Daß das elektiv tingierbare Eminentia-Bündel zu den neurosekretorischen Bahnen des vorderen Hypothalamus gehört, zeigt auch eine von F. E. Wilson, 1965, p. 73, operierte *Zonotrichia leucophrys gambelii*. Nach einseitiger Ausschaltung der neurosekretorischen Bahn proximal von der Eminentia mediana waren die gleichseitigen Palisadenzüge bis zur Medianebene nicht mehr mit Paraldehydfuchsin anfärbbar.

II. Elektronenmikroskopischer Teil

Nach Bern und Nishioka, 1965, sowie Bern u. a., 1966, sind die *Elementargranula* der *Palisadenschicht* wesentlich *kleiner* als die Einschlüsse des Hinterlappensystems. Hinsichtlich der Größe und Dichte des ersteren bestehen ausgeprägte Artunterschiede. Die Herkunft des kleingranulären Eminentia-Materials ist ungeklärt.

Aus technischen Gründen wurden die eigenen elektronenmikroskopischen Untersuchungen nicht bei *Zonotrichia leucophrys gambelii* sondern bei *Passer domesticus* durchgeführt. Die lichtmikroskopische Anatomie des Hypothalamus von *Passer domesticus* entspricht grundsätzlich dem bei *Zonotrichia leucophrys gambelii* geschilderten Bild. Untersucht wurden alle die Regionen, die die wesentlichsten Fasersysteme der Eminentia mediana (s. oben) und ihre Ursprungszellen enthalten.

1. *Elementargranula im Hypophysenhinterlappen* (Abb. 4A) *und in der Palisadenschicht der Eminentia mediana* (Abb. 4B, C). Im Gegensatz zu den typischen, meist 1500−2000 Å großen Granula im Hypophysenhinterlappen und dem caudalen, im Infundibularstamm verlaufenden Abschnitt der neurosekretorischen Bahn, messen die *Elementargranula* in der *äußersten* (dem Capillarnetz benachbarten) *Palisadenformation* nur etwa 800−1000 Å. Viele dieser Granula haben bei *Passer domesticus* − in Übereinstimmung mit Bern und Nishioka, 1965 − einen elektronendichten Kern. Neben diesem Körnchentyp kommen auch noch leere Bläschen mit einem Durchmesser von 300−600 Å vor. Größere elektronendichte Granula (Durchmesser um 2000 Å) sind in einer relativ geringen Zahl lediglich in den inneren, schon der Hinterlappenbahn enger benachbarten Zonen der Palisadenschicht und der retikulären Formation (C in Abb. 1) anzutreffen (Abb. 4D).

2. *Elementargranula im Bereich des Nucleus infundibularis* (Abb. 5A−D). In den Perikaryen des *Nucleus infundibularis* und in den feinen marklosen *Nervenfasern* dieses Areals finden sich in unserem Material 800−1000 Å, zum Teil aber auch sogar bis 1700 Å große elektronendichte Granula. Sie werden in der Golgi-Zone der Nervenzellen (Abb. 5D) gebildet. Damit zeigen auch diese („Gomorinegativen") Zellen eine sekretorische Aktivität (Monoamine ? vgl. Fuxe, 1964).

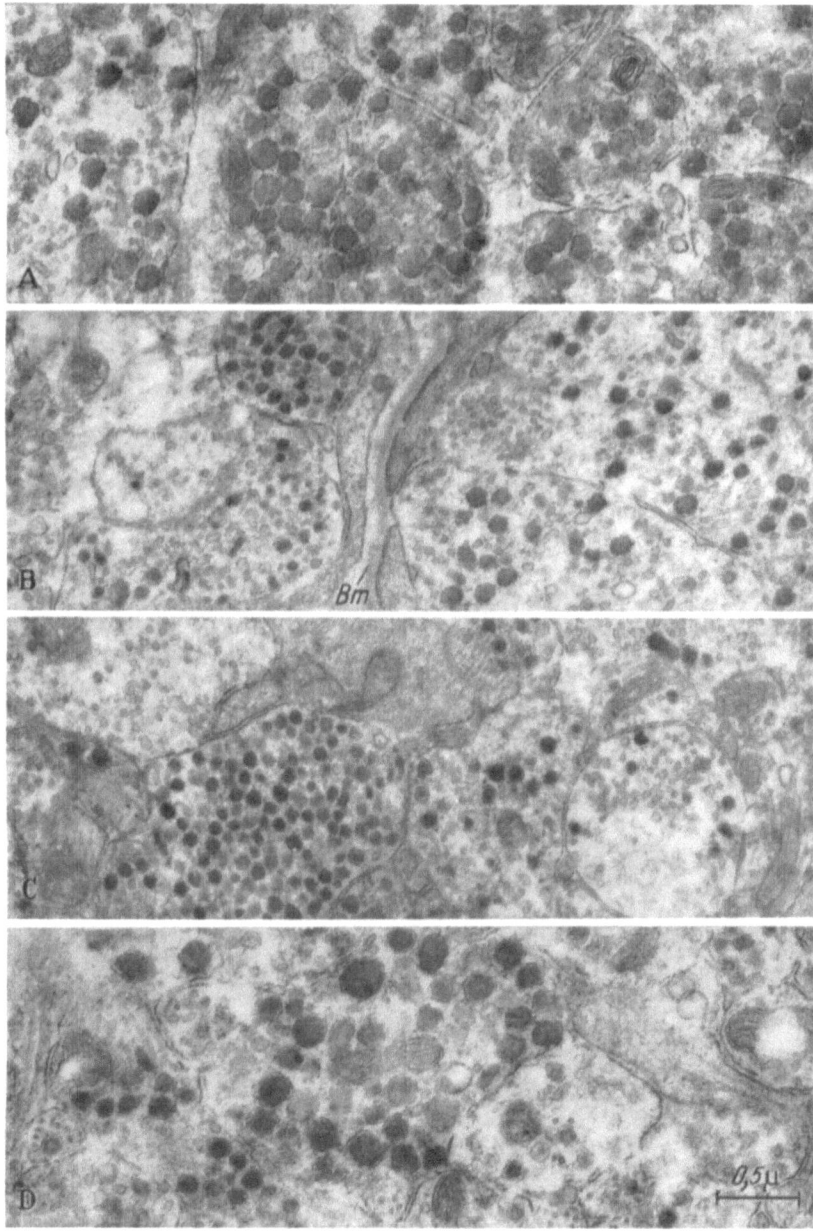

Abb. 4 A—D. Vergleich der verschieden großen *Elementargranula* (s. Text) im *Hypophysen-hinterlappen* (A) und drei verschiedenen Schichten der *Eminentia mediana* (B—D). *Passer domesticus.* — Glutataldehyd (5%) — O_4O_4 (1%). Epon (LUFT) 6:4. Kontrastierung mit Blei-monoxyd. Elmiskop I Siemens. Vergr. 22000fach. A Hypophysenhinterlappen. B Äußerste Lage der Palisadenschicht; Bm-Basalmembran (vgl. D_β in Abb. 1). C Innere Lage der Pali-sadenschicht (vgl. D_α in Abb. 1). D Nachbarschaft der neurosekretorischen Bahn (vgl. C in Abb. 1)

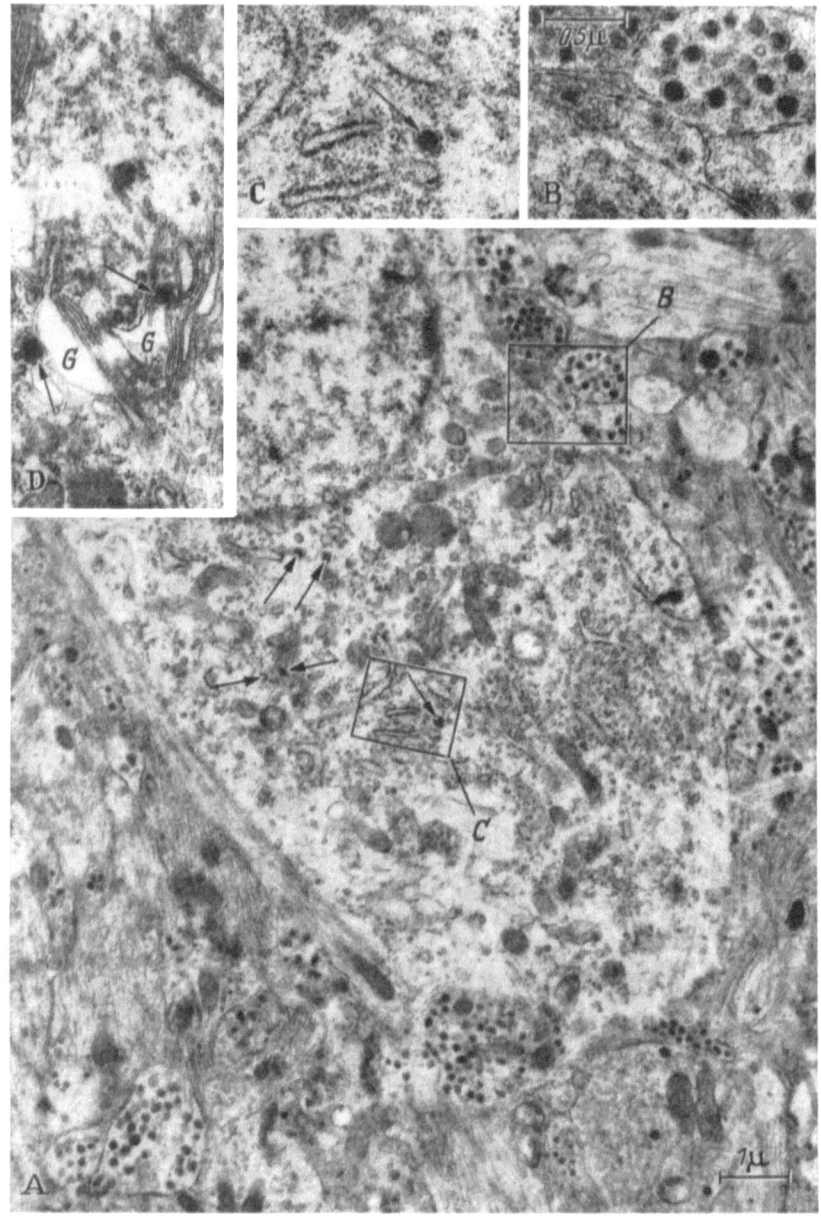

Abb. 5 A—D. Vergleich verschieden großer *Elementargranula* (s. Text) im *Nucl. infundi-bularis* (A—D), im *proximalen* Teil der *neurosekretorischen* Bahn (E—F) und in den Perikaryen des *Nucl. supraopticus* (G—H). *Passer domesticus.* (Technik wie in Abb. 4). Vergr. A 9000fach; B—F 22000fach. — A Nervenzelle des Nucl. infundibularis mit anliegenden granulierten Faserquerschnitten (Vergr. B) und vereinzelten elektronendichten Granula (↑) im Perikaryon (u. a. Vergr. C). D Elektronendichte Granula (↑) in der Golgi-Zone (G) einer anderen Nervenzelle des Nucl. infundibularis
E—F. Zwei eng benachbarte Nervenfasern mit (E) größeren (etwa 2000 Å) und (F) klei-neren (etwa 1000 Å) Elementargranula im proximalen Teil der neurosekretorischen Bahn. G—H Elementargranula in neurosekretorischen Nervenzellen des Nucl. supraopticus (lateraler Abschnitt); ↑ beachte das elektronendichte Material in den Zisternen des Golgi-Apparates (G)

An einzelnen Perikaryen des Nucleus infundibularis wurden synaptische Strukturen beobachtet.

3. *Elementargranula im proximalen Teil der neurosekretorischen Bahn* (Abb. 5 E bis F). Im *proximalen,* von der Sehnervenkreuzung und dem Tractus opticus bedeckten Teil der *neurosekretorischen Bahn,* der noch rostral von der Eminentia

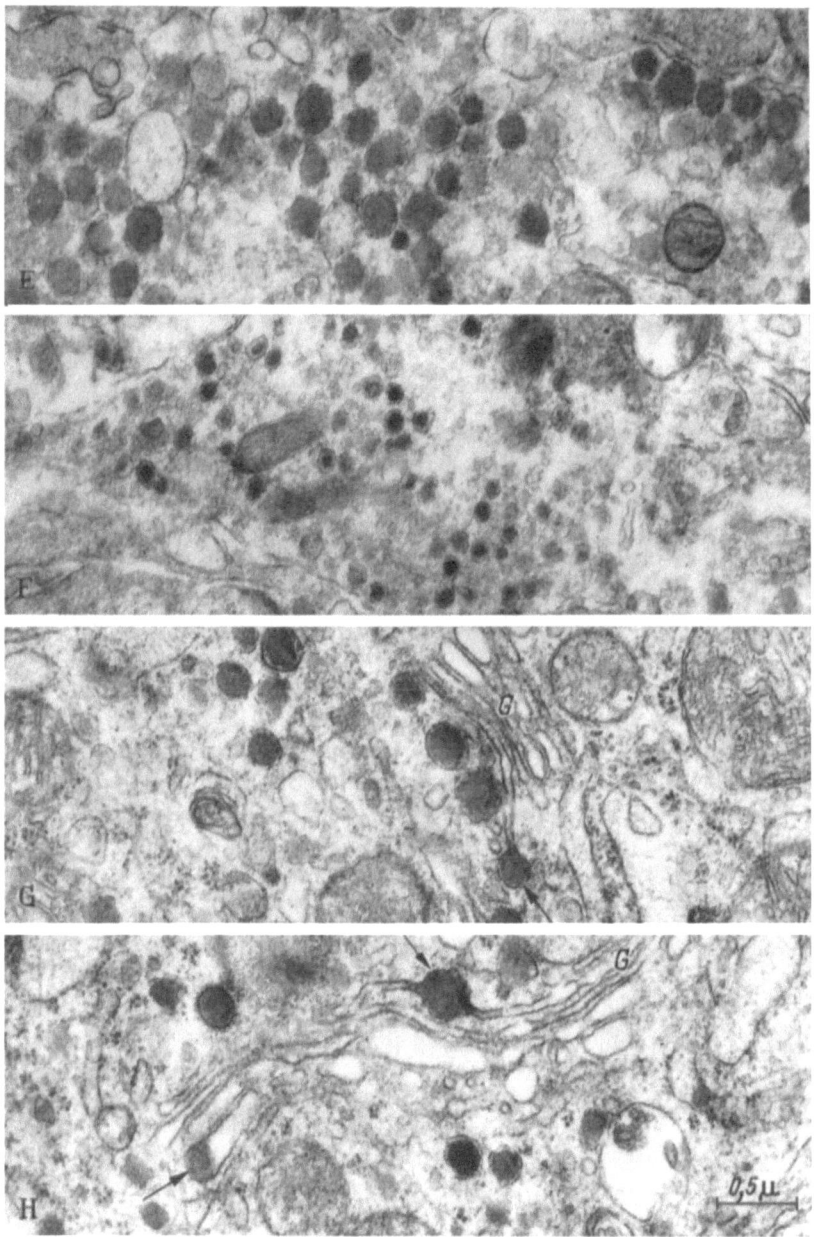

Abb. 5 E—H

mediana liegt, beobachtet man neben Faserquerschnitten mit 2000 Å großen
Granula (Abb. 5E) auch solche mit einem Elementargranula-Typ von 1000 Å
Durchmesser (Abb. 5F).

4. *Elementargranula im Nucleus supraopticus* (Abb. 5G—H). In den *Perikaryen*
des *Nucleus supraopticus* (medianer und lateraler Kernabschnitt) wurden neben
etwa 1500—2000 Å großen, z. T. noch in den Zisternen des Golgi-Apparates befind-
lichen Granula, auch kleinere Körnchen dargestellt. An der Oberfläche einzelner
Zellen sind axo-somatische Synapsen zu erkennen. In den Faserquerschnitten des
Neuropils, das die neurosekretorischen Perikaryen umschließt, sind 900—1400 Å
große elektronendichte Elementargranula recht häufig. Ob diese kleineren Granula in besonderen Elementen der neurosekretorischen Kerngebiete oder in den
Nervenzellen eines anderen Systems gebildet werden, ist unbekannt. Der diffuse
Nucleus supraopticus der Spatzenvögel hat auch noch andere, bisher nicht elektronenmikroskopisch untersuchte Abschnitte. Ein Ultrastrukturbefund fehlt auch
am Nucleus paraventricularis und an den eigenartigen neurosekretorischen Zellen
im Bereich des Tractus entopeduncularis.

Diskussion

Diese Befunde (1.—4.) zeigen, daß bei *Passer domesticus* der proximale Teil der
neurosekretorischen Bahn auch Faserelemente mit feineren Granula enthält als
der Hypophysenhinterlappen. Solche Granula finden sich auch in dem Neuropil,
das den Nucleus supraopticus umhüllt. Im Hinblick auf dieses feinkörnige Material
bestehen die folgenden Deutungsmöglichkeiten: 1. Granula des Hinterlappensystems, die noch nicht ihre endgültige Größe erreicht haben, 2. ein besonderes
kleinkörniges Neurosekret für die Eminentia mediana, 3. durch Fragmentation aus
den 2000 Å Granula entstandene Körnchen, 4. monoaminhaltiges Fasersystem, das
in tieferen Regionen des Hirnstammes entspringt und innerhalb der neurosekretorischen Kernareale terminale Verzweigungen bildet (vgl. Fuxe u. a., 1966/67).
Diese Frage kann nicht beantwortet werden.

Da etwa 1000—1500 Å große Granula sowohl in den Perikaryen des Nucleus
infundibularis als auch der Nachbarschaft des Nucleus supraopticus zu beobachten
sind, ist es im Bereich der *Palisadenformation* der Eminentia mediana *nicht* möglich, allein auf Grund der *Granulagröße* auf die genaue *Herkunft* dieses Materials zu
schließen. In den Perikaryen und Ausläufern der stark verzweigten *Ependym-* und
Gliazellen der Eminentia mediana wurden allerdings keine Elementargranula beobachtet. Systematische, für eine weitere biostatistische Auswertung geeignete Mes-
sungen müssen jetzt an dicht aufeinanderfolgenden Stufen des gesamten supra-
optico-paraventriculären und des tubero-infundibulären Systems vorgenommen
werden. Der Schwerpunkt neuer Studien muß außerdem stärker auf spezifische
histochemische Identifizierungsverfahren (u. a. die Methodik von Falck, 1962)
ausgerichtet werden.

Schlußbemerkung

Die mitgeteilten Befunde zeigen, daß das 1961 von uns entworfene *neuroanato-
mische Schema* des Zwischenhirn-Hypophysensystems von Spatzenvögeln grundsätzlich nicht revisionsbedürftig ist. Welchen funktionellen Einfluß das supra-
opticoparaventriculäre System auf den Hypophysenvorderlappen ausübt, ist

allerdings unklar und muß in weiteren experimentellen Untersuchungen geprüft werden.

Für die technischen Vorbereitungen danke ich meinen Mitarbeitern Frau T. Bias, Frl. B. Gerken, Frl. H. Jahn, Frl. H. Kirschstein, Herrn W. Kramer, Frl. M. Langbein, Frau Dr. Vaupel von Harnack und Frl. I. Völker.

Zusammenfassung

Licht- und elektronenmikroskopische Untersuchungen am Zwischenhirn-Hypophysensystem einiger Spatzenvögel zeigen, daß elektronendichte *Elementargranula* nicht nur in den Perikaryen des *Nucleus supraopticus*, sondern auch in den Zellen des *Nucleus infundibularis* gebildet werden. Da etwa 1000 Å große Granula nicht nur im Bereich der Tuberkerne, sondern auch im proximalen Teil der neurosektorischen Bahn und sogar im Neuropil des Nucleus supraopticus anzutreffen sind, läßt sich die *Herkunft* der 800—1000 Å großen elektronendichten *Granula* in der *Palisadenschicht* der Eminentia mediana *nicht* aufklären. In die Palisadenschicht der Eminentia mediana der Vögel dringt außer dem Tractus tuberoindundibularis auch noch ein Bündel *elektiv färbbarer* Fasern ein. Die letzteren, die wohl als ein *zweiter* Typ der („klassischen") *neurosekretorischen* Fasern aufgefaßt werden können, sind feiner als die zum Hypophysenhinterlappen strebenden Faserelemente.

Literatur

Benoit, J., et I. Assenmacher: Rapport entre la stimulation sexuelle préhypophysaire et la neurosécrétion chez l'oiseau. Arch. Anat. micr. Morph. exp. 42, 334—386 (1953).
— — The control by visible radiations of the gonadotropic activity of the duck hypophysis. Rec. Progr. Hormone Res. 15, 143—164 (1959).
Bern, H. A.: Hormonogenic properties of neurosecretory cells. (Vortrag, 4. Internationales Symposium über Neurosekretion, Strasbourg 1966; in diesem Band).
—, and R. S. Nishioka: Fine structure of the median eminence of some passerine birds. Proc. Zool. Soc., Calcutta 18, 107—119 (1965).
— — L. R. Mewaldt, and D. S. Farner: Photoperiodic and osmotic influences on the ultrastructure of the hypothalamic neurosecretory system of the White-crowned Sparrow, *Zonotrichia leucophrys gambelii*. Z. Zellforsch. 69, 198—227 (1966).
Braak, H.: Eine Methode zur räumlichen Darstellung des neurosekretorischen Zwischenhirn-Hypophysensystems. Mikroskopie (Wien) 17, 344—347 (1962).
Falck, B.: Observations on the possibilities of the celluar localization of monoamines by a fluorescence method. Acta physiol. scand., Suppl. 197, 1—26 (1962).
Farner, D. S., A. Oksche, and L. Lorenzen: Hypothalamic neurosecretion and the photoperiodic testicular response in the White-crowned Sparrow, *Zonotrichia leucophrys gambelii*. Neurosecretion. Memoirs of the Society for Endocrinology No. 12. (Ed. H. Heller and R. B. Clark), p. 187—197. London-New York: Academic Press 1962.
Fuxe, K.: Cellular localization of monoamines in the median eminence and the infundibular stem of some mammals. Z. Zellforsch. 61, 710—724 (1964).
—, and T. Hökfelt: The influence of central catecholamine neurons on the hormone secretion from the anterior and posterior pituitary. (Vortrag, 4. Internationales Symposium über Neurosekretion, Strasbourg 1966; in diesem Band).
Kobayashi, H.: Histochemical, electron microscopic and pharmacologic studies on the median eminence. Proceedings of the Second International Congress of Endocrinology 1964. Excerpta Medica International Congress Series No. 83, p. 570—576 (1965).
Oksche, A.: The fine nervous, neurosecretory, and glial structure of the median eminence in the White-crowned Sparrow. Neurosecretion. Memoirs of the Society for Endocrinology No. 12. (Ed. H. Heller and R. B. Clark), p. 199—208. London-New York: Academic Press 1962.

Oksche, A., W. Mautner u. D. S. Farner: Das räumliche Bild des neurosekretorischen Systems der Vögel unter normalen und experimentellen Bedingungen. Z. Zellforsch. **64**, 83—100 (1964.)

Sloper, J. C., and C. W. M. Adams: The hypothalamic elaboration of posterior pituitary principle in man. Evidence derived from hypophysectomy. J. Path. Bact. **72**, 587—602 (1956).

Sterba, G.: Zur cerebrospinalen Neurokrinie der Wirbeltiere. Verhandl. dtsch. Zool. Ges. Jena, S. 383—440 (1965).

—, u. K.-P. Wellner: Biochemische Korrelation der Pseudoisocyaninreaktion zum Nachweis von Neurosekret. Naturwissenschaften **50**, 334—335 (1963).

Taguchi, S., H. Kobayashi, and D. S. Farner: Observations on the uptake of ^{35}sulfur by the hypothalamo-hypophysial system of the White-crowned Sparrow (*Zonotrichia leucophrys gambelii*) following intraventricular injection of ^{35}S DL-cysteine. Z. Zellforsch. **69**, 228—245 (1966).

Vitums, A., S. Mikami, A. Oksche, and D. S. Farner: Vascularization of the hypothalamo-hypophysial-complex in the White-crowned Sparrow, *Zonotrichia leucophrys gambelii*. Z. Zellforsch. **64**, 541—569 (1964).

— K. Ono, A. Oksche, D. S. Farner, and J. R. King: The development of the hypophysial portal system in the White-crowned Sparrow, *Zonotrichia leucophrys gambelii*. Z. Zellforsch. **73**, 335—366 (1966).

Wilson, F. E.: The effects of hypothalamic lesions on the photoperiodic testicular response in White-crowned Sparrow, *Zonotrichia leucophrys gambelii*. Doctoral Diss. Washington State University, Pullman 1965.

Wingstrand, K. G.: The structure and development of the avian pituitary, p. 3—316. Lund: Gleerup 1951.

A Double Innervation of the Paraventricular Organ in Various Vertebrates

B. Vigh

Department of Histology and Embryology, Medical University of Budapest

In 1920 Kappers described the paraventricular organ in fishes and in reptilia as an ependymal organ localized at the lateral wall of the third cerebral ventricle. Since that time several researchers detected the paraventricular organ from fishes up to mammals in numerous species (Charlton, 1928; E. Legait, 1942; Fleisch-hauer, 1957, 1960; H. Legait, 1959; Diepen, 1962; etc.). Starting from the morphological picture the function of the organ was considered by the most authors to be a secretory one. But, in relation to the function direct examinations are lacking.

In our earlier investigations (Vigh et al., 1962; Vigh, 1964) we studied the Gomori positive material found at the territory of the paraventricular organ in different vertebrates. We observed that, besides of the neurosecretory Herring-bodies mentioned by numerous authors in the paraventricular organ, another Gomori positive substance can be found in some species which is similar to the ependymosecretion of the subcommissural organ.

In our present work, the following problems were studied: 1. the relation of the neurosecretory fibres to the paraventricular organ, and 2. the connection of the paraventricular organ and of the small nerve cells mentioned by E. Legait, H. Legait and Fleischhauer.

1. The relation of the neurosecretory fibres and of the paraventricular organ was examined in tailed amphibia (Triturus cristatus, Triturus vulgaris). In the newt some of the cell processes of the preoptic nucleus extend to the third ventricle. A part of these processes reaches the lumen of the third ventricle within the paraventricular organ.

We have studied these neurosecretory fibres after having influenced the water household. 73 newts were divided into four groups: The *first group* was exposed to the effect of drying in such a way that the animals were located on filter paper which was changed repeatedly. The animals of the *second group* were kept in a solution of 1 and 2 per cent of sodium chloride for different time, while those of the *third group* in distilled water. After dehydration in 1 per cent of sodium chloride the *fourth group* was rehydrated in aquarium water for different time. The control animals of each group were kept in normal aquarium water.

In the animals kept in 1 per cent of sodium chloride for $1^{1}/_{2}$ hours an increase of the Herring bodies' number could be observed in the paraventricular organ. After six hours of treatment Gomori positive material appeared in the ventricle's lumen, too. The free Gomori positive granules in the cerebrospinal fluid were situated near to the ventricular end of the neurosecretory cell processes. A similar picture can be found in the newt dehydrated on filter paper. The animals kept in 2 per cent sodium chloride died. The newts rehydrated after dehydration showed a decrease of the Herring-bodies in the paraventricular organ. We did not find any significant change between the control animals and those kept in distilled water. All these dates suggest that there is a considerable migration of neurosecretory material across the paraventricular organ into the cerebrospinal fluid during the alteration of the water household.

2. In the second part of our investigations the nerve cells situated near the paraventricular organ and which had been mentioned by some authors were studied in different vertebrates. We found that these cells which form a distinct cell group are present from fishes up to mammals (Vigh, Teichmann, Aros, 1967). The cells are not identical with any neurosecretory cell group, they contain no Gomori positive material. We consider this cell group to be a neuronal part of the paraventricular ependymal organ, and we called it "nucleus organi paraventricularis". The nerve cells are in close connection with the special ependyma of the paraventricular organ. In reptilia and birds there are numerous bipolar nerve cells in this nucleus. In our investigations made with silver impregnations (Vigh and Majorossy, 1967) we found that forming bulb-like nerve endings the processes of the nerve cells protude between the ependymal cells into the ventricle's lumen. With the fluorescence microscopic method monoamines are demonstrable in the nerve cells Teichmann, Vigh, Aros, 1967, while with electron microscope (Röhlich et al., 1967) catecholamine granules could be observed.

The results of our investigations show the followings: The paraventricular organ, an ependymal organ of the hypothalamus, possesses a double nervous connection: the one is presented by the neurosecretory cells, the other by a special group of nerve cells called by us "nucleus organi paraventricularis". After alterating the water household a considerable amount of neurosecretory material is emptied through the paraventricular organ into the cerebrospinal fluid. In the "nucleus organi paraventricularis" monoamines are produced. The type of the connection between the "nucleus organi paraventricularis" and the ependyma suggests a sensory function of the paraventricular organ.

References

Charlton, H. H. (1928): Glande-like ependymal structure in the brain. Proc. Kon. Akad. Wettensch. Amsterdam 31, 823—836.
Diepen, R. (1962): Der Hypothalamus. In: Handbuch der mikroskopischen Anatomie des Menschen. (Ed. Möllendorf-Bargmann), Bd. 4/7. Berlin-Göttingen-Heidelberg: Springer.
Fleischhauer, K. (1957): Untersuchungen am Ependym des Zwischen- und Mittelhirns der Landschildkröte (Testudo graeca). Z. Zellforsch. 46, 729—767.
— (1960): Fluorescensmikroskopische Untersuchungen an der Faserglia. I. Beobachtungen an den Wandungen der Hirnventrikel der Katze (Seitenventrikel, III. Ventrikel). Z. Zellforsch. 51, 467—496.
Kappers, C. U. A. (1920/21): Die vergleichende Anatomie des Nervensystems der Wirbeltiere und des Menschen. I., II. Haarlem: De Erven F. Bohn.
Legait, E. (1942): Les organes épendymaires du troisième ventricule. L'organe sous-commissural, l'organe subfornical, l'organe paraventriculaire. Thesis, Nancy.
Legait, H. (1959): Contribution a l'étude morphologique et expérimentale du systéme hypothalamo-neurohypophysaire de la poule Rhode-Island. Thesis, Nancy.

Röhlich, P., and B. Vigh (1967): Electron microscopic study of the paraventricular organ in the house sparrow (Passer domesticus). Z. Zellforsch. (in press).

Teichmann, I., B. Vigh, and B. Aros (1967): Histochemical studies on Gomori-positive substances. IV. The Gomori-positive material of the paraventricular organ in various vertebrates. Acta biol. hung. (in press).

Vigh, B. (1964): Ependymosecretion (Ependymal neurosecretion). Comparative histological investigation of the Gomori-positive secretion of the ependymal cells. Manuscript in Hungarian. Budapest: Library of the Medical University.

— B. Aros, P. Zaránd, I. Török, and T. Wenger (1962): Ependymal neurosecretion. II. Gomori-positive secretion in the paraventricular organ and the ventricular ependyma of different vertebrates. Acta morph. hung. 11, 335—350.

—, and K. Majorossy (1967): The nucleus of the paraventricular organ and its fiber connections in the hen (Gallus domesticus). Acta biol. hung. (in press).

— I. Teichmann, and B. Aros (1967): The "nucleus organi paraventricularis", a neuronal part of the paraventricular ependymal organ of the hypothalamus. A comparative morphological study in various vertebrates. Acta biol. hung. (in press).

Histochemical Studies of the Different Gomori-positive Substances in the Subcommissural Organ

I. Teichmann

Institute of Histology and Embryology, Medical University of Budapest

It is well known that Gomori's chrome haematoxylin and aldehyde fuchsin stain electively not only the neurosecretory material (Bargmann, 1949; Halmi and Davies, 1953; Gabe, 1953; etc.) and the ependymosecretion of the sub-commissural organ (Stutinsky, 1950), but also numerous other substances as e.g. elastic fibres, hyaline cartilague, the granules of mast cells, lipofuscin, lysosomes, etc. (Teichmann et al., 1966, 1967). Therefore, Gomori's methods cannot be considered to be a specific histochemical reaction. The "Gomori-positivity" of a material gives only some informations with regard to the content of acid groups, which may be bound by the basic dyes. So, we found it desirable to study various Gomori-positive substances with histochemical methods.

In our earlier works (Teichmann et al., 1964, 1965, 1966; Teichmann, 1967), we examined the following Gomori-positive materials: In the rat we studied the substance of the endolymphatic sac, the granules of the ependyma in the "recessus organ" and of the median eminence as well as the granules of the periventricular glial cells, and in the frog the Gomori-positive material of the ependymal wall of the third cerebral ventricle and of its hypendymal glial cells. In the earthworm we investigated the neurosecretory system, the Gomori-positive granules of the glial cells and the Gomori-positive cells observed in the connective capsule of the nervous system (Teichmann et al. in preparation).

In our present work we have studied the Gomori-positive material of the subcommissural organ with histochemical methods. The histochemistry of the subcommissural ependymosecretion was already described by several authors in various species (e.g. Bargmann and Schiebler, 1952; Wislocki and Leduc, 1952; Oksche, 1962; Talanti, 1958; etc.). The ependymosecretion is generally considered to be a mucopolysaccharide-protein complex.

We have studied the subcommissural organ in the guinea pig (see also Vigh et al., 1967), and we observed that there is histologically not only one material, but there are three different Gomori-positive substances. The *one Gomori-positive material (A_1)* consists of very fine moderately stainable granules which show no distinct outlines. This substance is diffusely localized in the cytoplasm of the ependymal cells. The *second material (A_2)* situated in the apical part of the cytoplasm is composed of granules ranging from 0,5 to 0,8 mikron in diameter. They possess sharp outlines and stain rather dark with Gomori's stainings. The *third Gomori-positive substance* can be found in the hypendymal glial cells. It is formed of somewhat bigger $(0,5-1,0\ \mu)$ granules than the A_2 material of the ependymal cells and stains in a purple red colour.

With the histochemical methods and stainings employed we have got the following results: Concerning the *Gomori-positivity* we found that all three substances can be demonstrated only after permanganate-sulphuric acid oxidation with chrome haematoxylin and aldehyde fuchsin. After oxidation with a less concentrated permanganate-sulphuric acid as used by Gomori for the demonstration of lipofuscin the A_1 material was negative with chrome haematoxylin, the A_2 granules were moderately stained and the glial granules were strongly positive. When oxidizing with peracetic acid the aldehyde fuchsin positivity was present in the two kind of granules, but not in the A_1 substance. The intensity of the staining appeared to be more moderate than after permanganate sulphuric acid oxidation.

The *reactions for proteins* or for protein-bound groups yielded the following results. With the tetrazonium reaction for proteins the A_1 material was positive, while the A_2 material was only moderately stained and the glial granules could not be demonstrated. The reaction for tyrosine was generally negative in the subcommissural organ. The DDD-method for the joint demonstration of SS- and SH-groups was stronger positive in the glial cells than in the ependymal cells. In the latter the fine A_1 substance was relatively stronger positive than the A_2 material. With Adam's and Sloper's alcian blue method for SS- and SH-groups there was a moderate positivity only in the A_2 granules while those of the glial cells stained strongly. After incubation in trypsin (1 mg/ml for 1 h) the Gomori-positivity of the subcommissural organ disappeared. Digestion with pepsin (2 mg/ml for 2 hrs) reduced the aldehyde fuchsin positivity strongly. Ribonuclease digestion (1 mg/ml 2 hrs) was without any effect on the three materials' Gomori-positivity.

The *reactions for polysaccharides* gave the following results: With the periodic acid Schiff reaction (PAS) all three substances were positive, but not equally. The fine A_1 material stained moderately with PAS, while the two other materials were strongly PAS-positive. After acetylation the PAS reactivity was negative, but it was positive after reactylation. Digestion with diastase did not change the intensity of the PAS reaction. With toluidine blue no metachromasia could be observed, except after sulfation. In the latter case the A_2 material and the glial granules showed induced metachromasia.

The *results* of the Sudan Black B staining *for lipids* were doubtful. With Berenbaum's acetonic Sudan Black for bound lipids the A_2 granules were moderately positive while with Luxol Fast Blue MBS for phospholipids no positivity could be obtained in the ependyma, nor in the hypendymal glial cells. The performic acid Schiff reaction for unsaturated lipids gave a negativ result in all three substances. But the peracetic acid alcian blue reaction was strongly positive in the granules of the glial cells.

Acid phosphatase activity was demonstrable in the whole cytoplasm of the subcommissural organ with favour of its apical part (method of PÓSALAKY-VAD ÁSZ', see in KISZELY-PÓSALAKY, 1964). In some cases pigment granules could be observed in the hypendymal glial cells of the adult guinea pig.

Summarizing our various results we may establish that the three materials which can be demonstrated histologically in the subcommissural organ show histochemical differences. The A_1 *material* situated diffusely in the cytoplasm of the ependyma seems to be a protein containing a small amount of polysaccharide.

The A_2 *granules* localized in the apical part of the cytoplasm is a mucopolysaccharide which appears to be bound to a moderate protein component, but which contains possibly bound lipids. The Gomori-positive granules of the hypendymal glial cells can be considered to be composed probably of a glycolipoprotein.

We think it possible that the A_1 and A_2 materials represent two different ependymosecretory substances. But it cannot be excluded that the A_2 granules demonstrate a condensed A_1 substance or lysosomes. Concerning the hypendymal glial cells their Gomori-positive granules may represent a phagocytized ependymosecretion, but it is more evident to consider them as to be in relation to the development of lipofuscin.

References

BARGMANN, W. (1949): Über die neurosekretorische Verknüpfung von Hypothalamus und Neurohypophyse. Z. Zellforsch. **34**, 610—634.

—, u. T. H. SCHIEBLER (1952): Histologische und cytochemische Untersuchungen am Subcomissuralorgan von Säugern. Z. Zellforsch. **37**, 593—596.

GABE, M. (1953): Sur quelques applications de la coloration par la fuchsine-paraldehyde. Bull. Micr. Appl. Ser. 2, **3**, 153—162.

HALMI, N. S., and J. J. DAVIES (1953): Comparision of aldehyde fuchsin staining, metachromasia and periodic acid Schiff reactivity of various tissues. J. Histochem. Cytochem. **1**, 447—459.

KISZELY, GY., u. Z. PÓSALAKY (1964): Mikrotechnische und histochemische Untersuchungsmethoden. Budapest: Akadémiai Kiadó.

OKSCHE, A. (1962): Histologische, histochemische und experimentelle Studien am Subcommissuralorgan von Anuren (mit Hinweisen auf den Epiphysenkomplex). Z. Zellforsch. **57**, 240—326.

STUTINSKY, F. (1950): Colloide, corps de Herring et substance Gomori-positive de la neurohypophyse. C.R. Soc. Biol. **144**, 1457—1460.

TALANTI, S. (1958): Studies on the subcommissural organ in some domestic animals. Ann. Med. exp. Fenn. **36**, 1—70.

TEICHMANN, I. (1967): Vergleichende histochemische Studien über die Gomori-positive Substanz des Ependyms und der hypendymalen Gliazellen im Frosch. Z. Mikr. Anat. Forsch. in Druck.

— B. AROS, B. VIGH u. S. KORITSÁNSZKY (1965): Histochemische Untersuchung Gomoripositiver Gliazellen im Regenwurm (Lumbricus terrestris, Eisenia foetida). Zool. J. Physiol. **71**, 552—557.

— — — (1966): Histochemical studies on Gomori-positive substances. III. Examination of the earthworm's neurosecretory system (Lumbricus herculeus, Eisenia foetida). Acta biol. hung. **17**, 329—357.

— B. VIGH, and B. AROS (1964): Histochemical studies on Gomori-positive substances in the endolymphatic sac of the rat. Acta biol. hung. **14**, 293—300.

— — — (1966): Histochemical studies on Gomori-positive substances. II. The Gomoripositive material of a special ependymal formation (recessus organ) in the ventral part of the third cerebral ventricle. Acta biol. hung. **17**, 13—29.

— — — (1967): Histochemical studies on Gomori-positive substances. IV. The Gomoripositive material of the paraventricular organ in various vertebrates. Acta biol. hung. (in press).

— — —, S. KORITSÁNSZKY (1965): Histochemical investigation of the periventricular Gomori-positive glial cells in the rat's hypothalamus. Acta morph. hung. Suppl. **13**, 47.

VIGH, B., P. RÖHLICH, I. TEICHMANN, and B. AROS (1967): Ependymosecretion (Ependymal neurosecretion). VI. Light and electron microscopic examination of the subcommissural organ of the guinea pig. Acta biol. hung. **18**, 53—66.

WISLOCKI, G. B., and E. H. LEDUC (1952): The cytology and histochemistry of the subcommissural organ and Reissner's fibre in rodents. J. comp. Neurol. **97**, 515—544.

Changes in the Hypothalamo-hypophysial System of Common Frogs under Osmotic Stress and in a Temperature Experiment

J. C. van de Kamer

Zoölogisch Laboratorium, Utrecht, the Netherlands

The hypothalamo-hypophysial system of the common frog was studied in our department by a research team of co-workers and students in biology. The purpose was twofold.

Firstly we wanted to analyse – histologically as well as cytochemically – a) the effect of osmotic stress, and b) the effect of high temperature on the system. The effect of a hypertonic salt solution upon the hypothalamo-hypophysial system was studied by placing the animals in a 1 % NaCl solution for 2–23 days. The frogs were kept in darkness at a constant temperature of 6° C. Similarly the effect of high temperature was investigated by keeping male common frogs in darkness at a constant temperature of 23° C for 1–9 weeks. Both experiments were carried out during the period January-February.

Secondly we wanted to bring younger students into touch with the scientific approach. As a matter of fact there are in such a common project several technical difficulties and problems of organization to overcome. I will only mention two of them.

1. For technical reasons it was necessary to fix by vascular perfusion all experimental animals on the same day, in order to bring the tissues simultaneously to paraffin. Consequently the animals had to be placed in experimental condition – for the salt experiment as well as for the high temperature experiment – at different times before the fixation day. Therefore there was a chance of the animals not being all in the same condition during the experiments. So we had to study control animals at different times in order to know if these controls showed the same level of accumulation of AF positive neurosecretory material.

2. To avoid subjective interpretation of the results, indices were made for the preoptic nucleus, the median eminence and the pars nervosa in which the quantity of aldehyde fuchsin (AF) positive material ranged from an empty to a maximally filled system. The index for the nucleus had 3 stages, that for the median eminence and pars nervosa 5 stages. An advantage of the use of these indices was that the quantity of secretion could now be set against time graphicially.

The results can be seen from the curves (Fig. 1). In the stress experiment the clearest effect is visible in the pars nervosa, where a progressive release of AF positive material could be observed. The animals reacted to their dehydration with an increasing release of antidiuretic hormone in order to keep as much water as possible inside the body. The salt load had no effect at all in the median eminence.

In the preoptic nucleus, however, a decrease in the quantity of secretion was observable during the experiment. This effect can be explained by assuming an augmented secretory activity in the nucleus, accompanied by an accelerated release of secretion via the fibres of the tract. Cyto- and histological criteria such as nuclear diameter as well as an augmented blood supply of the nuclear region give support to this supposition. Clearly the augmented synthesis cannot be kept in balance with the release, and this results in a continuing increasing release during the experiment.

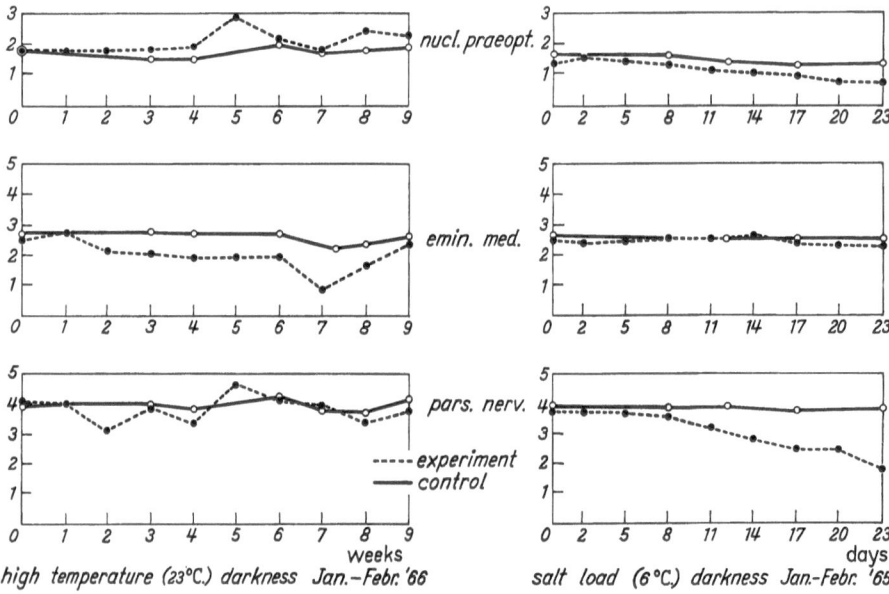

Fig. 1. Graphs showing the effect of high temperature (on the left) and salt load (on the right) upon the quantity of AF-positive material in the preoptic nucleus, the median eminence and the pars nervosa of Rana temporaria. Ordinate: indices values based on the quantity of AF-positive material (5: maximal, 0: minimal). Abscissa: time in weeks for the temperature experiment, in days for the salt load experiment. Solid lines: control animals. Broken lines: experimental animals

In the high temperature-experiment, however, the reverse is true; no clear release in the pars nervosa, only oscillations around the control level, and a clear and progressive release of AF positive material in the median eminence. As high temperature stimulates spermatogenesis in Rana temporaria (van Oordt, 1956) this effect suggests a correlation between the diminishing quantity of AF positive material in the median eminence and spermatogenesis. Preliminary analysis of the testes of the animals kept at high temperature showed a stimulation of spermatogenesis from the 7th week of the experiment on (Goos, unpublished results).

The quantity of neurosecretion in the preoptic nucleus augmented twice during the experiment. The first time after 5 weeks, the second at the end of the experiment. The balance in the perikarya between synthesis and release has in both cases moved to the synthetical phase. This means that the release of neurosecretory material in the median eminence is compensated by a new synthesis in the preoptic nucleus, and that there is not a complete balance between synthesis and extrusion.

Histochemical differences could be determined between the AF positive neuro-secretory substance in the pars nervosa and the inner zone of the median eminence on one hand, and in the outer zone of the median eminence on the other hand. Whereas all parts reacted strongly with aldehyde fuchsin (AF), only the pars nervosa and the inner zone reacted with Alcian blue and PAS; in the outer zone the PAS reaction was negative and the Alcian blue reaction but weakly positive. These differences were not the result of different total quantities of neurosecretion

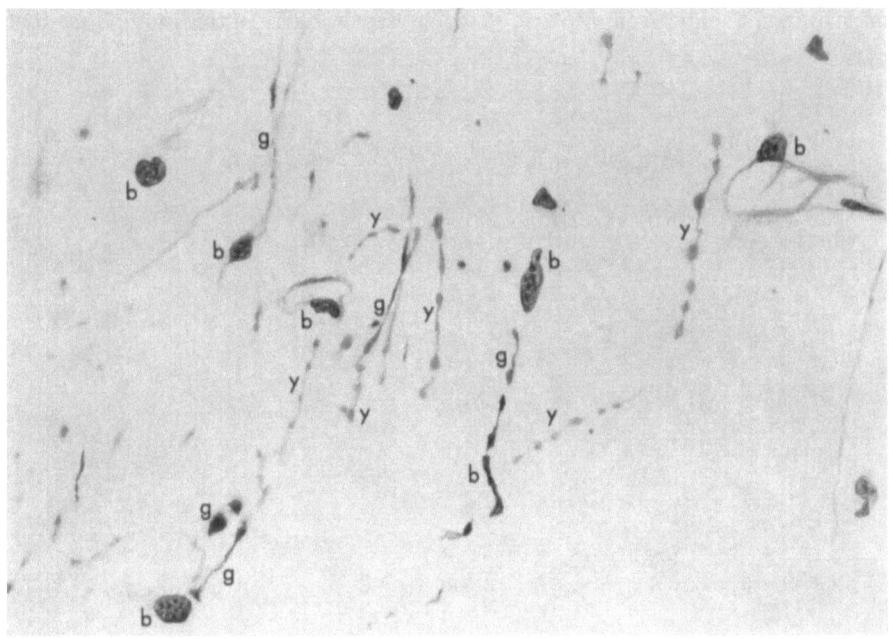

Fig. 2. Drawing of a parasagittal section through the hypothalamus of Rana temporaria near the preoptic nucleus. Combined Alcian yellow-Alcian blue method after Peute. Notice the yellow fibres (y), the bluish green fibres (b) and blue nuclei (b), and the yellow fibres which change their content into green

in inner and outer zone respectively, as granules of the same diameter reacted differently. These data suggest, therefore, the presence of at least two types of AF positive fibres.

Moreover, following the sectioning of fibres of the preoptic tract in the in-fundibular floor, behind the optic chiasm, and the subsequent accumulation of neurosecretory material in the cut fibres, the number of AF positive fibres was much larger than that of PAS positive and tyrosine positive fibres. This points also to the presence of two types of AF positive fibres in the tract, one PAS and tyrosine positive, the other PAS and tyrosine negative. The presence of two types of AF positive fibres raised the question whether also two types of perikarya might be distinguishable in the preoptic nucleus. Research on this point is in progress.

Another point which I would like to mention here, is the gradual increasing PAS positivity of the fibres of the tract going from the preoptic nucleus to the pars nervosa. Moreover, section of the fibres of the tract in the in fundibular floor at different distances from the optic chiasm, showed, going caudally, increasing PAS positivity of the accumulations in the fibres. Both facts suggest that during the transport of neurosecretory material, carbohydrates are added to the fibres and that possibly inside the fibreswellings a chemical transformation of neurosecretion occurs.

To bring out the presence of two types of AF positive fibres and a possible transformation of the neurosecretion more clearly, our co-worker PEUTE used the staining method of RAVETTO with Alcian blue and Alcian yellow for demonstration of different acidic groups in acid mucopolysaccharides. In this method sections

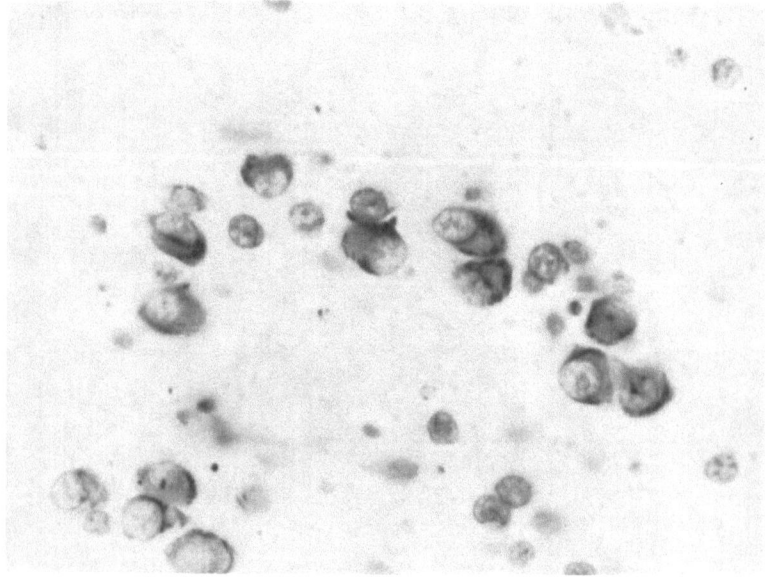

Fig. 3. Part of the preoptic nucleus of Rana temporaria. Combined Alcian yellow-Alcian blue method after Peute. Notice the yellow cytoplasm (central), and the bluish material (peripheral) in the perikarya

are first brought into an Alcian blue solution at pH 0.5, in which the strong acidic groups only are stained blue, secondly they are brought into an Alcian yellow loution at pH 2.3, in which the weak acidic groups only stain yellow. This methods applied to oxidized sections of the hypothalamus did not provide satisfactory results, as in the Alcian yellow bath all the blue dissolved and the slides stained totally yellow. In the modification of the method nb PEUTE the oxidized sections were placed in an Alcian yellow solution at pH 1.—, in which the strong acid groups stained yellow, and in which the weak acidic groups were not dissociated, and therefore did not stain. Thereafter the slides were put into an Alcian blue solution of pH 2.5, in which the weak acidic groups dissociated, and therefore stained blue. Consequently the final result of the method was a blue staining of weak acidic groups (formed by oxidation out of carbohydrates) and a yellow staining of the strong acidic groups (formed by oxidation of cystin).

This method applied to sagittal hypothalamic sections revealed the presence of separated yellow and bluish-green fibres in the neighbourhood of the perikarya of the preoptic nucleus as well as yellow fibres which locally showed green swellings (Fig. 2).

In the perikarya the superficial layer of the cell (the Nissl-region) stained bluish-green indicating weak acidic groups (the nucleic acids) together with strong acidic

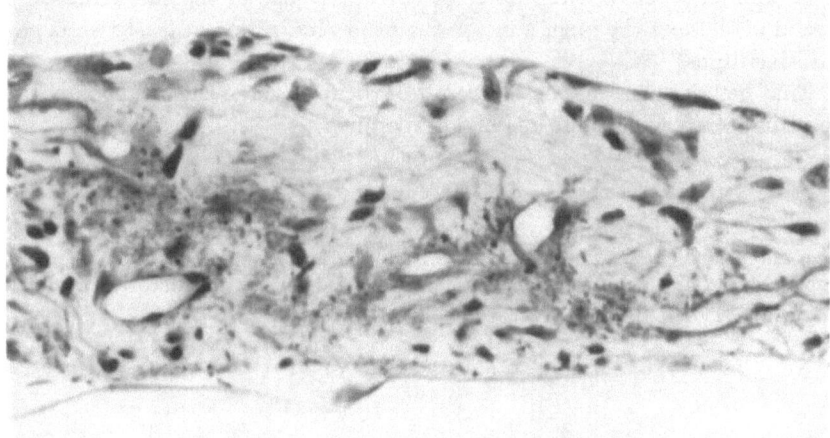

Fig. 4. Median eminence of Rana temporaria. Fibre endings in the outer zone green (ventral); the fibres of the preoptic-neurohypophysial tract in the inner zone yellow (dorsal). Combined Alcian yellow-Alcian blue method after Peute

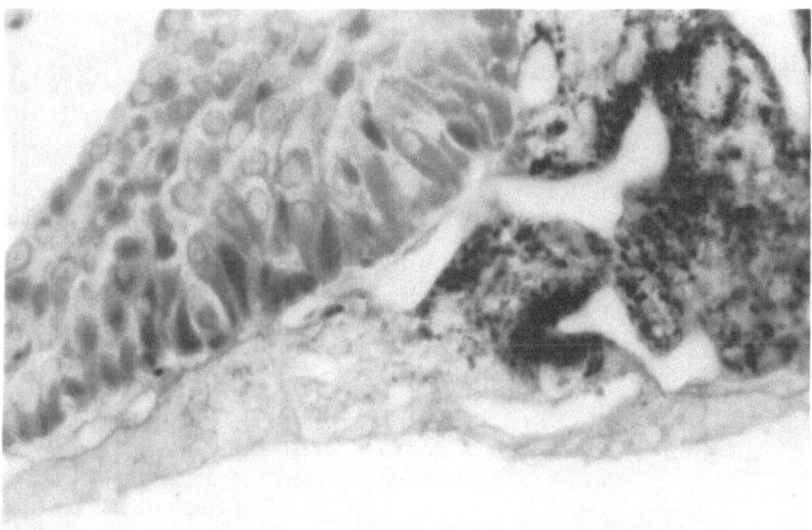

Fig. 5. Part of the neurohypophysis of Rana temporaria. Fibres of the preoptic-neurohypophysial tract yellow (upper right), on entering the neurohypophysis switching to deep blue green (to the left). Combined Alcian yellow-Alcian blue method after Peute

products, whereas the central part stained yellow pointing to strong acidic products only (Fig. 3). The axons originating from the perikarya always stained yellow.

Moreover, in the inner zone of the median eminence only yellow fibres are present, whereas in the outer zone the fibres stain yellowish green (Fig. 4).

7*

Furthermore the yellow stained fibres in the inner zone show a very clear and marked colour switch to blue green on entering the pars nervosa (Fig. 5).

These facts suggest:

1. A transformation of secretion inside the fibres.

2. A difference between the fibres of the outer zone of the eminentia on one hand, and of those of the inner zone on the other, indicating at least two types of AF positive fibres.

3. That before the release or as a result of the release the chemical composition of the neurosecretory substance is highly modified.

References

van Oordt, P. G. W. J.: The role of temperature in regulating the spermatogenetic cycle in the common frog (Rana temporaria). Acta Endocr. **23**, 251—264 (1956).

Ravetto, C.: Alcian blue-Alcian yellow: A new method for the identification of different acidic groups. J. Histochem. Cytochem. **12**, 44 (1964).

Observations sur l'appareil neurosécrétoire des stades larvaires d'alytes obstetricans intacts ou hypophysectomisés

P. DISCLOS

Laboratoire de Biologie animale S.P.C.N. Faculté des Sciences de Bordeaux (Prof. BOUNHIOL)

Matériel et méthodes. Ces observations portent sur des têtards, les uns nés au printemps avec métamorphose en été, les autres nés à l'entrée de l'automne et normalement hivernant. L'étude des voies neurosécrétoires extrahypophysaires a été principalement réalisée sur des animaux hypophysectomisés. L'ablation de l'hypophyse entraine une mise en charge progressive de tout l'appareil neurosécrétoire le rendant, après une longue évolution (8 à 12 mois de vie larvaire), particulièrement favorable à l'observation. Les techniques employées sont: la fuchsine paraldéhyde de GABE, classique et éprouvée, et la méthode de STERBA, fluorescence secondaire après coloration à la pseudoisocyanine. (Observations en lumière bleue: filtre 1,5 BG 12/Arrêt K 530 ou indifféremment en U.V purs 1 UGl/K 430. Dispositif photographique *Leitz orthomat*, film rapide ASA 135.) Les principales difficultés rencontrées pour l'observation en fluorescence sont le décollement des coupes et le peu de durée de la fluorescence. Cependant la méthode de STERBA se révèle plus sensible que la méthode classique à la fuchsine paraldéhyde (pour son auteur: 10 fois plus sensible). Elle présente un intêret certain bien que la fluorescence se manifeste également autour des vaisseaux sanguins et dans les tissus conjonctifs (cartilages ou fibres élastiques).

Observations. A. *Animaux d'été.* Une ponte prélevée sur les pattes du mâle fournit le matériel nécessaire à cette étude. Une partie de la ponte est décortiquée et fixée quelques 30 à 40 heures avant l'éclosion du reliquat. Ces très jeunes animaux mesurent déjà 1 cm et pèsent 0,023 g. La topographie du cerveau de ces animaux est d'ailleurs assez différente de celle des animaux plus agés. Le télencéphale notamment est très court; le système cavitaire intracéphalique est réduit. Le lobe nerveux est cependant déjà garni de grains de neurosécrétion FPA[1], assez finement poussiéreux, non coalescents. La FPA ne nous a pas permis de voir des cellules du noyau préoptique en charge. En fluorescence, on distingue de très fins chapelets granuleux en direction de l'hypophyse, un peu en dessus du nerf optique. On a pu repérer chez quelques animaux seulement 3 cellules du N.P.O très finement couronnées de grains fluorescents. Aucun trajet en direction du téléncéphale n'est visible; par contre on distingue nettement des chapelets de granules dans le plancher du mésencéphale et dans la réticulée mésencéphalique et bulbaire, sans pouvoir individualiser le faisceau à son départ. Sans oxydation permanganique préalable, tous ces chapelets disparaissent. Seuls restent fluorescents le conjonctif

---

[1] FPA: fuchsine paraldéhyde.

et quelques grains dans la moelle épinière et le télencéphale principalement. La finesse des granules et la fugacité de la fluorescence rend difficile la prise de vue, même avec un film rapide (temps de pose de l'ordre de 3 à 4 minutes). Azzali, 1952, montre que chez *Rana agilis* le lobe nerveux se charge en neurosécrétions chez le têtard de 11,3 mm et que le têtard de 37,3 mm possède un N.P.O bien chargé. Le têtard de *Rana agilis* de 11,3 mm est un animal morphologiquement plus évolué

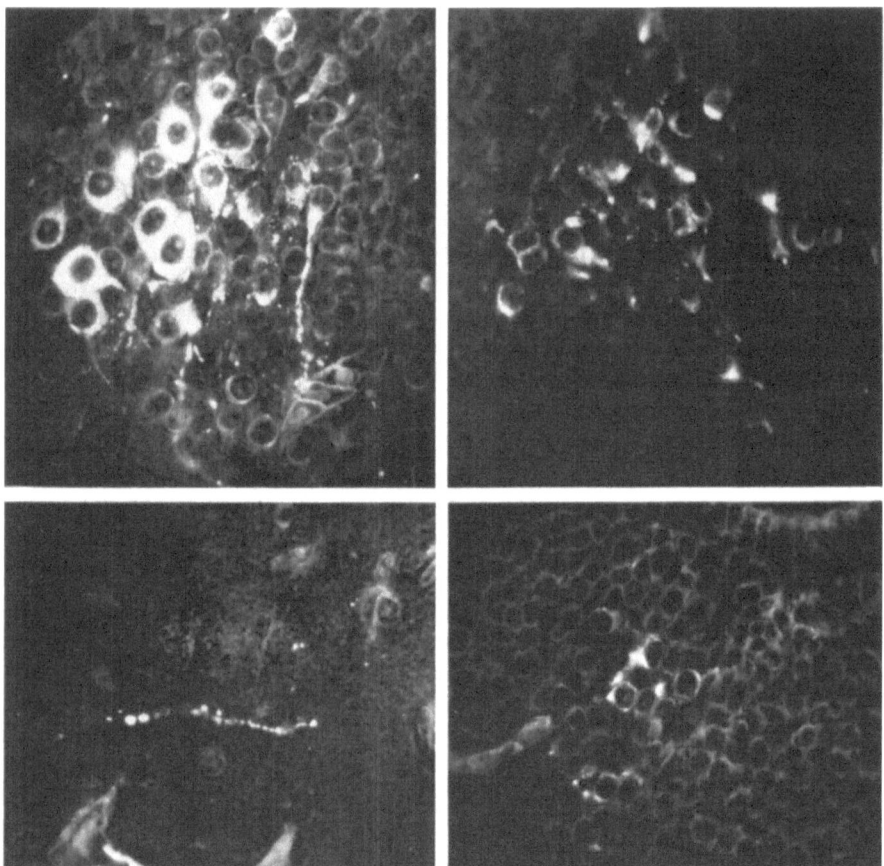

Fig. 1. Fluorescence à la pseudoisocyanine. A gauche — Hypophyséoprives — en haut: centre neurosécrétoire préoptique; en bas: chapelet de granules dans le mésencéphale. A droite — Centre neurosécrétoire de témoins nés à l'automne — en haut: âgé de 8 mois (comparer avec l'hypophyséoprive de même âge à gauche); en bas: 3 semaines après la naissance

que le têtard d'Alytes de 10 mm bien qu'étant, en valeur absolue, un animal plus jeune (développement lent de l'*Alytes*). Il a en effet perdu ses branchies externes et nage librement. Le têtard d'Alytes de 10 mm possède encore des branchies saillant à l'extérieur par un orifice médian et il est enveloppé dans ses membranes (dessin planche 2). A la naissance (fixation dans l'heure qui suit l'éclosion l = 1,5 cm; p = 0,055 g) la FPA montre un lobe nerveux déjà bien chargé et quelques fins trajets dans la lame infundibulo-hypophysaire. En fluorescence, les trajets dans le diencéphale, toujours très tenus, sont plus nombreux, les couronnes cernant les cellules du noyau préoptique sont légèrement plus importantes. Le nombre des cellules fonctionnelles (et repérées) s'est accru (5 à 6). Par la suite (fixation à 1, 3, 5, 8, 15, 21 jours) l'importance de la voie hypothalamo-hypophysaire s'affirme. Un faisceau de fibres neurosécrétoires en direction du télencéphale apparait. Les chapelets fluorescents sont toujours présents dans le mésencéphale et le bulbe.

B. *Animaux d'automne*. Les premières observations portent seulement sur des animaux âgés de 3 semaines. La neurohypophyse apparait déjà assez chargée en neurosécrétions. Les cellules du N.P.O ne montrent que peu d'affinité pour la

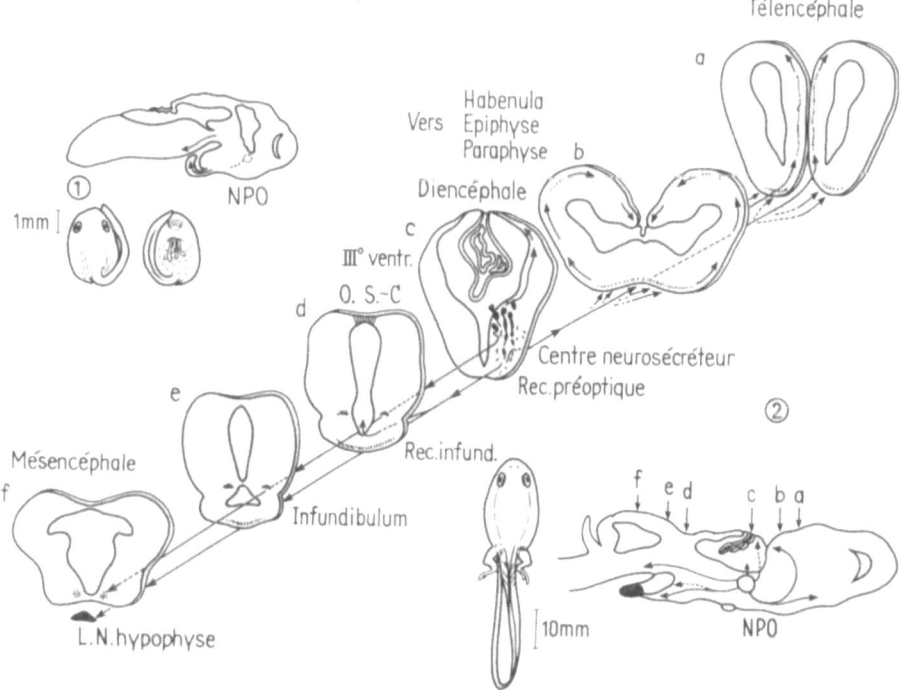

Fig. 2. Diagrammes des voies neurosécrétoires chez le têtard d'*Alytes*. 1. Très jeune larve 30 à 40 H. avant l'éclosion normale spontanée. Dessin de l'animal. Coupe semi-schématique parasagittale de l'encéphale. 2. Diagrammes établis à partir d'un témoin hivernant âgé de 8 mois et d'un hypophyséoprive de même âge. Coupes transversales et parasagittales. *Rec.* Recessus, *Infund.* infundibulaire, *O. S-C.* organe sous-commissural

F.P.A. Par contre la fluorescence met en évidence de fines couronnes de matériel neurosécrété autour des cellules du N.P.O. Le départ des axones est quelquefois visible. Ceux-ci semblent se diriger exclusivement vers l'hypophyse. Il n'y a pas de neurosécrétions dans le reste de l'encéphale (sauf peut-être dans le mésencéphale). Ces images suggèrent qu'à l'automne les phénomènes sécrétoires sont légèrement moins intenses qu'en été, cependant il est difficile de conclure sans avoir pu observer les animaux à leur naissance. Après 45 jours de vie larvaire, le faisceau préopticohypophysaire est bien souligné sur tout son trajet. Les voies extra-hypophysaires restent peu marquées. A l'approche de la métamorphose (8 mois de vie larvaire) les charges en matériel F.P.A$^+$ sont déjà beaucoup plus fortes. Au départ du N.P.O on distingue 2 grandes directions d'écoulement des granules: vers l'hypophyse et en avant vers le télencéphale. En fluorescence, on suit plus avant le faisceau hypothalamo-télencéphalique. Le faisceau hypothalamo-hypophysaire, bien marqué, est chargé de très nombreux granules finement pulvérulents. Une forte accumulation de granules fluorescents au niveau de l'éminence médiane laisse supposer un départ de matériel neurosécrété vers l'hypophyse antérieure et les capillaires qui se situent à ce niveau. Un faisceau beaucoup plus grêle se prolonge jusqu'à la neurohypophyse très chargée de grains plus moins coalescents. On peut repérer quelques axones en direction mésencéphalique.

C. *Animaux d'automne hypophyséoprives.* La mise en charge de l'appareil neuro-sécrétoire est progressive. On ne constate que peu de différence entre témoins et opérés âgés de 3 semaines ou 45 jours. Après 8 mois de vie larvaire, la charge de tout l'appareil neurosécrétoire est très marquée, mais les plus belles images ont été observées après 12 mois de vie larvaire. On peut alors esquisser une carte des voies neurosécrétoires hypophysaires et extra — hypophysaires. La charge du N.P.O est considérable. De larges flaques de matériel neurosécrété (corps de HERRING), s'accumulent dans l'hypothalamus. Un très important contingent de fibres se dirige vers le télencéphale, s'élargit à l'entrée de ce dernier et pénètre dans les 2 lobes télencéphaliques dans la région septale, remontant dans celle-ci de part et d'autre de la cloison interventriculaire. Un faisceau d'axones suit la paroi épendymaire, un peu en deçà des cellules de la paroi ventriculaire remontant en direction de l'habenula et de l'épiphyse. Cependant aucune image de neurosécrétion n'est visible dans ces régions par l'une ou l'autre de ces 2 méthodes. En effet, les parois du plexus choroïde, comme les méninges et les conjonctifs présentent une certaine fluorescence qui ne permet pas de conclure à la présence de micro-grains de neurosécrétat. Quelques cellules caliciformes F.P.A$^+$ font saillie dans la cavité du troisième ventricule (accumulation dendritique de matériel F.P.A$^+$, les axones n'apparaissent pas chargés). Des axones semblent se détacher du faisceau préoptico-hypophysaire vers le recessus infundibulaire avec des images de passage dans ce recessus (hydrencéphaloerinie ou artéfact de fixation ?). Quelques axones paraissent s'arrêter dans le noyau tubérien hypothalamique. Un faisceau d'axones quitte le N.P.O en position haute, en direction du mésencéphale où on retrouve quelques importants chapelets de granules, ainsi que dans le bulbe (particulièrement visible en fluorescence). On note une accumulation assez considérable de matériel neurosécrété en bout d'infundibulum simulant une neuro-hypophyse autour de capillaires sanguins qui abondent dans cette région. Signalons enfin de belles images fluorescentes données par l'organe souscommissural qui disparaissent si on néglige le temps d'oxydation au permanganate.

Conclusion. Ces observations ont été faites à l'occasion d'autres recherches. Il convient de les rapprocher de celles faites par STUTINSKY, BARRY et surtout chez les Amphibiens et les Reptiles par E. et H. LEGAIT. Ces auteurs ont, en effet, reconnu chez les Amphibiens adultes, anoures et urodèles (Rana, Triturus), les voies hypothalamo-télencéphaliques, habénulaires, et signalé des faisceaux en direction des noyaux non neurosécrétoires de l'hypothalamus, noté des images de l'hydrencéphalocrinie dans le troisième ventricule, ainsi qu'une régénération d'un pseudo lobe nerveux. Ils n'ont pas repéré de faisceaux neurosécrétoires dans le mésencéphale et le bulbe chez les amphibiens, mais par contre en ont montré l'importance chez les Reptiles (Natrix — Lacerta).L' Alytes présente ces faisceaux, même très jeune (30 H. avant la naissance «normale») et bien avant qu'apparaissent les faisceaux télencéphaliques. En fait la grande sensibilité de la méthode par fluorescence de STERBA (facilitée par l'observation sur fond noir de grains brillants) permet de déceler des neurosécrétions avant qu'elles ne soient visibles optiquement par la F.P.A. La signification de ces voies extrahypophysaires ne peut être précisée, mais, signalons que par ablation du télencéphale nous avons obtenu des imagos beaucoup plus petits que leurs témoins intacts dans des délais sensiblement identiques. (Rôle éventuel de télencéphale dans la croissance et les fonctions végétatives).

L'Alytes, animal déjà remarquable par son embryogénèse, semble donc présenter à côté des traits communs aux anoures un certain nombre de caractères reconnus jusqu'ici comme appartenant à des animaux plus évolués, tels les Reptiles: importantes voies télencéphaliques et surtout présence de voies neurosécrétoires postérieures.

Bibliographie

BARRY, J.: Recherches morphologiques et expérimentales sur la glande diencéphalique et l'appareil hypothalamo-hypophysaire (1959), 135 p. Thèse Fac. Sc. Besançon.

LEGAIT, E., et H. LEGAIT: Les voies extra hypophysaires des noyaux neurosécrétoires hypothalamiques chez les batraciens et les reptiles. Acta anat. (Basel) **30**, 429—433 (1957).

LEGAIT, H.: Les voies extra hypothalamo-neurohypophysaires de la neurosécrétion diencéphalique dans la série des vertébrés. p. 42—51. In: Zweites Internationales Symposium über Neurosekretion. Lund 1957. Berlin-Göttingen-Heidelberg: Springer 1958.

STERBA, G.: Fluoreszenz-mikroskopische Untersuchungen über die Neurosekretion beim Bachneunange (Lampetra planeri. Bloch). Z. Zellforsch. **55**, 763—789 (1961).

— Grundlagen des histochemischen und biochemischen Nachweis von Neurosekret (Trägerprotein der Oxytozine) mit Pseudoisozyanmen. Acta histochem. **17**, 268—292 (1964).

STUTINSKY, F.: Contribution à l'étude du complexe hypothalamo-hypophysaire. Thèse Fac. Sc. Paris 1955.

Activation of the Preoptico-Hypophysial Neurosecretory System through Olfactory Afferents in Fishes[1]

Andrzej Jasinski[2], Aubrey Gorbman, and Toshiaki Hara[3]

Department of Zoology, University of Washington

Introduction

The nature of the afferent pathways to the hypothalamic preoptic nuclei is a matter of importance, since neurosecretory axons from these nuclei extend to the pituitary gland. If we can define precisely the afferents to the preoptic nuclei, then better understanding of pituitary regulation by external factors may be expected. It is known, for example, that changes in the osmotic value of the internal and external environment affect the amount of stainable neurosecretory material in the preoptic or supraoptic nuclei of a variety of vertebrates (Sawyer and Roth, 1953; Legait, 1959; Oksche et al., 1959; Philibert and Kamemoto, 1965; Hild, 1951; Tramezzani and Uranga, 1954). Furthermore, injections of hypertonic solution into the blood by Cross and Green, 1959; Brooks et al., 1962 and by Koizumi et al., 1964, evoked changes in electrical activity of neurones in the supraoptic nucleus. From such work it is inferred that the hypothalamic neurones are themselves osmoreceptive, or that they are synaptically related to an osmoreceptor, and that they are involved in a reflex regulation of tonicity of body fluids, probably through release of antidiuretic hormones.

In reviewing facts characterizing the control of the preoptic nucleus, we have been struck by the relationship that appears to exist between the olfactory system and the preoptic or supraoptic nucleus. Easily traced neurone pathways exist between the olfactory tracts and preoptic nuclei (reviewed by Kappers, Huber, and Crosby, 1936). Recently Kandel, 1964, has shown in the goldfish that electrical stimulation of the olfactory tract evokes single unit spikes in the preoptic nucleus. Sundsten and Sawyer, 1961, have made the very interesting observation in the rabbit that administration of hypertonic solutions not only causes electrical changes in the supraoptic nucleus, it also evokes electrical changes in the olfactory bulb.

Teleologically, it is difficult to understand the utility of an olfactory-preoptic relationship, if, indeed, it exists at all. It is even more difficult to understand why the olfactory bulb should be specifically sensitive to changes in the internal osmotic environment. For these reasons we have undertaken further study of functional properties of the olfactory-preoptic link, specifically to find whether such

[1] This study was aided by a grant from the National Institute of Health (NB 04887).

[2] Present Address: Hoyer Department of Comparative Anatomy, Jagiellonian University, Cracow, 50 Krupnicza Str., Poland.

[3] Present Address: Department of Zoology, University of Tokyo, Tokyo, Japan.

innervation can activate neurosecretory activity. In the experiments described here, we have addressed ourselves to the question of whether chemical stimulation of the olfactory epithelium or electrical stimulation of the olfactory tract affects neurosecretion in the preoptic nucleus or in the axonal regions deriving from this nucleus. There has resulted clear evidence of a rapid and potent effect of such treatment upon hypothalamic neurosecretion. Further interest in these data resides in the fact that except for experiments by COOKE, 1964, with the pericardial organ in the crab, no direct evidence has been available relating direct stimulation of a neurosecretory neurone to release of its neurosecretory product. The rapid changes described here in electrically stimulated neurosecretory neurones would seem to apply to this general question.

Material and Methods

Eighty five goldfish, *Carassius auratus* L., ranging from 12 to 15 cm in length, were used. They were kept in a concrete tank at room temperature (21–23° C) and fed daily with commercial compressed fish-meal food. Part of the water was changed at approximately daily intervals. After anaesthesia with MS-222 (tricaine methane sulphonate, Sandoz), the fish were immobilized by intramuscular injections of Flaxedil (gallamine triethiodide), in a dose of 4 mg/kg. They were then wrapped in wet cloth and held in a shaped metal block holder resting in a lucite water chamber. A continuous flow of dechlorinated water was passed into the mouth through a glass tube fed by an elevated water reservoir (120–140 ml/min); this water, after passing over the gills, drained into the water chamber.

The brain was exposed by removing the dorsal portion of the skull with scissors. The meningeal tissue surrounding the brain was removed by gentle sponging. The anterior part of the brain pan, forming a suitable experimental chamber, was filled with mineral oil.

In several animals the olfactory mucosa was stimulated by means of infusion of 0.1 % NaCl solution through the nasal cavity; the responses in single units of the nucleus preopticus were recorded through using bipolar stainless steel electrodes, 1 mm apart, insulated to the tip. The recording electrodes were placed directly on the preoptic nucleus which is easily made visible by removal of the anterior choroid plexus and placing a drop of mineral oil in the exposed third ventricle.

The effect of control operations upon the hypothalamo-hypophysial system was studied in several groups of animals (Table 1): 1. untreated fishes, 2. sham operated (exposure of the brain), fixed immediately after operation, or with specified delays; 3. sham operated and electrically stimulated (electrodes placed on the abdominal surface), fixed without delay; 4. fishes exposed to tap water or distilled water infused through the nasal cavity (1 or 10 min, fixed with no delay).

For electrical stimulation the right olfactory tract was lifted in the mineral oil and contact was made with bipolar silver electrodes (0.15 mm in diameter, 1 mm apart). Rectangular pulses with various durations and amplitudes were delivered with a Grass S4 stimulator via an isolation unit. Other characteristics of the electrical stimulation are included in Table 3.

For chemical stimulation of the olfactory mucosa, a continuous flow of solution (15 ml/min) was infused into the left nasal cavity through glass tubing under slight hydrostatic pressure from an elevated reservoir. The solution used was 1.0, 2.5, or 5.0 % NaCl dissolved in distilled water. The data regarding chemical stimulation are included in Table 3.

Immediately after experimentation, or after a specified delay, the animals were killed by decapitation, the brains were exposed and immersed in Bouin's solution

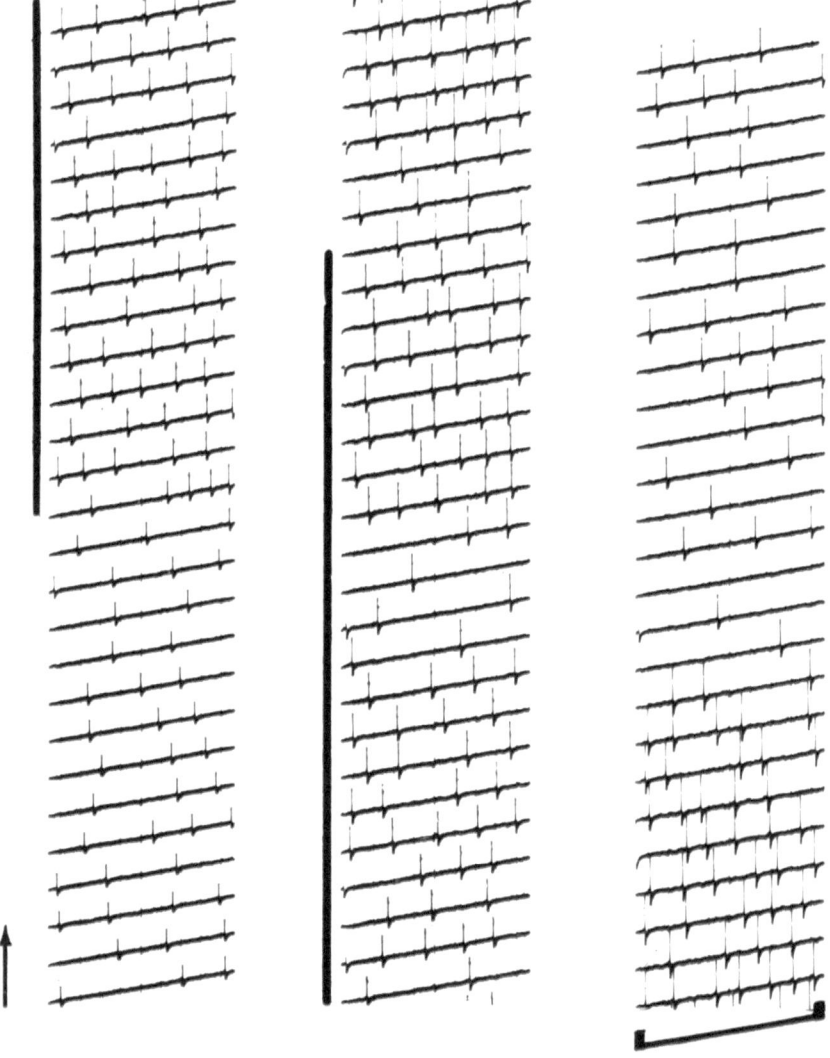

Fig. 1. Response of single neuronal units in the nucleus preopticus to infusion of 0.1% NaCl solution through the nasal cavity. Arrow indicates that the recording begins at the lower left and progresses upwards to the top. The same record then continues from the bottom of the next strip to the right. The thick black line indicates the time during which the actual flow of salt solution took place. Note the increase of unitary discharges during and immediately after stimulation

for 2–3 days. Protocols indicate variable times selected between electrical or chemical stimulation and sacrifice of the animals (0 to 90 min). Embedding was in paraplast and transverse sections (7 or 10 μ) were made. For staining of the hypothalamo-hypophysial complex Gomori aldehyde fuchsin was used.

The effects of control and experimental operations upon the hypothalamo-hypophysial complex (degranulation) was estimated accordingly to the arbitrary scales described below.

  Nucleus preopticus
   o) normal[1] appearance; perikarya filled with AF-stainable granules
   +) minimal degranulation
   ++) a few degranulated cells; remaining cells stained lighter
   +++) about 50 % of the cells remain stainable or about half of granules remain in perikarya
   ++++) a few cells remain stainable or only a few granules are present in the perikarya
   +++++) complete degranulation
  Juxta-somal axons
   o) normal appearance; axons deeply stained, Herring bodies present, usually in abundance
   +) minimal degranulation, Herring bodies present
   ++) axons stained more weakly than normal; none, or very few Herring bodies present
   +++) axons almost invisible, Herring bodies absent
  Hypothalamo-hypophysial tract
   > o) axons more heavily loaded with granules than normal
   o) normal appearance
   +) slight degranulation
   ++) a few granules visible
   +++) complete degranulation
  Neurohypophysis
   o) axonal endings and/or Herring bodies in abundance
   < o) noticeable depletion

Observations

The pattern of single unit discharges was clearly altered by exposing the olfactory epithelium to 0.1 % NaCl solution infused slowly through one of the openings of the nasal sac. Altered discharge patterns of about twenty such units were successfully recorded after obtaining a relatively stable pre-stimulation pattern. In some instances (Fig. 1) the rate of discharge was increased, the increased rate persisting for about 30 seconds after cessation of a one-minute infusion of 0.1 % NaCl. In some instances the pattern was unaffected, and in a few cells the pattern was inhibited. However, whether inhibited or stimulated, responsiveness of preoptic cells to chemical stimulation of the olfactory receptors

---

[1] By "normal" is meant the condition found in untreated control animals.

confirms the anatomical data, and the electrical experiments of KANDEL, 1964, in showing a functional connection between the olfactory system and the preoptic neurosecretory cells.

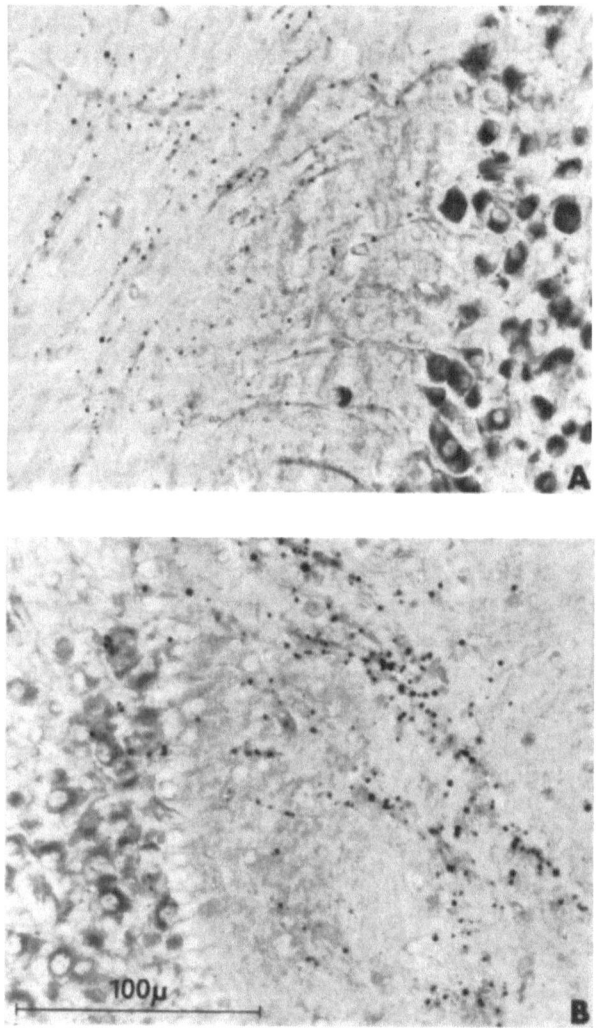

Fig. 2 A and B. Nucleus preopticus (pars parvocellularis), and juxta-somal axons in control and salt-immersed animals. Bouin, AF, cross sections (10 μ). A No 48. Animal untreated; AF-stainable material present in the cell bodies in abundance; numerous Herring bodies associated with juxta-somal axons. B No 58. Animal immersed for 6 days in 1% NaCl solution; extensive loss of neurosecretory material from the perikarya and the juxta-somal axons, whereas Herring bodies persist

Control Series (Table 1)

Untreated animals. Five untreated animals were studied for establishment of the typical or "normal" appearance of the hypothalamo-hypophysial complex (Table 1). The conditions in this group of animals were taken as a basis for the evaluation of the amount of neurosecretory substance found within the different regions of the hypothalamo-hypophysial complex (Fig. 2 A) in treated specimens.

Various control operations were maintained to detect the possible depletion of AF-stainable material in the hypothalamo-hypophysial complex brought about by operations preceeding the actual experimentation.

Sham operations (with or without delay in fixation) produced only a slight degranulation in the nucleus preopticus and juxta-somal axons. Similar minimal changes resulted when electrical stimulation of the abdomen was done in addition to the sham operations.

Water perfusion through the nostrils, with the exception of one specimen (N⁰ 89), produced no significant differences from untreated animals. Like the latter, they were therefore used as standard controls (Fig. 3).

Table 1. *Effect of control operations upon the preoptico-hypophysial system in goldfish*

Specimen number	Mode of operation	Degree of degranulation[1]				
		NPO Pars magnocellularis	NPO Pars parvocellularis	Juxta-somal axons	H-H tract	N H
46	Untreated	o	o	o	o	o
47	Untreated	o	o	o	o	
48	Untreated	o	o	o	o	o
52	Untreated	+	+	o	o	o
53	Untreated	o	o	o	o	o
39	Sham operated	+	++	++	o	
40	Sham operated	o	+	+	o	o
41	Sham operated[2]	++	++	++		
42	Sham operated[3]	+	++	+		
43	Sham operated and elect. stim.[4]	o to +	o to +	+	o	o
44	Sham operated and elect. stim.[4]	+	++	++	o	
45	Sham operated and elect. stim.[4]	o to +	o to +	+	o	
78	Sham operated and elect. stim.[4]	o	+	o	o	
79	Sham operated and elect. stim.[4]	o	o	o	o	o
80	Sham operated and elect. stim.[4]	++	++	o	o	o
87	Water perfusion through nostrils[5]	o	o	o	o	o
88	Water perfusion through nostrils[5]	o	o	o		
89	Water perfusion through nostrils[6]	+++	+++	++	+	
90	Water perfusion through nostrils[6]	o	o	o	o	
49	Immersion in 1% salt sol. – 2 days	o to +	+ to ++	>o	o	
50	Immersion in 1% salt sol. – 2 days	o to +	o to +	o	o	< o
51	Immersion in 1% salt sol. – 2 days	o	+	o	o	
54	Immersion in 1% salt sol. – 5 days	++	+++	o	>o	< o
55	Immersion in 1% salt sol. – 5 days	+	++	o	>o	< o
56	Immersion in 1% salt sol. – 6 days	++	+	o	>o	o
57	Immersion in 1% salt sol. – 6 days	++	+	o	o	o
58	Immersion in 1% salt sol. – 6 days	++	+	++	o	
59	Immersion in 1% salt sol. – 7 days	to +	o	o	o	

[1] The meanings of the symbols used in these columns is explained in the text.
[2] Fixed after 30 min delay.
[3] Fixed after 60 min delay.
[4] Stimulated abdomen: 60″, fixed without delay; 4 v, 3 msec, 10 CPS.
[5] Time of perfusion: 1 min, fixed without delay.
[6] Time of perfusion: 10 min, fixed without delay.

Immersion in 1 % NaCl Solution (Table 1)

The immersion of goldfish in 1 % NaCl solution for various, but relatively longer, periods of time did affect the appearance of the neurosecretory system, though to a moderate extent. After two days of immersion only minimal or slight degranulation occurred in the nucleus preopticus. More intensified degranulation followed five and six days of immersion in salt water (Fig. 2B). Parallel effects were noticed in the neurohypophysis, together with a greater than normal accumulation of AF-stainable granules in the hypothalamo-hypophysial tracts. One specimen kept for seven days in 1 % NaCl solution showed no changes in comparison with untreated animals.

Electrical Stimulation (Table 2)

In most of the animals the olfactory tract was stimulated 60 seconds and fixation was without delay. The usual voltage, pulse duration (in milliseconds), and frequency (cycles per second) of the electrial stimulus were 2, 3, and 10, respectively. In those experiments in which there was a delay between the end of electrical stimulation and killing and fixation, the delay was 15, 30, or 90 minutes. Although electrical stimulation was applied only to the right olfactory tract, changes were seen in the cells of the nucleus preopticus on both sides of the diencephalic ventricle.

Nucleus preopticus. Figure 4 summarizes graphically the degree of degranulation evoked in the cells of the nucleus preopticus by electrical stimulation of the olfactory tract. Generally similar effects after electrical stimulation were found in the pars parvocellularis and magnocellularis. When differences did appear, they usually did not exceed more than one "grade" in the evaluatory scale.

It is clear that even a relatively short stimulation (60 seconds) may cause complete degranulation in the NPO. However, considerable variation was found in this group of animals and all major grades of degranulation were found. In the group of 60 second-stimulated goldfish, the average degree of degranulation was only moderate. Generally, in the specimens killed immediately at the end of the electrical stimulation there was more degranulation than in those fixed after a delay. In the small number of 60 second-stimulated fish in which degranulation was minimal, the delay was the longest: 30 to 90 minutes. Examples of wide variations in response to brief electrical stimulation are included in Fig. 5.

Electrical stimulation of the olfactory tract over intervals longer than one minute (1.5—4 min) produced clear, consistent, and relatively uniform effects in the nucleus preopticus. However, the longest period of applied stimulation (10 min) did not always evoke the strongest effect (Fig. 4). With the prolonged stimulus as well as with the shorter one, delay in fixation influenced the quantity of AF-stainable granules present in the perikarya of the NPO. Such delay usually was associated with less complete degrees of degranulation. Accordingly, it is clear that the delay between the electrical stimulus and fixation permitted a certain degree of recovery. In contrast with the relatively prompt degranulation following even a short electrical stimulus of about one minute, it seems that the time required for full recovery of the depleted neurosecretory cells is measurable at least in hours.

Juxta-somal axons. Normally the juxta-somal axons extending from the nucleus preopticus are relatively broad, deeply stained, and readily traceable (Fig. 5A). Usually a large number of Herring bodies is closely associated with the axons.

Table 2. *Activation of the preoptico-hypophysial system in goldfish following electrical stimulation of the olfactory tract*

Specimen number	Stimulation Voltage/pulse duration in msec/CPS	Time Stimulation	Time Fixation delay, minutes	Degree of degranulation[1] NPO Pars magnocellularis	NPO Pars parvo cellularis	Juxta-somal axons	H-H tract	N H
2	2,1,100	15″	30′	++	++	++	+	
1	2,1,100	30″	30′	++	+++	+++	++	
28	2,1,100	30″	30′	++	++	+	○	
3	2,1,100	60″	0	++	+++	+		
7	2,3,100	60″	0	+++++	++++	+++	++	
18	4,3,10	60″	0	++++	++	+		
29	2,1,100	60″	0	++	+++	○		
30	2,3,100	60″	0	++	+++	+	○	○
66	4,3,10	60″	0	++	++	++	+	○
67	4,3,10	60″	0	○	○	○	>○	○
68	4,3,10	60″	0	+++	ⅠⅠⅠ	○	○	○
69	4,3,10	60″	15′	++++	++++	++	+++	>○
70	4,3,10	60″	15′	++	++	+	○	○
71	4,3,10	60″	15′	++	++	+	○	○
72	4,3,10	60″	30′	+	+	+	○	
75	4,3,10	60″	90′	+++	+++	++	+	<○
76	4,3,10	60″	90′	+	+	○	○	
77	4,3,10	60″	90′	++	++	+	○	
19	4,3,10	1.5′	0	++++	+++++	+++	++	○
35	4,3,10	1.5′	0	+++	+++	++		
20	4,3,10	2′	0	+++++	+++++	+++	+	○
36	4,3,10	2′	0	+++	+++	++	○	
21	4,3,10	2.5′	0	+++	+++	++	○	○
37	4,3,10	2.5′	0	++++	++++	+++		<○
22	4,3,10	3′	0	+++	+++	+	+	
23	4,3,10	4′	0	+++	+++	++	+	○
38	4,3,10	4′	0	+++	+++	++	○	
8	2,3,10	10′	0	+++	++++	+++	+++	
9	4,3,10	10′	0	++	++	++	○	
10	4,3,10	10′	0	++++	++++	+++	++	○
24	4,3,10	10′	0	++++ to +++++	+++++	++	++	
11	4,3,10	10′	15′	+++++	+++++	+++	+++	
25	4,3,10	10′	15′	+++ to ++++	++++	+++	○	<○
31	4,3,10	10′	15′	++++	++++	++	○	○
12	4,3,10	10′	30′	++++	++++	+++	+	
32	4,3,10	10′	30′	++	+++	+	○	○
33	4,3,10	10′	60′	+++	+++ to ++++	++	○	○
34	4,3,10	10′	90′	++ to +++	++ to +++	+++	○	○

[1] The meaning of the symbols used in these columns is explained in the text.

This initial portion of neurosecretory pathway appears clearly to be responsive to electric stimulation. In only relatively few instances was there a lack of response, or only a slight response was noticed. This response, in most specimens consisted of the disappearance of Herring bodies and a more or less complete loss of stainability in axons.

Judging from the rate of disappearance of AF-stainable material after brief electrical stimulation, the passage of the neurosecretory granules through the

juxta-somal axons is rapid. In most of the animals, regardless of duration of the
stimulus or length of delay before fixation, extensive or complete decrease of
Herring bodies and AF-stainable granules was found. Whenever stainability of

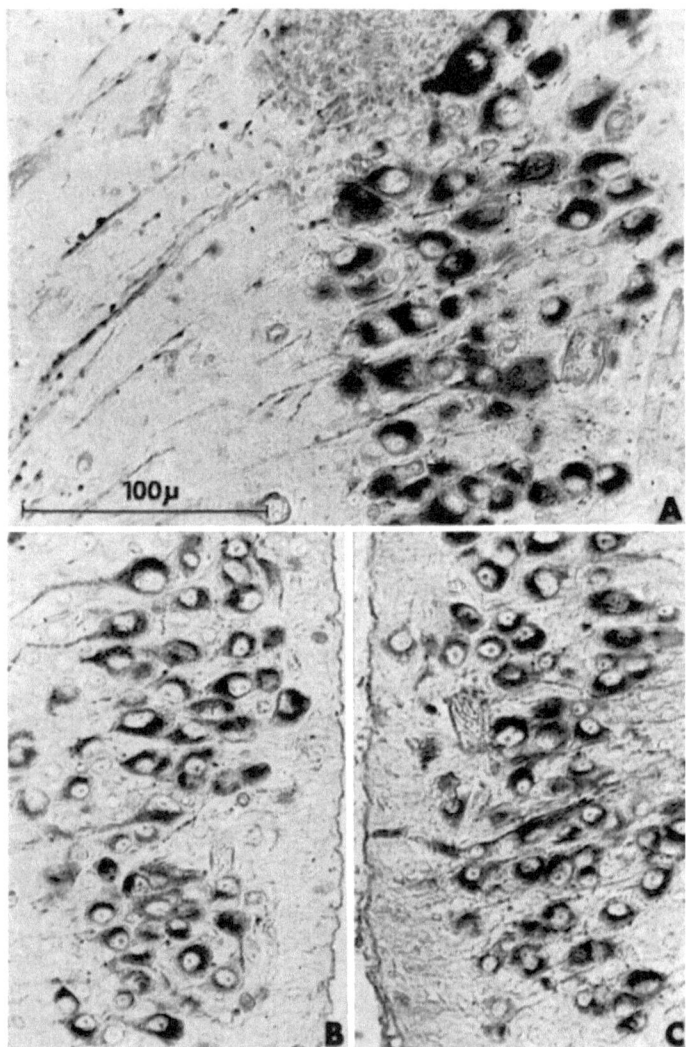

Fig. 3 A—C. Normal appearance of the nucleus preopticus — control animals killed and
fixed immediately after 1 minute of water perfusion through the nasal cavity. Bouin, AF,
cross sections (7 μ). A No 87. Pars magnocellularis and the juxta-somal axons with the associated Herring bodies. B No 88. Pars magnocellularis. C No 88. Pars parvocellularis

the juxta-somal axons differed in comparison with the more distal hypothalamo-
hypophysial tract, the juxta-somal axons were always more weakly stained.

Hypothalamo-hypophysial tract. In approximately half of the animals with
stimulated olfactory tracts partial, or even complete, discharge of AF-stainable
granules was found in more distal parts of the neurosecretory axons, in the hypo-

thalamo-hypophysial tracts. In a few animals the hypothalamo-hypophysial tract was granulated to a more than normal extent (Fig. 6).

Neurohypophysis. In none of the stimulated specimens (Fig. 7) was there any remarkable change in the amount of the neurosecretory substance in the primary rami of the neurohypophysis. However, it was clear that such olfactory stimuli, which were sufficient to evoke hypothalamic changes also diminished the amount

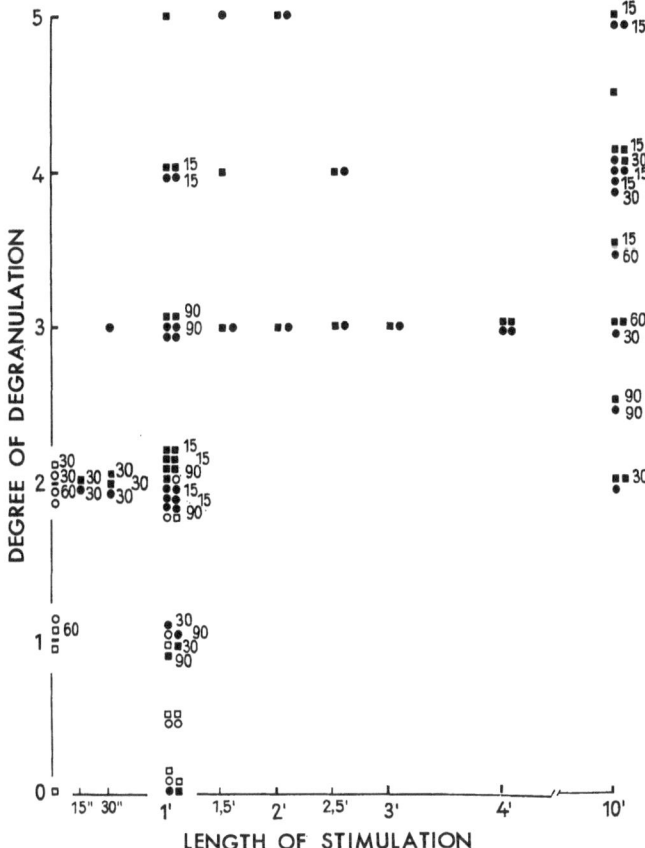

Fig. 4. Graphical summarization of the degree of degranulation evoked in the cells of NPO by electrical stimulation of the olfactory tract. Progressive degranulation is expressed on the ordinate scale from 0 to 5, according to an arbitrary series of criteria described in the text. Solid blocks, pars magnocellularis, specimens stimulated electrically; empty squares, pars magnocellularis, control specimens (with or without electrical stimulation delivered to the abdomen); filled circles, pars parvocellularis, specimens stimulated electrically; empty circles, pars parvocellularis, control specimens. Numbers next to a symbol indicate minutes delay in fixation of the particular specimen

of stainable material in the axonal endings and/or Herring bodies scattered between the cells of the pars intermedia. Under the experimenal conditions employed here complete loss of stainable axonal endings and/or Herring bodies in the neurointermediate lobe was never found.

In summary (Fig. 8) four typical groups, characterizing the nature of the morphological modifications induced in hypothalamic neurosecretory cells by electrical stimulation, may be recognized in this study:

8*

1. Changes in the secretory neurones are minimal or not significantly different from the normal state.

2. Perikarya and the juxta-somal axons are partially degranulated while the hypothalamo-hypophysial tract and neurohypophysis contains a normal amount of AF-stainable product.

3. All components of the neurosecretory cells are affected to some degree. Perikarya contain only a few stainable granules; the juxta-somal axons and hypothalamo-hypophysial tract are deprived of some or most of their stainable

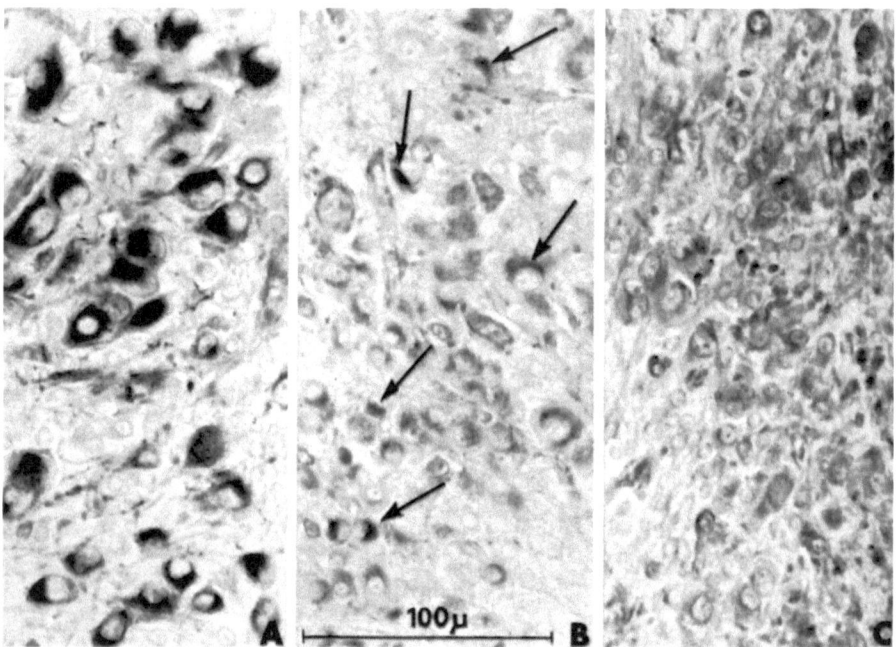

Fig. 5 A—C. Degranulation in the cells of the nucleus preopticus evoked by electrical stimulation of the olfactory tract. Bouin, AF, cross sections (A, B: 7 μ, C: 10 μ). A No 70. Most dorsal portion of the pars magnocellularis. Slight degranulation. Stimulated 60 seconds, fixed after 15 minute delay. B No 69. Pars magnocellularis. Strong effect; only in some cells (arrows) a few granules remain stainable. Stimulated 60 seconds, fixed after 15 minute delay. C No 7. Pars magnocellularis. Complete degranulation. Stimulated 60 seconds, fixed without delay

material; slight degranulation in the neurohypophysis may or may not be also noticeable.

4. The only AF-stainable substance remaining is in the neurohypophysis. Perikarya, the juxta-somal axons, and hypothalamo-hypophysial tract are depleted of visible neurosecretion; sometimes a few granules are present in the axons of the hypothalamo-hypophysial tract.

It is worth noting that in the specimens only minimally affected by the olfactory electrical stimulus, the neurosecretory granules were often displaced into the preaxonal region of the perikarya instead of being more evenly distributed in the cell body. The most common phenomenon during the initial stage of degranulation was a selective loss of AF-stainable granules from the cell bodies of certain cells. That is, cells tightly packed with granules could be found in close proximity to depleted cells. Many cells with dendrites extending to or projecting into the third ventricle were present in the NPO (Fig. 9). Often they were comparatively broad and filled with granules. This phenomenon was also common in animals stimulated chemically as well as in control specimens.

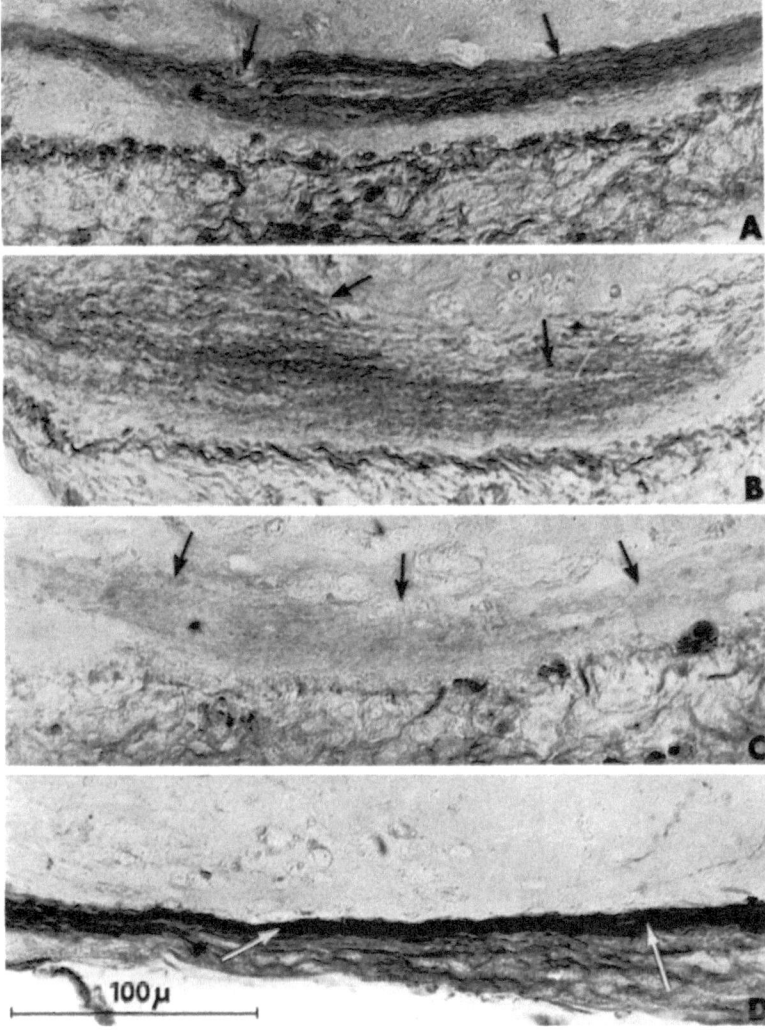

Fig. 6 A—D. The appearance of the hypothalamo-hypophysial tracts (arrows) in animals with electrically stimulated olfactory tracts. Bouin, AF, cross (7 µ). A No 38. Normal appearance. Stimulated 4 minutes; fixed without delay. B No 33. Normal appearance. Stimulated 10 minutes; fixed after 60 minute delay. C No 69. Complete degranulation. Stimulated 60 seconds; fixed after 15 minute delay. D No 67. Axons heavily loaded with AF-stainable granules. Stimulated 60 seconds; fixed without delay

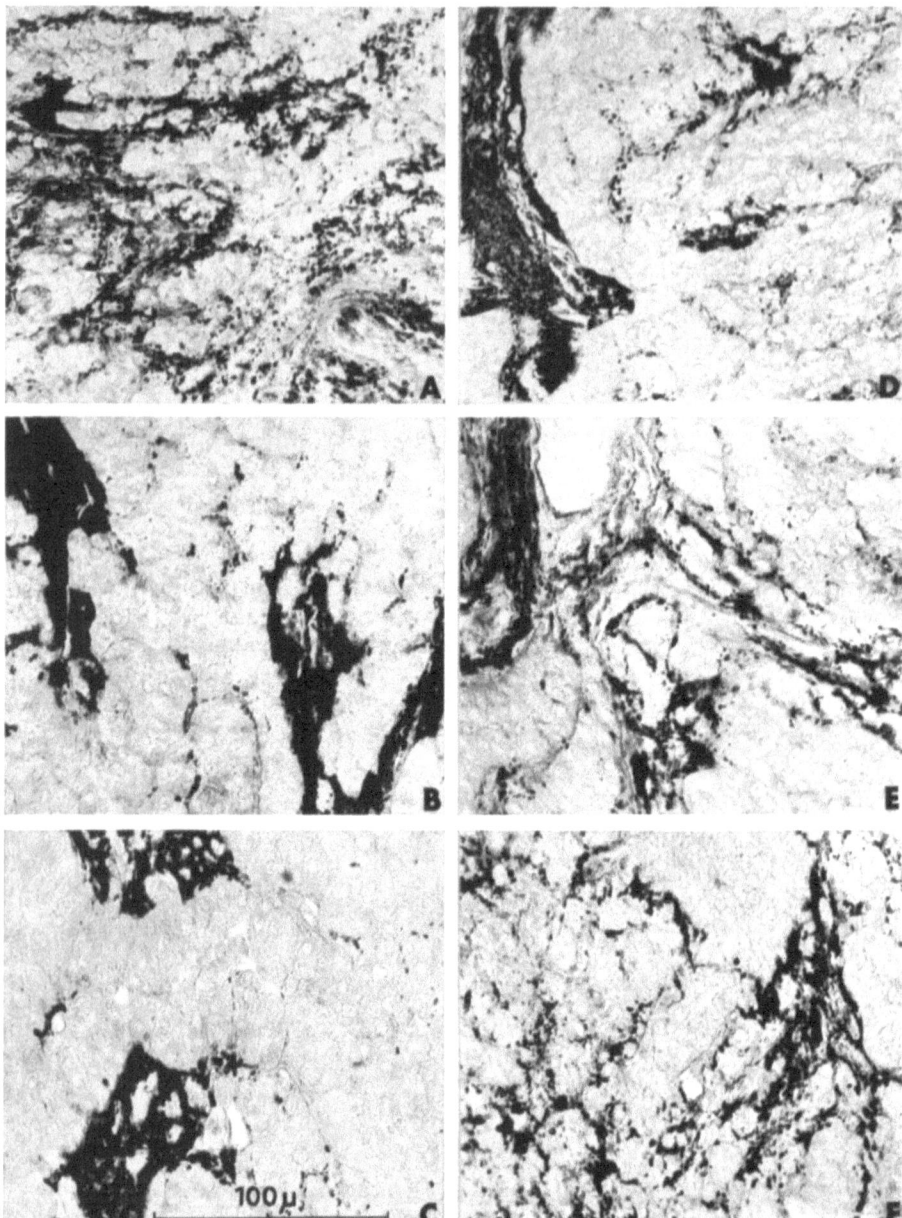

Fig. 7 A—F. Neuro-intermediate lobe of the pituitary. Bouin, AF. A No 48. Control animal (untreated). Axonal endings and/or HB present in abundance. B No 54. Control animal kept in 1% NaCl solution 5 days. Main ramifications of neural tissue are full of AF-stainable material whereas relatively few terminal portions of the axons are stained. C No 69. Animal stimulated electrically 60 seconds; fixed after 15 minute delay. Effect like that in animal No 54. D No 37. Animal stimulated electrically 2.5 minutes, fixed without delay. Slight degranulation. E No 31. Animal stimulated electrically 10 minutes, fixed without delay. Slight degranulation. F No 34. Animal stimulated electrically 10 minutes, fixed after 90 minute delay. Slight degranulation

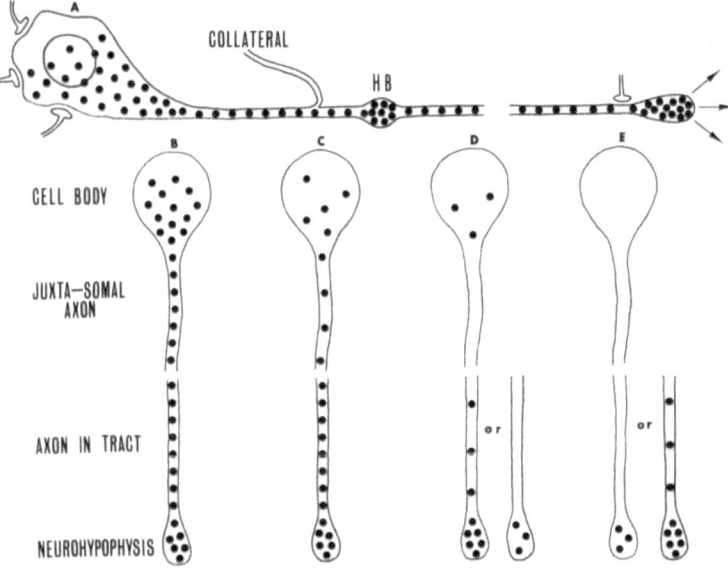

Fig. 8 A—E. Schematic representation of a typical neurosecretory cell of the goldfish nucleus preopticus (A) indicating the pattern of afferent innervation, the presence of recurrent collaterals (KANDEL, 1964), Herring bodies, axon-axonal terminations (KOBAYASHI and OOTA, 1964; KOBAYASHI et al., 1965) and secretion laden axonal endings. Four principal patterns of distribution below, showing the range of response (degranulation) to electrical stimulation delivered to the olfactory tract. Each drawing represents the entire hypothalamo-hypophysial system

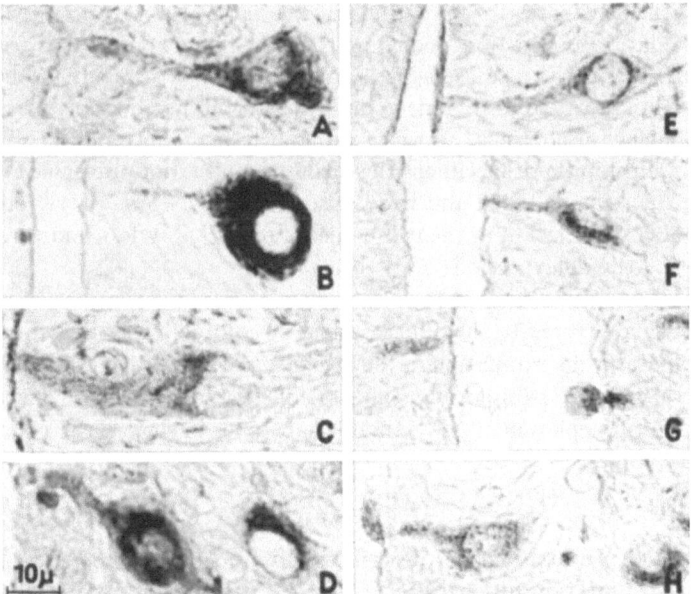

Fig. 9 A—H. Neurosecretory cells from the nucleus preopticus with dendrites extending to (A—F) or projecting into (G—H) the third ventricle

Chemical Stimulation (Table 3)

In some specimens the olfactory epithelium was stimulated by perfusion of NaCl solution through the left nasal sac. The concentration of the solution, duration of perfusion, and time delay in fixation are summarized in Table 3. As in animals stimulated electrically, the effects of chemical stimulation upon the cells of the NPO was bilateral even though the stimulus was not.

Table 3. *Activation of the preoptico-hypophysial system in goldfish following perfusion of the salt solution through the nasal cavity*

Specimen number	Concentration of NaCl solution	Time		Degree of degranulation[1]				
		Perfusion	Fixation delay	NPO Pars magnocellularis	NPO Pars parvocellularis	Juxta-somal axons	H-H tract	N H
84	2.5%	10'	0	+	÷	>o	o	<o
85	2.5%	10'	0	++	++	++	o	<o
86	2.5%	10'	0	++	++	o	o	<o
17	2.5%	30'	0	+++++	+++	+++		
13	5.0%	30'	0	++++	+++ to ++++	+++	+++	<o
14	2.5%	30'	30'	+++++	+++++	+++	+++	
4	1.0%	30'	60'	++	++	++	o	
15	2.5%	60'	0	+++++	+++++	+++		
5	1.0%	60'	60'	+++	+++	+++	+++	
16	2.5%	120'	0	++++	++++	+++		
6	1.0%	120'	60'	++	+++	++	o	

[1] The meaning of the symbols used in these columns is explained in the text.

Following such chemical stimulation over a period of ten minutes, only a slight degranulation in the cell bodies of the NPO appeared, but a significant effect of stimulation was also seen in the neurohypophysis. Stimulation applied over a thirty minute period, or longer, induced an intense degranulation in the cells of the nucleus preopticus, as well as in the juxta-somal and hypothalamo-hypophysial axons (in these specimens the pituitaries were not preversed). It is also clear that in the animals killed and fixed after a relatively long delay (one hour), the amount of degranulation in the cell bodies is remarkably less, indicating some recovery during the delay period.

Thus, chemical stimulation of the olfactory mucosa, in contrast with results of electrical stimuli delivered to the olfactory tract, required a relatively longer time to evoke comparable degranulation in the perikarya of neurosecretory cells. On the other hand, this type of stimulation is no less effective, and seemingly it causes an even more uniform depletion of AF-stainable substance in the entire hypothalamo-hypophysial complex.

Discussion

The results of the experiments described here appear to demonstrate a functional activating relationship between olfactory stimulation and hypothalamic neurosecretion in the goldfish. If this is accepted as demonstrated, then the reports by ARVY and GABE, 1954; ARVY et al., 1954; TUURALA, 1957; FRIDBERG and

OLSSON, 1959, and by others of degranulation of hypothalamic neurosecretory systems following immersion of fish in sea water or saline solutions must be re-evaluated. Neurosecretory phenomena like those following prolonged saline immersion could be evoked by us also by briefly infusing relatively weak salt solutions into the nasal sac (or by electrical stimulation of the olfactory tract). Accordingly, it is quite possible that the immersion experiments do not represent an osmotic response in the strict sense, but rather the effect of salt on the olfactory receptor in fish.

It is perhaps specious to argue whether in our experiments the olfactory epithelium is acting as an osmoreceptor or whether specific chemoreception for sodium and/or chloride ions is involved. The effective nasal concentration of NaCl for neurosecretory depletion during a 10-minute exposure is 1 %, or perhaps even less, since still lower concentrations were not tested by us. Furthermore, we have found in other experiments (unpublished) that 0.1 % sodium chloride evokes potential patterns (EEG) in the olfactory bulb which cannot be distinguished from those evoked by sucrose, amino acids, or other organic materials at similar molar concentrations. Thus, it is difficult to avoid the conclusion that weak NaCl, acting in a manner resembling other olfactory active agents, can evoke neurosecretory activity and derivative phenomena.

An interesting but yet unanswered question is whether olfactory stimulants other than NaCl can provoke the neuroendocrine depletion which we have here described for NaCl and for electrical activation. The ability of hypertonic immersion to deplete hypothalamic neurosecretion in fishes has been referred to above.

In mammals injection of hypertonic solutions not only results in such neuro-secretory release (LEVEQUE and SCHARRER, 1953; DE GROOT, 1957), but it also produces measurable increases in antidiuretic (ADH) hormone levels in the blood (CHAMBERS et al., 1945; GINSBURG and BROWN, 1957; ANDERSON, 1957). Although our experiments have shown that release of neurosecretion probably occurs after appropriate olfactory stimulation in goldfish, it remains to be proven that olfactory stimuli can lead to release of neurohypophysial hormone peptides like ADH. This possibility deserves experimental testing. There are several experimental findings linking olfactory and hypothalamic functions in mammals which seem curious because their utility is difficult to understand, or they are unexpected. For example, SAWYER, 1963, recently has reviewed a number of experiments in which hypothalamus-activating substances like adrenaline and histamine, even when applied directly to the hypothalamus, produce at the same time EEG changes which are strongest in, or emanate from the olfactory bulbs. Various authors have reported in mammals a pheromone-like naso-genital relationship in which male odors affect the sexual cycle of the female, presumably through the hypothalamus (see WHITTEN, 1956; DIXON, 1959; also SCHARRER and SCHARRER, 1963).

Finally, we should mention again the discovery by SUNDSTEN and SAWYER, 1961, that hypertonic saline-injected rabbits have an activated EEG in the olfactory bulb at the same time as stimulation of neurones in the supraoptic nucleus is recorded. Thus, evidence exists showing that activation between the olfactory and hypothalamic neurosecretory systems may proceed in either direction.

Because it can serve as a kind of single event "time marker", the rapidity of depletion of hypothalamic neurosecretion after electrical stimulation makes it possible to study the dynamic aspects of neurosecretory granular movement and replenishment. This could be useful in further work designed specifically to trace the movement of neurosecretory granules through the axon and to estimate the rate of such movement. Even in our experiments, not specifically directed to this question, several conclusions are suggested:

1. Generally, as increasing degrees of depletion of neurosecretory material were observed in the hypothalamic neurones, the first depleted region was the perikaryon- followed by the juxta-somal axons, the tracts, and finally the region of endings in the neurointermediate lobe. This suggests that the slowest process is release from axonal terminal, and that movement of granules through the other parts of the neurone is relatively more rapid.

2. In animals in which delay was permitted between the end of electrical stimulation and killing and fixation of the brain, re-accumulation of neurosecretory material generally occurred. The extent of re-accumulation, with broad variability, was greater as the length of delay until fixation increased. Periods of 15 minutes generally were insufficient to permit much change, but delay periods of 60 to 90 minutes usually permitted restoration of nearly normal levels of AF-stainable granulation. It may be questioned whether such observations made on surviving Flaxedil-treated goldfish with an exposed brain tell us much about this phenomenon in normal goldfish. Nevertheless, these data provide the first real evidence relating to rates of release and regeneration of neurosecretory material.

3. In animals in which delay before fixation permitted some restoration of depleted neurosecretory material, it is of great interest that the apparent patterns of distribution of this material did not differ from those seen immediately after stimulation. That is, the axonal endings always contained some neurosecretory material, and as more AF-stainable granules reappeared, they were found to accumulate in the tracts, the axons, and finally in the cell bodies (Fig. 8). This suggests that if the neurone cell body is the site of granule synthesis, AF-granules leave the cell body almost as rapidly as manufactured to accumulate progressively from the axon terminal backward. Hence, the entire neurosecretory neurone – not just the ending – is used for neurosecretory storage, and movement of granules toward the ending seems to be a relatively rapid phenomenon. An alternative explanation is that stimulation merely changes the stainability of the neurosecretory granules and we are observing here only regional changes in such stainability. Electron microscopy might settle this question.

References

ANDERSON, B. (1957): Polydipsia, antidiuresis and milk ejection caused by hypothalamic stimulation. In: The Neurohypophysis (Ed. H. HELLER), p. 131—140. London: Butterworths Scientific Publications.

ARVY, L., M. FONTAINE et M. GABE (1954): Action des solutions salines hypertoniques sur le système hypothalamo-hypophysaire, chez Phoxinus laevis Agass. et chez Anguilla anguilla L.C.R. Soc. Biol. (Paris) 148, 1759—1761.

—, et M. GABE (1954): Modifications du système hypothalamo-hypophysaire chez Callionymus lyra L. et Ammodytes lanceolatus Les. au cours des variations de l'équilibre osmotique. C. R. Ass. Anat. 41, 843—849.

BROOKS, C. McC., J. USHIYAMA, and G. LANGE (1962): Reactions of neurons in or near the supraoptic nuclei. Amer. J. Physiol. 202, 487—490.

CHAMBERS, G. H., E. V. MELVILLE, R. S. HARE, and K. HARE (1945): Regulation of the release of pituitary by changes in the osmotic pressure of plasma. Amer. J. Physiol. 144, 311—320.

COOKE, I. M. (1964): Electrical activity and release of neurosecretory material in crab pericardial organs. Comp. Biochem. Physiol. 13, 353—366.

CROSS, B. A., and J. D. GREEN (1959): Activity of single neurones in the hypothalamus: effect of osmotic and other stimuli. J. Physiol. 148, 554—569.

DE GROOT, J. (1957): Neurosecretion in experimental conditions. Anat. Rec. 127, 201—217.

DIXON, T. J. (1959): Studies on oviposition behaviour of Syrphidae (Diptera). Trans. roy. Entomol. Soc. London, 111, 57—80.

FRIDBERG, G., and R. OLSSON (1959): The praeoptico-hypophysial system, nucleus tuberis lateralis and the subcommissural organ of Gasterosteus aculeatus after changes in osmotic stimuli. Z. Zellforsch. 49, 531—540.

GINSBURG, M., and L. M. BROWN (1957): The effects of haemorrhage and plasma hypertonicity on the neurohypophysis. In: The Neurohypophysis (Ed. H. HELLER), p. 109—130. London: Butterworth Scientific Publications.

HILD, W. (1951): Experimentell-morphologische Untersuchungen über das Verhalten der „neurosekretorischen Bahn" nach Hypophysentieldurchtrennung, Eingriffen in den Wasserhaushalt und Belastung der Osmoregulation. Virchows Arch. path. Anat. 319,526—546.

KANDEL, E. R. (1964): Electrical properties of hypothalamic neuroendocrine cells. J. Gen. Physiol. 47, 691—717.

KAPPERS, C. U. A., G. C. HUBER, and E. C. CROSBY (1936): The Comparative Anatomy of the Nervous System of Vertebrates, Including Man. vol. 1—2. New York: Macmillan Company.

KOBAYASHI, H., and Y. OOTA (1964): Functional electron microscopy of the vertebrate neurosecretory storage-release organs. Gunma Symp. endocr. 1, 63—79.

— T. HIRANO, and Y. OOTA (1965): Electron microscopic and pharmacological studies on the median eminence and pars nervosa. Arch. Anat. micr. 54, 277—294.

KOIZUMI, K., T. ISHIKAWA, and C. McC. BROOKS (1964): Control of activity of neurons in the supraoptic nucleus. J. Neurophysiol. 27, 878—892.

LEGAIT, G. (1959): Contribution a l'étude morphologique expérimentale du système hypothalamo-neurohypophysaire de la Poule Rhode-Island. Thèse d'Agrégation de l'Enseignement Supérieur, Univ. Catholique de Louvain, Nancy.

LEVEQUE, T. F., and E. SCHARRER (1953): Pituicytes and the origin of the antidiuretic hormone. Endocrinology 52, 436—447.

OKSCHE, A., D. F. LAWS, F. I. KAMEMOTO, and D. S. FARNER (1959): The hypothalamohypophysial neurosecretory system of the white-crowned sparrow, Zonotrichia leucophrys gambelli. Z. Zellforsch. 51, 1—42.

PHILIBERT, R. L., and F. I. KAMEMOTO (1965): The hypothalamo-hypophysial neurosecretory system of the ring-necked snake, Diadophis punctatus, Gen. comp. Endocr. 5, 326—335.

SAWYER, C. H. (1963): Mechanisms by which drugs and hormones activate and block release of pituitary gonadotropins. Proceed. First Internat. Pharmacol. Meeting. Vol. I, p. 27—46. Oxford-London-New York-Paris: Pergamon Press.

SAWYER, W. H., and W. D. ROTH (1953): Neurohypophyseal function in dehydrated and adrenalectomized rats as indicated by hormone assay and neurosecretory activity. Fed. Proc. 12, 125.

SCHARRER, E., and B. SCHARRER (1963): Neuroendocrinology. New York-London: Colombia University Press.

SUNDSTEN, J. W., and C. H. SAWYER (1961): Osmotic activation of neurohypophysial hormone release in rabbits with hypothalamic islands. Exp. Neurol. 4, 548.

TRAMEZZANI, J. H., and J. URANGA (1954): Variations de la substance Gomori-positive et action antidiurétique de la neurohypophyse des crapauds hydratés ou déshydratés. C.R. Soc. Biol. 148, 1665.

TUURALA, O. (1957): Über den Einfluß der osmotischen Belastung auf die Neurosekretion der Kleinfische Gasterosteus aculeatus L. und Phozinus laevis L. aus dem Brachwasser des Finnischen Meerbusens. Ann. Acad. Sci. fenn. A, IV, Biol. 36, 1—9.

WHITTEN, W. K. (1956): Modification of the oestrus cycle of the mouse by external stimuli associated with the male. J. Endocrinol. 13, 339—404.

Pathological Aspects of the Concept of Neurosecretion with Special Reference to the Pathogenesis of Diabetes Insipidus

J. C. SLOPER, M. A. KARIM*

Pathology Department of Charing Cross Hospital Medical School, University of London, England

M. A. RICHARDS**

Department of Medicine, Royal Veterinary College London, England

This is the first occasion at these symposia in which a paper has been devoted to the pathological aspects of neurosecretion. This we propose to do, drawing particular attention first, to the bearing the concept of neurosecretion has on the study of the selective vulnerability of different parts of the central nervous system; and second, to the problem of the pathogenesis of diabetes insipidus. Although our main concern is the pathogenesis of the human disease, our studies involve also the dog, rat and mouse. It should perhaps be emphasised that this tendency to limit the number of species examined is forced on the pathologist, for he is obliged to define the normal with considerable care, no mean problem in a species such as man, whose life span is over 70 years. He is obliged, too, to take particular care in the exclusion of naturally-occurring diseases, for example, forms of nephritis, in the animals which he uses for experiments. This surely is a problem which must bedevil the work of the comparative endocrinologist, although little reference has been made to it here, save by Dr. BERN. This emphasis on animal work should not, incidentally, obscure the great contribution of human pathologists to the clarification of neurohypophysial function. It was, for example, a necropsy made by VON GAUPP in 1944 which led the latter first to suggest that the nerve-fibres of the posterior pituitary secreted antidiuretic hormone. This was no idle speculation, for he and ERNST SCHARRER had written in 1935 one of the earliest papers on the possible endocrine activity of neurones of the supraoptic nucleus.

In 1952 I was studying this same problem, namely, the pathogenesis of human diabetes insipidus, and learnt first from VASQUEZ-LOPEZ about the concept of neurosecretion then emerging from BARGMANN, 1951, and his colleagues in Kiel. VASQUEZ-LOPEZ, 1942, as a devoted pupil of del Rio Hortega, and thus of RAMON Y CAJAL, had devoted many years to the study of the neurohypophysis as a sensory organ. His acceptance of BARGMANN's work was so whole-hearted that I, too, was soon convinced.

* Under Colombo Plan Fellowship.
** Present address: Nutritional Research Laboratory, Petfoods Ltd., Melton Mowbray, Leicestershire, England.

It was clear, however, that the concepts then advanced, and the methods of study then available, were inadequate for satisfactory pathological investigations. In particular, it seemed improbable that particles of neurosecretory material (N.S.M.) 2 or more micra in diameter could pass down the tractus hypophyseus, possibly enveloping nerve fibres; it seemed odd too that such particles should represent an inert glycolipoprotein bearer substance unrelated to the hormone. It was clear, in fact, that the techniques then in use, while a vast improvement on those hitherto available, nevertheless stained so many other intraneuronal inclusions elsewhere in the nervous system, that they were of dubious value in the study of pathological states. This applied especially to man, whose ageing neurones are filled with a variety of lipoprotein inclusions.

With a view to overcoming these difficulties, we set about developing new methods for these investigations. I make no apology for this insistence on the importance of methodology, a point which I believe Gomori also used to stress. Gomori in fact never studied neurosecretion, although two methods he developed for the study of pancreatic islet granules were modified for the study of BARG-MANN's N.S.M. namely, the acid permanganate chrome-alum haematoxylin (C.A.H.) and acid permanganate aldehyde-fuchsin (A.F.) techniques. A brilliant cytochemist and the originator of many techniques, he would, I feel, have been very distressed by the terms "Gomori positive and negative" which some still appear to apply to N.S.M.

Methods

(i) Cytochemistry. We showed first, that BARGMANN's C.A.H. N.S.M. contained a component probably rich in protein-bound cystine; and second, that this material could represent either the posterior pituitary principles, (SLOPER, 1954 and SLOPER, 1966) or some closely linked precursor or carrier polypeptides. Our attempts to establish this point *in vitro* were, like I suspect ACHER's in 1957, vitiated by the tendency of polypeptides to be dissolved out of our preparations. RODECK, 1959, however, using formol-fixed agar as a vehicle, overcame this *in vitro* problem in BARGMANN's laboratory, and established that vasopressin and oxytocin could indeed be stained *in vitro* by the techniques available for N.S.M. In practice, we have found that only two techniques are suited to experimental studies, both of which demonstrate protein-bound cystine. These are the thioglycollate − ferric ferricyanide (see SLOPER, 1955) and the performic acid alcian blue techniques and their modifications (ADAMS and SLOPER, 1956). BARRNETT's, 1954, thioglycollate-dihydroxydinaphthyldisulphide method is, in this respect much too sensitive.

It must be stressed, however, that these methods mean little unless accompanied by respectively unreduced or unoxidised controls and by sections treated with trypsin. Any basic dye, for example, can be substituted for Alcian blue but the dye should be used at pH 1 or lower. We currently employ a Victoria blue resorcin-fuchsin mixture. STERBA's, 1961, substitution of the fluorescent dye, pseudo-isocyanin, for Alcian blue seems a promising step. His interpretation of its specificity, however, worries me; for he believes that this technique specifically demonstrates carrierpolypeptide, in that the sulphydryl groups revealed by oxidation in this polypeptide are differently-spaced from those similarly revealed in the octapeptide posterior pituitary hormones. If spacing is critical, surely *in vitro* studies should be performed in solid formol-fixed agar, following Rodeck, rather than in aqueous solutions ? Moreover, it would be of interest to repeat these experiments with pure octapeptide hormones as test substances. Sterba, 1964 and Wellner in fact used as their test substances a posterior pituitary extract capable of causing contraction of the mouse uterus; the limitations of this as an assay technique are reviewed by Sawyer, 1966.

Equally, it must be insisted that the cytochemical techniques we have introduced have marked shortcomings. It is essential that more specific methods should be developed, based possibly on the use of fluorescent antibodies prepared against vasopressin or its precursors, and comparable in sensitivity with the superb methods developed by the late Hillarp and his colleagues for demonstrating monoamines.

(ii) Radioisotopes and Flow Rate. Our second problem was to devise a means of studying the dynamics of neurosecretion, and this we achieved by demonstrating that the pattern of uptake of sulphur by the hypothalamo-hypophysial system of the rat, after the subarachnoid injection of ^{35}S-dl cysteine, was consistent with the Bargmann-Scharrer concept of neurosecretion (Sloper, 1958). In six separate experiments we showed that this pattern was reproducible, that is, that isotopes rapidly accumulated in the supraoptic nuclei (S.O.N.) of the rat, but took some 10 hours to accumulate in the infundibular process. This allowed us to postulate a possible rate of flow along the tractus hypophyseus of some 0.2 mm per hour; and to suggest that we had here a method of biosynthesising labelled vasopressin. This was ultimately and elegantly achieved in the dog by Sachs, 1960.

We next showed in rats given hypertonic saline that, although the S.O.N. was depleted of cystine-rich N.S.M., the pattern of radioisotope uptake by the S.O.N. was consistent with high synthetic activity. Moreover, the rate of uptake of isotope by the similarly depleted infundibular process was consistent with an increased rate of secretion. We thus had evidence strongly supporting the theory of *submicroscopic* flow of neurohormone, a theory we had advanced at Lund in 1957.

(iii) Ultrastructure. Meantime, ultrastructural studies made by Palay, 1957, indicated that granules some 1,000 Å in diameter were the packages in which N.S.M. was transported; this concept although criticised by Green and Maxwell, 1959, is endorsed by our own electronmicrographic studies on the dog (Sloper and Bateson, 1965).

We have, however, largely avoided the use of the electronmicroscope in pathological studies, because there is as yet no cytochemical technique available for the demonstration of, for example, the cystine-rich component of N.S.M. in the electron dense contents of neurosecretory vesicles (N.S.V.).

(iv) Cell-Division. To study cell-division in neuroglia, neurohypophysial interstitial cells, and neurone-precursors, we inject tritiated thymidine intraperitoneally 4 times successively at six hourly intervals. This technique is unlikely to miss transient peaks of mitotic activity in the mouse; it gives a measure of those cells which were preparing for mitosis at the time of injection of labelled thymidine.

(v) Hormone Bioassay. The *bioassay* techniques used by our collaborators, namely, Dr. J. Lee, G. Bissett, and Dr. J. Jones, currently include those which involve the intravenous injection of antidiuretic extracts into cytostomised anaesthetised rats; and the measurement of milk-ejection in the rabbit.

Findings

Reaction to Injury

(i) Administration of Hypertonic Saline. Animals given hypertonic saline pose several pathological problems. First, does the entire neurone increase in size, a form of work hypertrophy? Second, is the depleted secretory neurone active or exhausted? Third, do these changes ever end in degeneration of the secretory neurones? These problems are of especial interest in neuropathology: for in an earlier era, dominated by electrophysiological concepts, there was little reason to correlate activity with alteration in chemical composition; features such as size and shape of neurones, the dispersal of Nissl substance in the perikaryon, or again, the appearance of swellings in nerve fibres, were interpreted as evidence of degeneration.

The early analyses of this problem we owe to SEYLE, HILLARP, ORTMANN and HILD. The underlying technical difficulties of measuring the depletion of N.S.M. were, however, never overcome, although partial success was achieved by DE GROOT and HARTFIELD, 1961, and SLOPER and KING, 1963. The variables, to which little attention has been paid, include: (i) the staining technique, (ii) thickness-variation in sections, (iii) adequate photometry and, (iv) variations in the size of the perikaryon or nerve fibre. Our additional problem was to assess the uptake of radio-isotope by the H.N.S. after the injection of labelled amino acids in a series of 6 groups of rats given 3 per cent saline for varying periods.

We concluded that there was evidence of enlargement of the perikaryon and nucleus and that the measurement of two diameters of each provided a good index of secretory activity. The infundibular process became enlarged, but whether this was due to a hypertrophy of nerve-ending or interstitial cell is still unknown. KARIM has recently established with tritiated thymidine that such cells continue to divide in the mouse in adult life, a point already known from mitotic counts (ORTMANN, 1951). Why this should be so is unknown. There is to my knowledge no evidence that an increase in the size and number of neuroglial cells occurs in the nervous system in association with increased cerebral activity; but this is undoubtedly what we must anticipate if neuro-secretory systems are distributed throughout the brain.

Second, we concluded that there was a probable depletion of N.S.M. in cell body and nerve ending, although if both enlarge, then the dispersal of N.S.M. might make this "depletion" more apparent than real. In terms, however, of radioisotope uptake after ^{35}S-cysteine injection, the whole system appeared to show increased activity. In particular, there was an apparent acceleration in the accumulation of labelled material in the infundibular process, a change we established with the aid of granule-counts in autoradiographs. Whereas others therefore had correlated the *presence* of N.S.M. with secretory activity, we suggested that it was its *absence* which was the better indication: and in 1960 we advanced the "bath" concept of the neurosecretory system. A bath represents the pituitary system: in the stressed animal the plug is out, the taps are full on, and the level of water (hormone) in the bath may be very low. The "depleted" enlarged secretory neurone is in short not exhausted, but is highly active. We have in fact never found evidence of degeneration in saline-treated animals.

On the other hand, in the course of our studies we noted, like Ortmann, the occasional persistence of large granules of N.S.M. in the infundibular process, the tractus hypophyseus, and the otherwise apparently depleted nuclear regions. It seemed to us that such accumulations, and indeed, similar accumulations in the fibres of the tractus hypophyseus might represent transient or permanent disturbances in what we have termed the normal submicroscopic flow of N.S.M. down the nerve fibre. Such aggregations we would distinguish sharply from those which characterise storage sites, such as the infundibular process in the normal animal.

This concept of the "constipation of the neurone" ("axoplasmic sludging" or "thrombosis") has important implications. If established, it suggests that we may have in the nervous system a cause of disease comparable, on a far smaller scale, with the disorders of blood vessels which dominate so many problems in medicine today. We have, however, found no means of producing such a condition in the H.N.S. although we have sought to do so, in particular by overhydrating rats, and then studying the pattern of uptake of labelled cysteine. It seems to me, however, that Fuxe, 1965, may have obtained this "sludging" in monoaminergic fibres in the nervous system of rats treated with cocaine.

(ii) Surgical Trauma. Our main contribution has been to show that the changes first observed by Hild, 1951, and Stutinsky, 1951, in animals, can also occur in man (Adams and Sloper, 1956; Sloper, 1962); that is, that following section of tractus hypophyseus there is the accumulation of (cystine-rich) N.S.M. on the cell-body side of lesions, and a retrograde accumulation of similar material along the nerve fibres as far as the perikaryon. Our series now includes 21 serially sectioned hypothalami from humans whose pituitary stalks have been severed for the relief of malignant disease, patients who have survived between 31 hours and 540 days of operation. In this series cytolysis and karyorrhexis are first apparent between 22 and 40 days of operation. What we still do not know is how long neurones thus injured can continue to elaborate polypeptides. Surviving neurones certainly retain this function: for Flament-Durand (see this volume) found with the ^{35}S-cystine technique that in 2 hypophysectomised rats, many surviving neurones retained secretory activity 30 days after operation; and that isotope accumulated some 10 hours after operation in the residual neurohypophysis in these animals.

With reference to late changes, Stutinsky (see review 1957), made a very considerable neuropathological advance when he showed that a structure full of N.S.M. developed in the median eminence of animals from which the posterior pituitary had been resected, a structure which appeared to function in many respects like a normal posterior pituitary (see Billenstien and Leveque, 1955). This remarkable discovery was no accident, for Stutinsky had since 1948 been studying the hypothalamic effects of hypophysectomy. The question arose as to whether this change in the appearance of the median eminence reflected the formation of a new organ, or the modification of an old. This was a matter of fundamental importance to the pathologist, for it is commonly held that in the normal mammal, neurones and their fibres have little capacity for such regeneration.

Now, if all the blood from the median eminence and upper stalk normally escapes from this region by pituitary portal veins, then the whole region should die after stalk-section: that is, a month or so later any neurones, neuroglia, connective tissue or vessels found in the site would have to be newly formed. Neither in STUTINSKY's nor MOLL's, 1957, rats, did this appear to occur; moreover, in our human series there were cases where, 20 and 40 days, for example, after stalk-section, some upper neurohypophysial tissue appeared to survive. This we explained by postulating that in these cases the blood escaped from the upper neurohypophysis by other channels than the pituitary portal vessels.

What then is the evidence that there is any new tissue in the "reformed" median eminence? To our mind, this is provided by the redistribution of nerve fibres, for example, the way in which argentaffin fibres in the median eminence of the hypophysectomised human can engulf islands of pars tuberalis.

Such fibres could be derived either from nerves which normally end in the median eminence — and we suggested from cell-counts that these came mostly from the caudal P.V.N.: or they could come from fibres which had budded either from injured nerves, or from new-formed secretory fibres. In either case there need be little more than a slight modification in the secretory architecture of the median eminence.

(iii) Chemical Injury. When it seemed that the main function of a neurone was the transmission of a nervous impulse, there was a tendency to distinguish neurones solely in terms first, of the rapidity with which they performed this function; second, of their situation and interconnections and endings; and perhaps third, in terms of their size. It was extremely difficult to account for their selective vulnerability, the way for example in which certain neurones in the cerebellum tended to be sensitive to poisoning by organic tin compounds, or part of the hypothalamus to poisoning by gold thioglucose. Now, however, that we are beginning to entertain the possibility that neurosecretory phenomena are widespread throughout the central nervous system, it seems to me that we can seek for a more plausible explanation for this selective vulnerability. We are no longer dealing with a myriad of similar cells; but rather with groups of neurones each of which may have a biochemical individuality. It seemed to us that neurones of the N.H.S. should, by virtue of their activity in the synthesis, transport, storage and secretion of neurohormones, be especially vulnerable to such chemical injury.

Our earliest experiments in this field were made with intraperitoneal injections of puromycin (100 mg), 4 times at half-hourly intervals, methionine sulphoximine (100 mg) and 3-acetyl pyridine (0.115 ml), into groups of 6 rats each weighing 100 gm. Of the drugs used, the first interferes with R.N.A. synthesis; the second with the incorporation of glycine into polypeptides; and the third, probably with carbohydrate metabolism. ^{35}S-cysteine was given by subraachnoid injection within 30 minutes of the administration of the second and third drugs, and 30 minutes after the first injection of puromycin. We found no cytological changes in the H.N.S., nor any abnormality in ^{35}S-uptake in animals killed 10 hours later. These were, however, preliminary and acute experiments. It may be that the local administration of, for example, puromycin, will be shown to interfere with vasopressin synthesis.

(iv) Ionising Radiation. We next studied the effects of ionising radiations, a matter of immediate clinical importance for it was widely believed that nervous tissue was relatively resistant to radiation. This belief was in urgent need of

adequate assessment, for various techniques had been devised to destroy the
adenohypophysis for the relief of, for example, carcinomatosis or incapacitating
diabetic neuropathy, techniques which involved the use of very high doses of
radiation in the immediate vicinity of the hypothalamus and optic chiasm. It
seemed at the time (Sloper, 1957) that the risk of chronic radio-necrosis was great,
particularly since Arnold, 1954, had claimed that in macaques the S.O.N. was
especially susceptible to damage, undergoing chronic radio-necrosis with doses as
low as 1500 rad (betatron-induced: 22 m.e.v.: 2.5 cm beam).

Our earlier work in this field was made with Dr. Webb Haymaker and involved
the study of the H.N.S. in two series of 77 and 48 macaques, which survived up to
6 days, whole body irradiation (2,500—30,000 rad, 140 Ba — 140 La), or whole
head irradiation (60 Co, 10,000 rad), (Haymaker et al., 1958; Vogel et al., 1958).
We found signs of acute radiation damage, but these were in no way peculiar to the
H.N.S.; and rather surprisingly, there was no evidence of any disturbance in the
distribution of N.S.M. For we had hoped that doses of this order might interfere
with "axonal" transport. More recent acute experiments made by Kratzsch et al.,
1962, in the rat do, however, suggest that irradiation can deplete the H.N.S. of
N.S.M.

Our later studies with Dr. Barbara King of the chronic effects of irradiation
involved the use of X-rays (250 kV thoraeus filter, dose rate 120 rad per minute).
In a series of 79 rats irradiated with between 620 and 5600 rad we used a beam of
0.95 cm diameter, checking by radiographs in each instance that this beam was
vertically centred through the H.N.S. Functional studies, involving the analysis of
the antidiuresis produced by nicotine in hydrated irradiated rats proved unsatis-
factory, probably because nicotine was given subcutaneously rather than by
intravenous injection. Inital experiments established that extracts made from
pituitaries irradiated in situ in the killed animal with 5,600 rad showed no diminution in antidiuretic activity. Conversely, pitressin (Parke Davis), made up in
solution and exposed to the air was partly inactivated by irradiation (54% by
2,625 r, 75% by 10,000 r, 90% by 24,000 r). These findings suggested that the
presumably labile disulphide groups in vasopressin might be protected from the
effects of radiation by tissue factors.

Chronic radionecrotic lesions were obtained in the rats given 1,340 rad or
greater doses, these lesions first appearing 170 days after radiation. A few lesions
were associated with hyaline arteriolar necrosis. Patchy and inconstant, they
sometimes involved the S.O.N. or P.V.N. as well as other irradiated areas. Few
animals survived more than a few days after 5,600 rad. Some survived long after
doses of 4,450 rad, and survivals of between 180 and 700 days were achieved with
doses below this. We had hoped to demonstrate a disturbance in ^{35}S-cysteine
uptake by the H.N.S. long before gross morphological damage became apparent.
In 4 rats, however, 1 killed at 7 days (1,340 rad), 1 at 28 days (4,450 rad), and 2 at
40 days (1,340 rad), no abnormalities were found; and in a further 16 rats killed
between 100 and 200 dys after irradiation with 1,340 rad or above, 10 hours after
radioisotope injection, the pattern of ^{35}S-uptake, save where there was overt
radionecrosis, was normal.

These experiments do not indicate any particular susceptibility of the H.N.S.
to the form of radiation used; nor again do they clarify the underlying problem,

namely whether it is the vessels, neuroglia or neurones which are first damaged by radiation. In regions which subsequently show chronic radionecrosis ARNOLD's experiments — and, incidentally, the pioneer work of MOGILNITZKY, 1930 — remain to be explained. Our own feeling is that, short of repeating ARNOLD's use of the betatron, the critical factor probably lies in the size of field irradiated.

(v) Ultrasound (3 MHz). Ultrasound can be used to cause minute areas of necrosis in nervous tissue (NELSON et al., 1959). With Dr. JONES we have studied the lesions in 3 rats produced by Dr. HARE and Professor WARWICK, of Guy's Hospital, by means of a beam (1.5 KW/sq. cm, 3 MHz) directed stereotactically at the median eminence.

Beams of ultrasound, lasting one second each, were focussed to give small areas of necrosis about 1 mm in diameter. Within these areas there was a complete loss of all structure, while at their edges there was a cellular reaction in which foam cells were especially conspicuous. In one rat two median contiguous areas of necrosis destroyed the larger part of the optic chiasma and median eminence; pars distalis and pars intermedia were unaffected, but the infundibular process showed a gross loss of nerve fibres and ontained very little N.S.M. Many neurones survived in the P.V.N. and some in the caudal part of the S.O.N.; some of these neurones contained N.S.M. This animal which survived 14 days (see Table 1) had developed a severe polyuria, but still secreted vasopressin following the injection of nicotine.

Table 1. *Effects of ultrasonically induced hypothalamic lesions on urine output in "Wistar" rats.* Unpublished data provided by Dr. J. JONES *and* Dr. J. LEE

Animals (Wistar Rats)	Survival Time (in days after lesion)	Urine Flow (ml/kg/hour)	Urine Osmolality (m Osm/kg.)	Percentage reduction of urine flow after intravenous nicotine (20 μ-g)	Percentage reduction of urine flow after intravenous vaso-pressin (10—20 μ-U)
Normal (18)	—	1.0—6.3	330—1460	75 (Mean)	58 (Mean)
Experimental	14	8.1	320	80	80
	13	8.6	370	No effect	30
	10	15.6	180	No effect	100

In a second rat, which survived 13 days, there were three contiguous areas of necrosis which destroyed the chiasma; a few neurones survived in the S.O.N. and P.V.N. and these showed evidence of cytolysis and nuclear pyknosis, and were entirely lacking in N.S.M. The atrophic infundibular process was devoid of N.S.M. In this animal the injection of nicotine elicited no secretion of vasopressin, but the injection of vasopressin causes only a minor reduction in urine flow, thus raising the possibility of the vasopressin resistance of the renal tubules. The third animal, which was killed on the tenth day, exhibited a vasopressin-sensitive polyuria; the pathological changes in the H.N.S. were similar to those in the second case, but unfortunately the pituitary was not examined.

From these preliminary observations it is clear that the use of ultrasound as a means of destroying the H.N.S. is likely to be of great value in neuroendocrine research, for it readily yields a posterior-lobectomised animal ("the Stutinsky

9*

preparation"). In particular, it is possible to avoid injuring the pituitary and possibly the portal vessels also; the local inflammatory response is relatively slight and there is little danger of the introduction of infection. An unexpected pathological feature was the appearance of unequivocal and gross evidence of neuronal degeneration within 14 days of injury. This presumably reflects the proximity of the damage to the cell bodies of affected neurones. Our observations are also indirectly relevant to the pathogenesis of diabetes insipidus. It will be noted that only in one case was there unequivocal evidence of a diminished output of vasopressin; in the other two some vasopressin was probably secreted, while in one of these the response to vasopressin injection was so poor as to raise the possibility of renal resistance to vasopressin.

(vi) Selective Vulnerability. These investigations of the reaction of the H.N.S. to various forms of injury, have at no point established the selective vulnerability of secretory neurones. This possibly reflects our failure to choose suitable forms of injury; but it is equally possible that it reflects the resistance of secretory neurones to injury. If this concept can be substantiated, it will be tempting to correlate it with the hypothesis that secretory neurones are, phylogenetically, the oldest of all.

Diabetes Insipidus

A major contribution of the concept of neurosecretion has been the clarification of the pathogenesis of diabetes insipidus. Until recently this syndrome was little understood; its nomenclature was confused and the relevant literature recorded many supposed cases which would not satisfy the simplest diagnostic criteria (see Blotner, 1958). The clarification of this problem is the more important because it seems probable that those varieties of diabetes insipidus in which there is hypothalamo-neurohypophysial dysfunction will serve as a model for other diseases in which there is also a disturbance in a neurosecretory mechanism.

(i) Classification. Many conditions can cause diabetes insipidus (see de Wardener, 1961). Our main purpose here is to analyse the extent to which neuro-

Table 2. *Anatomical sites relevant to the pathogenesis of diabetes insipidus*

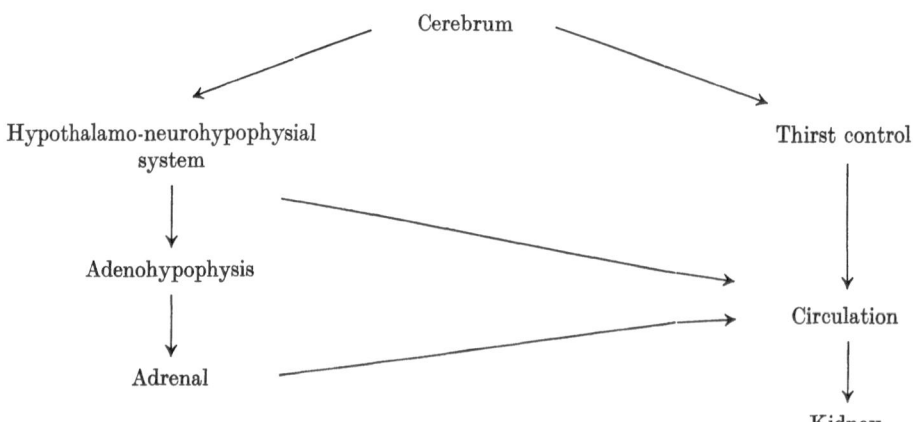

secretory function has been studied in those variants of this syndrome (Table 2) in which the basic dysfunction appears to lie in:

    (i) Increased thirst

    (ii) Diminished production of vasopressin

    (iii) Diminished action of vasopressin on the kidney

    (iv) Excessive inactivation of vasopressin.

We propose to report also the first recorded cases of vasopressin inactivation diabetes insipidus, with active hepatitis.

(ii) Diagnostic Criteria. To establish the *syndrome* we require measurements of water intake and urine output; and of the osmolality of the urine, or again of its specific gravity, provided adequate evidence is provided of the absence of sugar and gross proteinuria.

Evidence of a *diminished production* of vasopressin is assessed in terms of the effect on urine osmolality of dehydration sufficient to cause a 3 to 5 per cent fall in body weight. Other methods, involving, for example, the intravenous injection of nicotine or hypertonic saline are acceptable. To determine whether vasopressin is able to modify *renal function* we inject vasopressin intramuscularly in subjects with free access to water, again assessing the urine osmolality. These methods will soon be replaced by the assay of vasopressin in the plasma, but techniques at present available are insufficiently sensitive. Our *pathological* criteria include the examination of serial sections of the hypothalamus and pituitary, and a more limited m croscopical examination of kidney, liver, adrenals thyroid.

The clinical methods we have applied with Professor DE WARDENER's help. The problem of the investigation of disorders of thirst we have not yet attempted; the recognition of such disorders is difficult, the more so because even normal subjects, when they have drunk large quantities of water, become, if transiently, resistant to vasopressin (see BARLOW and DE WARDENER, 1959).

(iii) Disorders of Thirst. These can be produced experimentally in a vauch of ways (FUZAMAS, 1966), for example in goats by electrical stimulation in the region of the P.V.N. (ANDERSSON and McCANN, 1955). An inheritable form of polydipsia has also been reported in certain rats (SILVERSTEIN et al., 1961) which, in females at least, is unassociated with significant vasopressin resistance or recognisable lesions in kidney or brain or pituitary.

A similar compulsive polydipsia has been described in humans (see BARLOW and DE WARDENER, 1959), a condition sometimes associated with a psychosis; no case has yet been analysed at necropsy.

(iv) Diminished Production of Vasopressin. a) Inherited. The most exciting discovery in this field is that of a strain of rats which appear to secrete oxytocin but little or no vasopressin, and to inherit this tendency as a recessive trait (VALIN et al., 1962; VALTIN and SCHROEDER, 1964). This is the first time in which an identifiable biochemical disorder of specific groups of neurones has been shown to cause an *inherited nervous disease.*

Dr. VALTIN has sent us heterozygous specimens of his strain, and we have confirmed his clinical and pathological findings on two homozygous animals. These are not easily separable in terms of water-intake or output, since some heterozygous animals have a polydipsia. Dr. KARIM, however, in conjunction with Dr. LEE, Dr. JONES and Dr. BISSETT (Table 3), has found that the distinction can be made

Table 3. *Familial diabetes insipidus in the "Brattleboro" strain of rats* (Valtin and Schroeder, 1962). Unpublished data provided by Dr. J. Jones and Dr. J. Lee

Pituitary Vasopressin (Oxytocin) Content (m-U/gland)	Urine		Percentage reduction of urine flow after intravenous nicotine (20 μ-g)	Percentage reduction of urine flow after intravenous vaso- pressin (10—20 μ-g)
	Flow (ml/kg/hour)	Osmolality (mOsm/kg)		
Non-diabetic (13 Brattleboro Rats) 100—500 (100—400)	1.0—7.1	320—1800	75 (Mean)	38 (Mean)
Diabetes Insipidus (9 Brattleboro Rats) Nil (60—240)	5.4—13.7	170—200	Nil	80 (Mean)

unequivocally by bisecting the posterior lobe of the pituitary of animals killed for pathological examination, and demonstrating in one fragment the presence of oxytocin but no vasopressor activity, a technique likely to prove indispensable in pathological studies. As Sokol and Valtin, 1965, have reported, neurones and their nuclei in the S.O.N. and P.V.N. appear large; cystine-rich N.S.M. is scanty here and in the infundibular process. Harrington and Valtin, 1965, have shown that, in terms of the pattern of uptake of labelled cysteine, these neurones are highly active. There are, however, morphological features which merit further study, in particular, the abundance of A.F. N.S.M. in nuclear regions and median eminence. Cystin-rich N.S.M. seems sparser, and we suspect that some material reacting with the aldehyde-fuchsin technique in these animals may be lipofuscin. In this respect it is of great interest that Orkand and Palay, 1966, have reported in the S.O.N. of affected animals abundant large electron-dense granules, that is, granules which presumably could be "lysozomes" or "lipofuscin". Ours are, however, preliminary observations and require further study.

A similar inherited diabetes insipidus may occur in man, but in the relevant cases (see Gaupp, 1941; Bravermann et al., 1965), neither the clinical nor pathological data fully satisfy the criteria mentioned above.

b) Acquired. The experimental work of many, and in particular, Fisher et al., 1935, make it clear that much of the H.N.S. must be destroyed for the production of the syndrome. In rats this has been carried out most thoroughly by Friedman and Friedman, 1965.

A number of human cases fulfil the criteria we have put forward, but it is exceptional to find that such a case has been adequately examined at necropsy. Blotner's, 1958, first case in fact satisfies most criteria, although it would be valuable to know in this case both the degree of urinary concentration elicited by vasopressin, and the state of the kidneys at necropsy. What, in fact, we must stress is not that diabetes insipidus has not been recognised but rather, that insufficient evidence is available to allow us to identify the specific disorder of function in individual cases.

We have, in fact, recently found that full investigations are rather easier to undertake in the dog, an animal in which Richards has recently identified 9 naturally occurring cases (see Table 4). The disease was known to occur in the dog, but was scantily documented.

Table 4. *Naturally occurring diabetes insipidus in the dog*

Number and variety of cases	Urine			
	Flow (ml/kg./hour)	Osmolality during free access to water (m Osm./kg)	Effect of Dehy-dration[1] (m Osm./kg)	Effect of intra-muscular vasopressin injection (5—10 i.u.)
Normal (3)	up to 1.1	> 300	1060—1180	665—110
"Hypothalamo-neurohypophysial" (6)	4.5—25.7	75—187	145—304 and 1160	665—1100 (mean value: 871)
"Nephrogenic" (1)	15.3	102	130	148
"Hepatic" (2)	6.4—7.2	51—58	345—552	405—790[2]

[1] Weight loss of between 3 and 5 per cent of initial body-weight, reached in up to 24 hours.

[2] Peak reached in $3-4^1/_4$ hours after injection of vasopressin, instead of $5^1/_2-24$ hours (mean time interval: 12 hours) in hypothalamo-neurohypophysial cases.

Two cases were pups where the condition could have been acquired *in utero*. Both showed a slight chronic encephalitis and meningitis, although the P.V.N. and S.O.N., in which less than 10 per cent of the normal number of neurones survived, showed no inflammation. In one pup the lateral ventricles were grossly dilated, although the communications between the ventricles were patent. Scanty aggregations of cystine-rich N.S.M. were present in the atrophied infundibular process.

Two adults showed a similar patchy perivascular and meningeal fibrosis, which again spared the nuclear regions, with an associated diminution in secretory neurones in the H.N.S.

In a fifth case serial sections finally revealed the cause of the inflammation, namely, *Toxocara canis* (RICHARDS and SLOPER, 1964). This parasite was embedded in granulation tissue in the median eminence; it has never before been described in the brain of its definitive host, although it is a known cause of human encephalitis. In two further cases adenohypophysial tumours, so called "invasive adenomas" had destroyed most of the H.N.S. The first tumour replaced the infundibular process, spared a thin rim of pars distalis, and bulged into and just invaded a greatly thinned and stretched median eminence in which there was some N.S.M. Very few neurones surved in P.V.N., but many, which contained abundant N.S.M., were present in the rostral and most lateral parts of S.O.N. These presumably accounted for the endogenous vasopressin secreted after dehydration. The second tumour appeared to originate in the rostral part of the adenohypophysis, sparing much of the pars distalis and the whole of the indundibular process. This latter, however, was grossly atrophied and devoid of N.S.M., since growth, extending into the hypothalamus, had destroyed the median eminence. Numerous secretory neurones survived in the rostral S.O.N. and P.V.N.

The value of a pathological study is especially evident in the second of these cases; for this subject when dehydrated achieved a urinary osmolality of 1,160 m/osm/kg (see Table 4), and the possibility thus arose that it might be suffering from a primary polydipsia rather than a diminished secretion of vasopressin. Pathological findings at necropsy, on the other hand, largely resolved this problem, by showing that much of the neurosecretory system was, in fact, destroyed: but that a number of actively secreting neurones survived.

(v) Vasopressin-resistant Diabetes Insipidus. BIGGART, 1937, was one of the first to draw attention to this condition, tentatively correlating it with lesions in the region of the tubero-infundibular or ventromedial hypothalamic nuclei. Subsequent interest stemmed from the discovery that many cases of inherited diabetes insipidus were vasopressin-resistant, most of these cases proving to be "nephrogenic", in the sense that there was supposedly a primary renal lesion (FORSSMAN, 1945; WILLIAMS and HENRY, 1947). Various pathological processes, including amyloidosis and sarcoidosis can be found in the kidney, while two cases reported by DARMADY et al., 1964, revealed, by dissection of nephrons, a shortening in the proximal convoluted tubules.

In only one reported case of vasopressin-resistant diabetes insipidus — an infant of three months, have the clinical and pathological criteria we have put forward been all but satisfied (CAMPBELL, 1961). No lesions were, in fact, seen in the kidney, while the neuronal vacuolation observed in the H.N.S. we would accept as normal: the question thus arises as to the cause of the vasopressin-resistance. It would be of the greatest interest in this case to know the histological state of the liver.

We can report a further case of "nephrogenic" diabetes insipidus. The dog was six years old, an age at which slight degrees of renal inflammation are common. In this case (see Table 4) however, the kidneys showed severe and diffuse medullary fibrosis, among which there were numerous foci composed of lymphocytes and histiocytes. Serial sections of H.N.S. revealed no abnormality and the examination of the other organs listed above showed no abnormality.

(vi) Vasopressin-inactivation Diabetes Insipidus Associated with Hepatitis. HANKISS in 1958 suggested that in a patient suffering from diabetes insipidus, polyuria diminished with the development of a hepatitis. The underlying mechanism was presumably a diminution in the capacity of the hepatic parenchyma to inactivate vasopressin, that is, the exact opposite of the syndrome we propose to report.

Shortly afterwards HANKISS et al., 1961, reported 9 cases of "vasopressin-inactivation" diabetes insipidus. These cases were unassociated with renal or hepatic disease and in the absence of clinical details in any individual case, the validity of the diagnosis is difficult to assess. On the other hand, this syndrome seems to be an entity, for we have encountered cases strongly suggestive of it in 2 dogs suffering from an active hepatitis. Function tests (see Table 4), gave results intermediate between our "nephrogenic" and "neurohypophysial" cases; thus dehydration elicited the secretion of some endogenous vasopressin, and the injection of vasopressin was followed by a peak urine osmolality which was low, and which was reached much earlier than in dogs with hypothalamo-neurohypophysial diabetes insipidus. In these dogs the H.N.S. proved entirely normal. On the other hand, in the kidneys of both there were small areas of chronic inflammation with in one case, occasional neutrophil leucocytes. These lesions were far less than in our "nephrogenic" case; but they make it difficult entirely to exclude a partial "nephrogenic" form of vasopressin resistance. Although renal function in terms of blood urea and urinary sediment was normal, there was in one case slight albuminuria, a common enough symptom in ageing dogs. Both dogs showed evidence, in terms of serum glutamic pyruvic transaminase (125 and 144 S.F. units) and alkaline phosphatase (120 K.A. units) suggestive of a hepatic dysfunction; and both cases proved at necropsy to have an acute and active chronic, widespread, but focal inflammation of the liver.

Similar diabetes insipidus has recently been observed by RICHARDS in a third dog; this animal survived, and six months later, with the return to normal (25 S.F. units) of serum glutamic pyruvic transaminase, water intake fell to almost normal (1.7 ml/kg/hr from 11.4 ml/kg/hr). This coincided with a marked improvement in the response to the injection of vasopressin (1,050 m/osm/kg at 7 hours from 580 m/osm/kg at 3 hours).

This possibly causative association between hepatitis and diabetes insipidus has never previously been recorded. Our cases recall the experiments of HELLER and URBAN, 1935, in which they showed that liver homogenates were particularly well able to inactivate antidiuretic hormone. It is tempting to suppose that enzymes tend to be relased either locally in the liver or in the circulation in acute hepatitis, and thus give rise to diabetes insipidus. Certainly we are now searching for the same syndrome in humans with hepatitis.

Acknowledgements. Grateful thanks are due to the Clinical Research Sub-Committee of Charing Cross Hospital for their continued support; to Professor DE WARDENER, of the Department of Medicine, and to Dr. LEE, and Dr. JONES of the Department of Physiology of the Charing Cross Hospital Medical School for their great help; to Professor WARWICK and Dr. J. HARE of the Anatomy Department, Guy's Hospital Medical School for the preparation of ultrasonic lesions; and to the Central Research Fund of London University for the provision of an osmometer.

References

ADAMS, C. W. M., and J. C. SLOPER: The hypothalamic elaboration of the posterior pituitary principles in man, the rat and dog. Histochemical evidence derived from performic acid — Alcian blue reaction for cystine. J. Endocrin. 13, 221 (1956).

ANDERSSON, B., and S. M. McCANN: Drinking, antidiuresis and milk ejection from electrical stimulation within the hypothalamus of the goat. Acta physiol. scand. 35, 191 (1955).

ARNOLD, A.: Effects of X-irradiation on the hypothalamus. A possible explanation for the therapeutic benefits following X-irradiation of the hypophysial region for pituitary dysfunction. J. clin. Endocr. 14, 859 (1954).

BARGMANN, W.: Zwischenhirn und Neurohypophyse; eine neue Vorstellung über die funktionelle Bedeutung des Hinterlappens. Med. Mschr. 5, 466 (1951).

BARLOW, E. E., and H. E. DE WARDENER: Compulsive water drinking. Quart. J. Med. 28, 235 (1959).

BARRNETT, R. J.: Histochemical demonstration of disulfide groups in the neurohypophysis under normal and experimental conditions. Endocrinology 55, 484 (1954).

BIGGART, J. H.: Anatomical basis for resistance to pituitrin in diabetes insipidus. J. Path. Bact. 44, 305 (1937).

BILLENSTIEN, D. C., and T. F. LEVEQUE: The reorganization of the neurohypophysial stalk following hypophysectomy in the rat. Endocrinology 56, 704 (1955).

BLOTNER, H.: Primary or idiopathic diabetes insipidus; a system disease. Metabolism 7, 191 (1958).

BRAVERMAN, L. E., J. P. MANCINI, and D. M. McGOLDRICK: Hereditary idiopathic diabetes insipidus. Ann. intern. Med. 63, 503 (1965).

CAMPBELL, W. F.: Vasopressin-resistant diabetes insipidus associated with cytological changes in the supraoptic and paraventricular nuclei. Lancet 1961 II, 522.

DARMADY, E. M., J. OFFER, J. PRINCE, and F. STRANACH: The proximal convoluted tubule in the renal handling of water. Lancet 1964 II, 1254.

DE WARDENER, H. E.: The Kidney. 2nd ed. London: Churchill, Ltd. 1961.

FISHER, C., W. R. INGRAM, and S. W. RANSON: Relation of hypothalamico-hypophyseal system to diabetes insipidus. Arch. Neurol. Psychiat. (Chic.) 34, 124 (1935).

Flament-Durant, J.: See p. 60 in this volume.

Forssmann, H.: On hereditary diabetes insipidus. Acta med. scand. Suppl. **159**, 1 (1945).

Friedman, S. M., and C. L. Friedman: Salt and water distribution in hereditary and in induced hypothalamic diabetes insipidus in the rat. Canad. J. Physiol. Pharmacol. **43**, 699 (1965).

Fuxe, K.: Evidence for the existence of monoamine neurons in the central nervous system. (Thesis, Karolinska Institutet, Stockholm.) Uppsala: Almqvist and Wicksells 1965.

Gaupp, R. von: Über den Diabetes insipidus. Z. ges. Neurol. Psychiat. **171**, 514 (1941).

— Ein weiterer Beitrag zur pathologischen Anatomie des Diabetes insipidus. Z. ges. Neurol. Psychiat. **177**, 500 (1944).

—, and E. Scharrer: Die Zwischenhirnsekretion bei Mensch und Tier. Z. ges. Neurol. Psychiat. **153**, 327 (1935).

Green, J. D., and D. J. Maxwell: Comparative anatomy of the hypophysis and observations on the mechanism of neurosecretion. In: Comp. Endocrin. p. 368 (Ed. A. Gorbman). New York: Wiley 1959.

Groot, J. de, and J. E. Hartfield: Quantitative changes in rat pituitary neurosecretory material in altered adrenocortical function. Acta Neurol. **22**, 177 (1961).

Hankiss, J.: Improvement of diabetes insipidus in hepatitis. N. Y. State J. Med. **58**, 2219 (1958).

— M. Keszthelyi, and B. Siro: A new type of diabetes insipidus due to increased hormone inactivation. Amer. J. Med. Sci. **242**, 605 (1961).

Harrington, A. R., and H. Valtin: Vasopressin effect on urinary concentration in rats with hereditary diabetes insipidus (Brattleboro strain). Proc. Soc. exp. Biol. (N.Y.) **118**, 448 (1965).

Haymaker, W., G. Laqueur, W. J. Nauta, J. E. Pickering, J. C. Sloper, and F. S. Vogel: The effects of barium 140-lanthanum 140 (gamma) radiation on the central nervous system and pituitary gland of macaque monkeys; a study of 67 brains and spinal cords and 77 pituitary glands. J. Neuropath. **17**, 12 (1958).

Heller, H., and F. F. Urban: The fate of the antidiuretic principle of postpituitary extracts in vivo and in vitro. J. Physiol. **85**, 502 (1935).

Hild, W.: Experimentell-morphologische Untersuchungen über das Verhalten der „Neurosekretorischen Bahn" nach Hypophysenstieldurchschneidung, Eingriffen in den Wasserhaushalt und Belastung der Osmoregulation. Virchows Arch. path. Anat. **319**, 526 (1951).

Mogilnitzky, B. N.: Zur Frage über den Zusammenhang der Hypophyse mit dem Zwischenhirn. Virchows Arch. path. Anat. **267**, 263 (1930).

Nelson, E., P. A. Lindstrom, and W. Haymaker: Pathological effects of ultrasound on the human brain — a study of 25 cases in which ultrasonic irradiation was used as a lobotomy procedure. J. Neuropath. exp. Neurol. **18**, 489 (1959).

Orkand, P. M., and S. L. Palay: The fine structure of the supraoptic nucleus in normal rats compared with that in rats with hereditary diabetes insipidus. Anat. Rec. (abstr.) **154**, 397 (1966).

Ortmann, R.: Über experimentelle Veränderungen der Morphologie des Hypophysen-Zwischenhirnsystems und die Beziehung der sog. „Gomorisubstanz" zum Adiuretin. Z. Zellforsch. **36**, 92 (1951).

Palay, S. L.: The fine structure of the neurohypophysis. Progr. Neurobiol. **2**, 31 (1957); (Korey, S. R., and J. I. Nurnberger eds.) New York: Hoeber 1957.

Richards, M. A., and J. C. Sloper: Hypothalamic involvement by "Visceral" Larva Migrans in a dog suffering from diabetes insipidus. Vet. rec. **76**, 449 (1964).

Rodeck, H.: Zusammenhänge zwischen Neurosekret und den sogenannten Hypophysenhinterlappenhormonen. III Mitt. Untersuchungen zur färberischen Darstellung von synthetischen Oxytocin. Z. ges. exp. Med. **132**, 122 (1959).

Sachs, H.: Vasopressin biosynthesis I. In vivo studies. J. Neurochem. **5**, 297 (1960).

Silverstein, E., L. Sokoloff, O. Mickelsen, and G. E. Jay: Primary polydipsia and hydronephrosis in an inbred strain of mice. Amer. J. Path. **38**, 143 (1961).

Sloper, J. C.: Histochemical observations on the neurohypophysis in dog and cat with reference to the relationship between neurosecretory material and posterior lobe hormone. J. Anat. (London) **88**, 576 (1954).

SLOPER, J. C.: Hypothalamic neurosecretion in the dog and cat with particular reference to the identification of neurosecretory material with posterior lobe hormone. J. Anat. (Lond.) 89, 301 (1955).
— The effect of ionising radiations on hypothalamus and pituitary. Cong. Intern. Neuropath. Acta Medica Belgica (Brussels) p. 279 (1957).
— The application of newer histochemical and isotope techniques for the localisation of protein-bound cystine or cysteine to the study of hypothalamic neurosecretion in normal and pathological conditions. 2nd Internat. Symp. on Neurosecretion (1957) p. 20 (BARGMANN, W., B. HANSTRÖM, and E. SCHARRER, eds.) Berlin-Göttingen-Heidelberg: Springer 1958.
— The hypothalamic neurosecretory cell: its normal characteristics, its reaction to injury and its capacity for regeneration in man and in a variety of animals. Symp. Zool. Soc. London, 9, 29 (1962).
— The experimental and cytopathological investigation of neurosecretion in the hypothalamus and pituitary. In the Pituitary Gland, Vol. III, p. 131 (HARRIS, G. W., and B. T. DONOVAN, eds.) London: Butterworths 1966.
—, and R. G. BATESON: Ultrastructure of neurosecretory cells in the supraoptic nucleus of the dog and rat. J. Endocrin. 31, 139 (1965).
—, and B. C. KING: Activity and degeneration in secretory neurones of the hypothalamus and posterior pituitary of the rat. J. Path. 86, 179 (1963).
SOKOL, H. W., and H. VALTIN: Morphology of the neurosecretory system in rats homozygous and heterzygous for hypothalamic diabetes insipidus (Brattleboro strain). Endocrinology 77, 692 (1965).
STERBA, G.: Floureszenzmikroskopische Untersuchungen über die Neurosekretion beim Bachneunauge (Lampetra planeri). Z. Zellforsch. 55, 763 (1961).
—, and K. P. WELLNER: Grundlagen des histochemischen und biochemischen Nachweises von Neurosekret (= Trägerprotein der Oxytozine) mit Pseudoisozyaninen. Acta Histochem. 17, 268 (1964).
STUTINSKY, F.: Sur l'origine de la substance Gomori-positive du complexe hypothalamo hypophysaire. C. R. Soc. Biol. Paris 145, 367 (1951).
— Recherches experimentales sur le complexe hypothalamo-neurohypophysaire. Arch. Anat. micr. Morph. exp. 46, 93 (1957).
VALTIN, H., and H. A. SCHROEDER: Familial hypothalamic diabetes insipidus in rats (Brattleboro strain) Amer. J. Physiol. 206, 425 (1964).
— — K. BENIRSCHKE, and H. W. SOKOL: Familial hypothalamic diabetes insipidus in rats. Nature (Lond.) 196, 1109.
VASQUEZ-LOPEZ, E.: Structure of the neurohypophysis with special reference to nerve endings. Brain 65, 1 (1942).
VOGEL, F. S., G. C. HOAK, J. C. SLOPER, and W. HAYMAKER: The induction of acute morphological changes in the central nervous system and pituitary body of macaque monkey by cobalt-60 (gamma) radiation. J. Neuropath. 17, 138 (1958).
WILLIAMS, R. H., and C. HENRY: Nephrogenic diabetes insipidus appearing during infancy in males and transmitted by females. Ann. int. Med. 27, 84 (1947).

Données nouvelles sur les mécanismes du contrôle hypothalamique gonadotrope

C. Kordon et A. Moszkowska*

Laboratoire d'Histophysiologie du Collège de France, Paris

Nos connaissances de la physiologie du contrôle hypothalamique de l'adénohypophyse ne nous permettent pas encore de tirer des conclusions valables quant aux fonctions respectives des divers types de fibres présents dans l'éminence médiane. Certains résultats physiologiques nous fournissent cependant des éléments de réponse sur les deux points suivants:

1. la hiérarchie des diverses structures hypothalamiques impliquées dans la régulation de l'adénohypophyse;

2. le rôle possible des monoamines dans les mécanismes de cette régulation.

Nous aborderons ici ces deux problèmes sous l'angle du contrôle hypothalamique des fonctions *gonadotropes*.

Centres hypothalamiques et contrôle des fonctions gonadotropes

On sait depuis longtemps que certaines interventions expérimentales sur l'hypothalamus — des lésions, des stimulations électriques, par exemple — sont capables d'induire des modifications plus ou moins durables des fonctions gonadotropes. Le problème se pose dès lors de savoir si ces interventions modifient *directement* ou *indirectement* la synthèse des médiateurs neurosécrétés; ou, en d'autres termes, si ces interventions affectent la *voie neurosécrétoire* ou seulement des centres qui retentissent secondairement sur l'activité de cette dernière.

Des destructions bilatérales de très petites dimensions, systématiquement localisées dans diverses régions de l'hypothalamus, chez plusieurs centaines de rats, nous permettent d'apporter une réponse à cette question. En effet, plusieurs lésions de régions différentes retentissent sur le contrôle des fonctions gonadotropes: les lésions *préoptiques basales* (fig. 1 A), décrites depuis longtemps par Dey, 1941, et par Hillarp, 1949, provoquent un oestrus permanent accompagné d'un développement massif des follicules ovariens et d'une hypersécrétion de FSH et d'oestrogènes. Des lésions, à la fois plus caudales et plus dorsales, situées dans l'*aire supraoptique* (fig. 1 B) provoquent également un oestrus permanent, mais sans hyperoestrogénémie. Des dosages d'hormones gonadotropes dans l'hypophyse (fig. 2), l'examen des ovaires sur coupes sériées et l'examen cytologique de l'adénohypophyse après ces divers types de lésions (Kordon, 1966) confirment que l'hypersécrétion de FSH est présente dans le premier cas et absente dans l'autre; l'évaluation du contenu de l'éminence médiane en FSH-RF, pratiquée dans les deux groupes d'animaux (Moszkowska et Kordon, 1960,

---

* Avec la collaboration technique de Mme. E. Pattou.

Tableau 1. *Modifications, sous l'effet de deux types différents de lésions hypothalamiques, de l'activité gonadotrope de l'hypophyse (appréciée par plusieurs critères distincts)*

lésions	Stock hypophysaire FSH		histologie ovarienne	activité FSH-RF dans l'éminence médiane	observations	diagnostic
	cytologie hypophysaire	dosage				
préoptique basale	cellules nombreuses et très granulées	+ +	développement folliculaire massif	forte		sécrétion et excrétion de FSH élevées
aire supra-optique	cellules involuées	normal	normal	normal		sécrétion et excrétion de FSH normales à subnormales

lésions	Stock hypophysaire LH		histologie ovarienne	activité LRF dans l'éminence médiane	observations	diagnostic
	cytologie hypophysaire	dosage				
préoptique basale	normale	subnormal (1)	0 corps jaune	non décelable	blocage réversible	libération de LH freinée
aire supra-optique	cellules involuées	?	0 corps jaune	non décelable	blocage non réversible	sécrétion de LH perturbée

(1) Taleisnik (S) et McCann (S.M.), Endocrinology 68, 263—272 (1961).

1965) révèle un taux exagéré de ce transmetteur dans le premier cas et un taux normal dans l'autre. Ces données sont résumées sur le tableau 1.

Nous pouvons en tirer une première conclusion: les lésions préoptiques basales qui exagèrent l'activité FSH-RF de l'hypothalamus, n'agissent pas en détruisant une structure neurosécrétoire chargée d'élaborer un facteur hypophysotrope. En effet, une telle structure ne pourrait alors élaborer qu'un «anti-FSH-RF» (puisque l'activité FSH-RF est plus élevée après la lésion qu'avant). Or, une telle hypothèse n'est actuellement étayée par aucun argument expérimental. Ces lésions préoptiques doivent donc détruire un centre hypothalamique intégrateur, et lever ainsi l'inhibition que ce centre exerce normalement sur la synthèse de FSH-RF.

Cette conclusion est en accord avec la théorie proposée par Flerko, 1957, et par Desclin et coll., 1962, qui ont montré que le centre préoptique basal était responsable de la rétroaction des oestrogènes sur la fonction FSH de l'hypophyse: après suppression de cette rétroaction, le taux d'oestrogènes s'élève d'une manière irrefrénée et bloque ainsi, secondairement, la libération «ovulante» de l'hormone LH. Nous avons obtenu, par une technique originale, une démonstration complémentaire de cette théorie (Kordon, 1966): Chez des sujets porteurs de lésions *préoptiques basales*, en oestrus permanent depuis deux semaines et présentant l'hypertrophie folliculaire caractéristique de cette préparation, nous avons pratiqué une deuxième lésion, *prémamillaire* (fig. 1 C) dont l'effet sur des sujets entiers est de diminuer la production de FSH et d'oestrogènes. Quarante-huit heures après la seconde lésion, quatorze animaux sur quinze présentèrent une ovulation. En revanche, lorsque la lésion prémamillaire est réalisée sur des sujets porteurs d'une lésion *supraoptique*, les animaux n'ovulent pas et présentent seulement la régression folliculaire caractéristique des lésions prémamillaires.

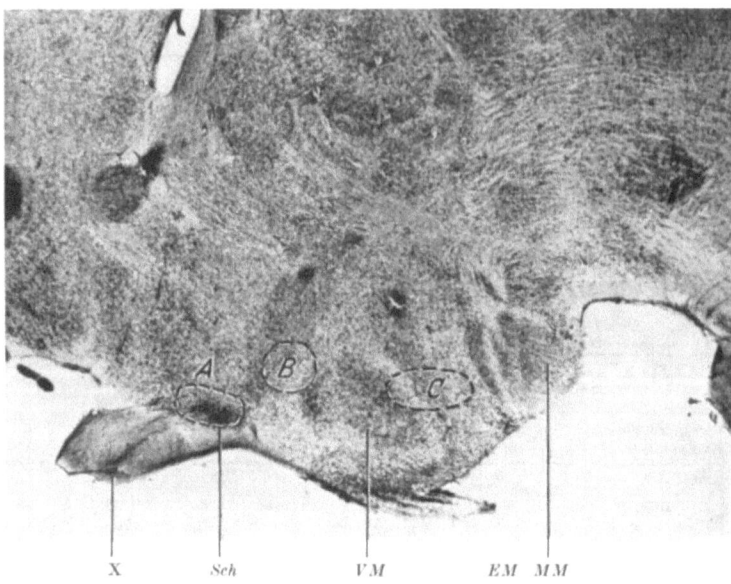

Fig. 1. Coupe sagitale paramédiane de l'hypothalamus du Rat. *EM*, éminence médiane; *MM*, noyau mamillaire; *Sch*, noyau suprachiasmatique; *VM*, noyau ventromédian; *X*, chiasma. Zones dont la lésion produit un effet gonadotrope: *A*, région préoptique basale; *B*, aire supraoptique; *C*, région prémamillaire. *Thionine*, x 13.

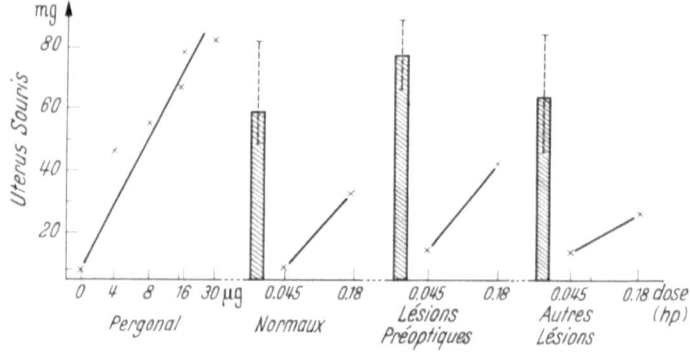

Fig. 2. Dosage de l'activité gonadotrope totale de l'hypophyse de Rats témoins et porteurs de lésions hypothalamiques (test de STEELMAN et POHLEY). Les rectangles hachurés représentent la contenu moyen d'une hypophyse (en microgrammes-équivalents du standard gonadotrope Pergonal)

Cette dernière expérience nous permet donc de confirmer l'analyse du tableau 1: les lésions *préoptiques basales* n'interfèrent pas directement avec la libération ovulante de LH; c'est l'hyperoestrogénémie provoquée par une libération excessive de FSH qui s'y oppose secondairement. Les lésions *supraoptiques*, elles, affectent directement et irréversiblement, l'approvisionnement de l'éminence médiane en LRF, d'où blocage définitif de l'ovulation.

Localisation des éléments neurosécrétoires du contrôle gonadotrope

Les éléments neurosécrétoires responsables de la synthèse des médiateurs hypophysotropes semblent donc difficiles à localiser par des techniques de lésion ou de stimulation électrique; d'autres tentatives en ce sens se sont déjà soldées par des échecs (OLIVECRONA, 1957). D'où viennent donc les médiateurs de type FSH-RF ou LRF ? Le problème semble actuellement difficile à résoudre. Tout au plus pourrait-on suggérer un rapprochement entre la région supraoptique du Rat, nécessaire, nous l'avons vu, à la présence de LRF dans l'éminence médiane (MOSZKOWSKA et KORDON, 1961, 1965; KORDON, 1966), et les noyaux neurosécrétoires AF-négatifs décrits par BARRY et coll.; 1964, et BARRY, 1966, chez le Cobaye, au niveau du tuber latéral; ces noyaux semblent, en effet, contenir du LRF en quantité appréciable. Mais en l'absence d'autres informations, ce rapprochement n'a pour l'instant qu'une valeur d'hypothèse.

Parmi les autres lésions hypothalamiques qui affectent les fonctions gonadotropes, celles de la région arquée perturbent l'approvisionnement de l'éminence médiane en neurosécrétat; mais cet effet paraît dû essentiellement à la convergence de fibres neurosécrétoires au voisinage du noyau arqué (KORDON, 1966).

Monoamines et régulation hypothalamique gonadotrope

A cet égard, les résultats de la littérature demeurent encore très fragmentaires. Des corrélations histophysiologiques ont été décrites entre le taux de certaines monoamines dans l'hypothalamus et la synthèse polypeptidique dans les voies neurosécrétoires (ARVY, 1964). L'ovulation peut être supprimée par des traitements dépléteurs de la sérotonine et de la noradrénaline (BARRACLOUGH et SAWYER, 1957; COPPOLA et coll., 1966).

Puisque, ainsi que nous l'avons montré plus haut, des centres hypothalamiques intégrateurs, non neurosécrétoires au sens strict, jouent un rôle important dans le contrôle de l'activité neurosécrétoire hypothalamo-adénohypophysaire, il n'est pas étonnant que les médiateurs monoaminergiques du système nerveux central soient étroitement impliqués dans les régulations neuroendocriniennes. Mais les monoamines n'interviennent pas seulement au niveau de la commande des synthèses neurosécrétoires. A l'autre extrémité de la voie hypothalamo-hypophysaire, certaines d'entre elles semblent capables d'agir sur la réponse hypophysaire aux transmetteurs hypothalamiques.

L'expérience suivante, réalisée par une technique *in vitro* mise au point par l'un de nous (MOSZKOWSKA, 1959), permet de mettre cette action en évidence dans le cas d'une indolamine (la 5-hydroxytryptamine ou 5-HT). Incubées en présence de fragments d'hypothalamus de Rat, des antéhypophyses de Rat libèrent beaucoup plus d'hormone gonadotrope dans le milieu que lorsqu'elles sont incubées seules (fig. 3). Il est d'ailleurs intéressant de relever que, dans ce cas, le bilan gonadotrope total (activité gonadotrope encore contenue dans la glande à la fin de l'incubation + activité excrétée dans le milieu) est nettement supérieur au contenu gonadotrope de la glande avant l'incubation, ce qui prouve que l'extrait hypothalamique n'agit pas seulement sur la libération ou l'excrétion des hormones déjà contenues dans la glande, mais stimule également l'activité sécrétoire de cette dernière. (MOSZKOWSKA et SCEMAMA, 1964; MOSZKOWSKA, 1965). L'adjonction de

5-HT au milieu d'incubation ne modifie pas la sécrétion de l'hypophyse incubée seule; en revanche, elle supprime complètement la réponse de la glande à la stimulation hypothalamique. D'autres indolamines, comme la mélatonine, n'affectent pas significativement la réponse hypophysaire aux transmetteurs hypothalamiques, (fig. 3) (MOSZKOWSKA, 1965).

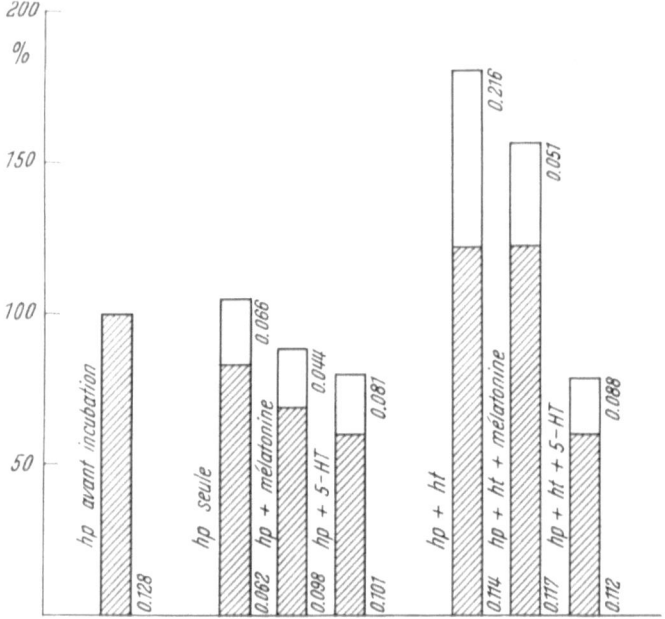

Fig. 3. Activité gonadotrope de l'hypophyse incubée dans diverses conditions expérimentales. hp, hypophyse; ht, hypothalamus; 5-HT, 5-hydroxytryptamine. Dosage par le test d'augmentation pondérale de l'ovaire de ratte impubère (les chiffres le long des rectangles représentent l'indice de précision du dosage)

Activite gonadotrope de l'hypophyse (hachures) et du liquide d'incubation (blanc) après 3 heures d'incubation dans differentes conditions experimentales.

En pour cent de l'activité d'une hypophyse ♂ adulte non incubée.

Conclusions

Des médiateurs monoaminergiques semblent donc pouvoir modifier *in vitro*, la réponse de l'hypophyse aux transmetteurs polypeptidiques hypothalamo-hypophysaires. Ces résultats n'ont pu être encore confirmés *in vivo*; cependant la présence de 5-HT dans l'éminence médiane (FUXE, 1964) de même que l'absence de réponse à des activations expérimentales de l'hypothalamus dans des conditions particulières comme la gestation (KORDON et PSYCHOYOS, 1966) permettent de supposer que les monoamines peuvent également affecter l'hypophyse *in situ*.

De telles interférences entre les effects de transmetteurs polypeptidiques et de monoamines devraient permettre de mieux comprendre la signification de l'innervation complexe de l'éminence médiane, par des fibres de dimensions, d'origines et, sans doute, d'activités pharmacologiques très différentes.

Bibliographie

ARVY, L. (1962): Histochemical demonstration of enzymatic activities in neurosecretory centres of some homoiothermic animals. Mem. Soc. Endocr. **12**, 215—225.

BARRACLOUGH, C. A., and C. H. SAWYER (1957): Blockade of the release of pituitary ovulating hormone in the rat by chlorpromazine and reserpine. Endocrinology **61**, 341.

BARRY, J. (1966): Neurosécrétion hypothalamique Gomori-négative et contrôle gonadotrope chez le Cobaye mâle. Symp. international sur la Neurosécrétion, Strasbourg.

— J. LEFRANC, J. LEONARDELLI et M. MAZZUCA (1964): Recherches histophysiologiques sur les cellules du noyau hypothalamique latérodorsal interstitiel du Cobaye. C. R. Ass. Anat. **121**, 231—234.

COPPOLA, J. A., R. G. LEONARDI, and W. LIPPMAN (1966): Ovulatory failure in Rats after treatment with brain norepinephrine depletors. Endocrinology **78**, 225—228.

DESCLIN, L., J. FLAMENT-DURAND, and W. GEPTS (1962): Transplantation of the ovary to the spleen in rats with persistent estrus resulting from hypothalamic lesions. Endocrinology **70**, 429—438.

DEY, F. L. (1941): Changes in ovaries and uteri in guinea-pigs with hypothalamic lesions. Amer. J. Anat. **69**, 61—87.

FLERKO, B. (1957): Le rôle des structures hypothalamiques dans l'action inhibitrice de la folliculine sur la sécrétion de l'hormone folliculo-stimulante. Arch. Anat. micr. Morph. exp. **46**, 159—172.

FUXE, K. (1964): Cellular localization of monoamines in the median eminence and the infundibular stem of some animals. Z. Zellforsch. **61**, 710.

HILLARP, N. A. (1949): Studies on the localisation of hypothalamic centres controlling the gonadotrophic function of the hypophysis. Acta endocr. (Kbh.) **2**, 11—23.

KORDON, C. (1966): Recherches sur le contrôle hypothalamique des fonctions gonadotropes femelles du Rat. Thèse de Sciences, Paris, 152.

—, et A. PSYCHOYOS A. (1966): Effet de lésions de l'hypothalamus antérieur sur l'implantation des blastocystes chez le Rat. J. Physiol. (Paris) **58**, p. 547.

MOSZKOWSKA, A. (1959): Contribution à la recherche des relations du complexe hypothalamo-hypophysaire dans la fonction gonadotrope. C. R. Soc. Biol. (Paris) **153**, 1945—1948.

— (1965): Quelques données nouvelles sur le mécanisme de l'antagonisme épiphyso-hypophysaire. Rôle possible de la sérotonine et de la mélatonine. Res. Suisse zool. **72**, 145—160.

—, et C. KORDON (1960): Action d'implants d'hypothalamus femelles lésés sur la fonction gonadotrope de l'hypophyse greffée. C. R. Soc. Biol. (Paris) **154**, 2021.

— — (1965): Contrôle hypothalamique de la fonction gonadotrope et variation du taux des G.R.F. chez le Rat. Gen. Comp. Endocr. **5**, 596.

—, et A. SCEMAMA (1964): Sécrétion et excrétion de l'antéhypophyse in vitro dans diverses conditions expérimentales. C. R. Soc. Biol. (Paris) **158**, 2038—2032.

OLIVECRONA, H. (1957): Paraventricular nucleus and pituitary gland. Acta physiol. scand., suppl., 136.

Cellular Processes Concerned with Vasopressin Biosynthesis, Storage and Release[1]

H. Sachs[2], R. Portanova[3], E. W. Haller[4], and L. Share[5]

Department of Physiology, Western Reserve University, School of Medicine
Cleveland, Ohio, USA.

The mammalian hypothalamo-neurohypophysial complex[6] contains a group of well defined neurons whose cell bodies lie in the anterior hypothalamus and whose axons extend into the neurohypophysis; they are responsible for the elaboration of the polypeptide hormones, oxytocin and vasopressin. These neurons fulfill the morphological and functional criteria of neurosecretory cells. The most distinguishing morphological features of these neuron sare that their axon endings (in the neural lobe) about on blood vessels rather than on other nerve cells, and that their axoplasm usually abounds with dense granules about 0.1 to 0.3 μ in diameter. These granules were presumed to contain the polypeptide hormones, oxytocin and vasopressin and therefore were termed "neurosecretory granules" (NSG) by morphologists. Since these NSG appeared to move in a proximo-distal direction, it was postulated that the synthesis of the hormones takes place in the perikaryon within the NSG, which then move in a protoplasmic flow along the axon to the region of the nerve endings. It is in this region that, in response to appropriate stimuli, the release of the NSG, or their contents, into the blood stream is thought to occur (2). The rudimentary features of this "neurosecretory process" are represented schematically in Fig. 1. Studies in our own and other laboratories have begun to outline some of the cellular mechanisms involved in the intermediate neurosecretory stages. In this manuscript, we report on some of our recent findings on the biosynthesis, storage, and release of vasopressin.

Vasopressin Biosynthesis

Over the past several years we have attempted to trace the path of vasopressin biosynthesis in the hypothalamo-neurohypophysial complex of the dog, and more recently of the guinea pig. In our studies, we have relied primarily on isotope methods. On the basis of labeling experiments carried out both *in vivo* and *in vitro*, we have proposed a precursor model for vasopressin biosynthesis (3, 4). According to this model, the biosynthesis of the peptide bonds in vasopressin

[1] Supported in part by grants from the National Institutes of Health, USPHS (AM-02650, HE-06035) and the Heart Association of Northeast Ohio.
[2] Supported by a Research Career Devolopment Award, No. 2 K 3 AM-14827.
[3] Recipient of USPHS Predoctoral Research Fellowship No. 6448 M 0406.
[4] Recipient of USPHS Predoctoral Research Training Grant 5T1-CM-899.
[5] Supported by a Research Career Development Award No. 5-K3-HE 1498.
[6] For a comprehensive discussion of this subject. See ref. 1.

would occur solely in the perikaryon, on ribosomes, via pathways common to the biosynthesis of other peptide chains (i.e., involving transfer RNA, messenger RNA, etc.). However, it is further proposed that the biosynthesis of vasopressin first leads to a bound, biologically inactive form (i.e., as part of a precursor molecule) and that the appearance of the biologically active octapeptide occurs at a time and place removed from the initial biosynthetic events. Conceivably, the release of the octapeptide from the precursor molecule would take place during the formation and maturation of the NSG. A number of experimental findings are in accord with the precursor model for vasopressin biosynthesis, some of which have been reviewed in a previous publication (3). The most convincing evidence in favor of the "precursor model" has come from labeling experiments carried out *in vitro* with guinea pig hypothalamo-median eminence (HME) tissue. As in the case of the *in vivo* isotope experiments, the incorporation of ^{35}S- or ^{3}H-labeled amino acids into vasopressin was preceded by a lag period of about one hour's duration. If the slices were removed from the initial incubation medium after the first hour of incubation, and reincubated in fresh buffer, labeled hormone appeared under conditions which precluded further *de novo* peptide bond synthesis (Table 1, exp. 1). Furthermore, the release of labeled vasopressin from a labeled precursor can take place in a cell free system. Homogenates containing labeled precursor were prepared from slices of guinea pig HME tissue which had been incubated with ^{35}S-cys-

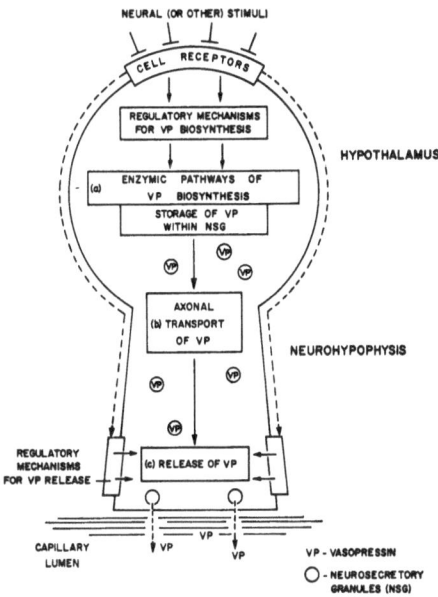

Fig. 1. Schematic representation of a number of intermediate stages involved in the neurosecretory function of the vasopressin producing cells of the mammalian hypothalamo-neurohypophysial complex (3)

teine or ^{3}H-tyrosine for one hour. Such homogenates did not contain significant quantities of labeled hormone; however, incubation of these homogenates at 37 C gave rise to ^{35}S- or ^{3}H-vasopressin (Table 1, exp. 2). Although the biosynthesis of labeled precursor (formed during the first hour of slice incubation) was inhibited by puromycin, the release of hormone from precursor was not inhibited by this drug. Boiling the labeled homogenates prior to incubation did, however, prevent the formation of labeled vasopressin. On the other hand, freezing and thawing did not appear to be deleterious, and in fact, labeled homogenates could be stored at —20 C for several weeks without appreciable loss of activity.

The possibility existed that newly synthesized (i.e., labeled) vasopressin was initially physically bound to protein or nucleic acid structures in a form not extractable by trichloroacetic acid (TCA), and that subsequent incubation rendered the labeled hormone extractable into TCA. In order to examine this possibility, homogenates containing labeled precursor (i.e., capable of releasing labeled vasopressin upon incubation) were again utilized. Degradation of the macro-molecular structures of such prelabeled homogenates with either pepsin or a mix-ture of deoxyribonuclease and ribonuclease failed to release labeled hormone. These experiments suggest that initially, newly formed hormone is not merely physically bound to some protein or nucleic acid molecules, but is an integral part of some precursor molecule.

It has been a consistent finding that after the continuous infusion of ^{35}S-cysteine into the third ventricle of dogs for 3 to 6 hours, the most highly labeled vasopressin molecules did not follow the ribosome rich fractions; instead, the newly formed hormone was associated with cellular structures that sedimented in a relatively low centrifugal field (8). The question whether such cellular fractions also contained labeled precursor was next examined. For these studies, homogena-

Table. 1 *Production of Labeled Vasopressin From Precursor Labeled in Vitro*

Guinea pig hypothalamo-median eminence
slices incubated in vitro with a labeled amino acid
↓
after 1 hour, slices removed from incubation media

one portion, added TCA and vasopressin isolated	one portion incubated (as slices or as an homogenate, or centrifugal fractions deriv-ed from the homogenate) for an additional 5 hours in fresh buffer containing puro-mycin and unlabeled amino acid

| *Counts/min/µg* | | | | *Counts/min/µg* | |
Exp.	*Vasopressin*	*Protein*		*Vasopressin*	*Protein*
1	0	106	(slices)	1248	104
2	0	78	(homog.)	826	83
3	0	—	a) particulate material (600 × g, 15 min)	244	—
			b) 600 × g supernatant	92	—

Exp. 1 and 2, guinea pig hypothalamic-median eminence slices were incubated with ^{35}S-cysteine (1.1 to 1.3 × 10^9 cpm), Exp. 3, with ^{3}H-tyrosine (1.2 × 10^9 cpm) for 1 hour; second incubation (right hand columns) was in the presence of puromycin (2 × 10^{-4} M) and either 5 × 10^{-3} M unlabeled cysteine (Exp. 1, 2) or tyrosine (Exp. 3), respectively. Exp. 3 slices (previously incubated for 1 hour with ^{3}H-tyrosine) were homogenized in 0.88 M sucrose and centrifuged at 600 × g for 15 min at 4 C; the pellet was washed successively with 3 por-tions of 0.88 M sucrose, suspended in potassium phosphate buffer, pH 7.4 (5), and incubated with an unlabeled homogenate of guinea pig hypothalamo-median eminence tissues; the 600 × g supernatant (Exp. 3b) was also incubated in the presence of an unlabeled homogenate as described above for the 600 × g pellet.

Vasopressin was isolated for specific activity determinations as previously described (4). In the same experiment, purified nuclei prepared according to the method of Maggio, Sieke-vitz and Palade (6) as modified by Bondy and Warlsh (7) was inactive, i. e., did not give rise to labeled vasopressin.

tes, prepared from slices of guinea pig HME tissue which had been incubated with a radioactive amino acid for one hour, were fractionated by means of ultra-centrifugation, and the fractions were incubated at 37 C (Table 1, exp. 3). It was found that particulate structures which sediment at low centrifugal speeds were the most active in the formation of labeled vasopressin. These observations are thus consistent with the *in vivo* labeling experiments (*8*). Whereas the initial biosynthetic steps appear to be ribosomal events (i.e., puromycin sensitive), the subsequent release and/or formation of vasopressin from some precursor takes place at other cellular loci.

Obviously, however, final proof of the precursor model must await the isolation and characterization of the precursor molecule.

Is Hormone Biosynthesis Attuned to the Secretory Activity of the Cell?

The availability of an *in vitro* system capable of hormone biosynthesis afforded the opportunity to examine the question whether those stimuli which affect the release of hormone also affect the biosynthetic events. Prolonged water deprivation is a powerful stimulus for the release of vasopressin. As a first approach, this stimulus was applied to the intact animal prior to removal of the HME tissues. It was a consistent finding (*9*) that HME slices taken from guinea pigs deprived of water for 4 days incorporated 2 to 5 times more radioactivity into vasopressin than HME tissues from guinea pigs with free access to water. Analogous results have been obtained with HME tissues of guinea pigs allowed to drink 2.5 % sodium chloride for a period of 10 days. The results of RNA studies (*10*), coupled with our own findings, suggest that the prolonged reception of nerve impulses effective in the release of vasopressin may also be translated into enhanced synthesis of specific RNA molecules involved in polypeptide hormone biosynthesis.

Storage and Release of Vasopressin

Many morphological studies (*1*) on the mammalian hypothalamo-neurohypo-physial complex have indicated that vasopressin is contained within membrane-bound vesicles (NSG) that range from 0.1 to 0.3 μ diameter. This concept was verified by the isolation and characterization of the NSG in our own (*11*) and in a number of other laboratories (*12, 13*). In the above investigations, differential and density gradient centrifugation techniques were employed for the isolation of NSG from neurohypophysial tissues. These techniques were subsequently applied to studies on the distribution of vasopressin among the subcellular structures of the nerve cell bodies located in the anterior hypothalamus (*14*). As might be expected, the combination of centrifugation and isotope experiments indicated that the bulk of the hormone was held within NSG. However, the perikaryon was shown to contain small but discreet pools of particulate-bound vasopressin aside from the NSG. Labeling experiments (see above) have implicated these "pools" in the early stages of hormone biosynthesis (*8*).

Recently we have directed our attention to a number of questions concerning the existence and nature of the pools of vasopressin in the neurohypophysis; these are:

1. Is there a readily releasable pool of hormone; and if so, what proportion of the total hormone content does this pool comprise?

2. Once such a pool is released, will the application of further stimuli lead to the further secretion of hormone, albeit at a lower rate?

In order to examine these questions, we have developed methods and experimental test systems whereby the hypothalamo-neurohypophysial cells (or their axons) could be stimulated in a reproducible manner and their response quantitatively measured. The results of a number of experiments carried out both *in vivo*

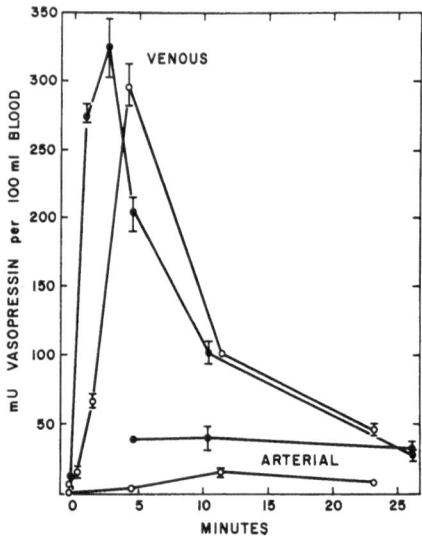

Fig. 2. Time course of discharge of vasopressin into the blood of dogs which have been rapidly bled and maintained at a blood pressure of 50 mm Hg. 0——0, dog No. 1; 0——0, dog No. 2

The experiments were performed as described (15); venous blood obtained from the superior vena cava; arterial blood from a femoral artery. Bleeding was initiated at zero time, vertical bars represent 95 per cent fiducial limits of potency estimate.

Points are plotted at the middle of the interval required to collect each 100 ml blood sample. These collection times in minutes were for dog No. 1: control sample, 0.36; post hemorrhage, 0.36, 1.0, 2.10, 2.4, and 1.38; for dog No. 2: control sample, 0.23; post hemorrhage, 0.93, 1.33, 1.1, 0.88 and 0.58.

and *in vitro* suggest that the neurohypophysis has a limited capacity to sustain a high rate of release of vasopressin in response to extensive stimulation applied over a relatively short time interval. The available evidence accords with the view that the pool of neurohypophysial vasopressin is heterogeneous and that there is a readily releasable pool which comprises about 10—20% of the total hormonal content of the neurohypophysis. Once this "readily releasable" pool of hormone has been discharged, the neurohypophysis, nevertheless, is still capable of releasing vasopressin in response to appropriate stimuli, but at a greatly reduced rate.

The results of experiments performed some years ago (Fig. 2) demonstrate that within a few minutes following hemorrhage of anesthetized dogs to a blood pressure of 50 mm Hg, vasopressin is released into the blood at a rate several thousand times pre-hemorrhage values (15). However, about 30 minutes after hemorrhage, the rate of release of hormone declines considerably. Analysis of the neurohypophysis and an estimation of the total output of vasopressin over the 30 minute post hemorrhage period revealed that only about 10—15 % of the total hormone in the gland was released.

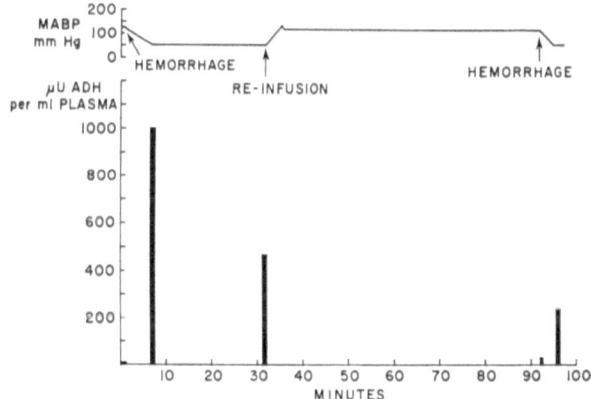

Fig. 3. Effect of repeated hemorrhage on plasma levels of vasopressin (ADH). The experiment was performed essentially as described for Fig. 2 expect that venous blood was obtained from an external jugular vein and the vasopressin in plasma was extracted and estimated by means of an antidiuretic bioassay according to Share (16). Ordinates: lower portion, microunits of antidiuretic hormone (ADH) per ml of plasma; upper portion, mean arterial blood pressure, mm Hg; abscissa: time in minutes

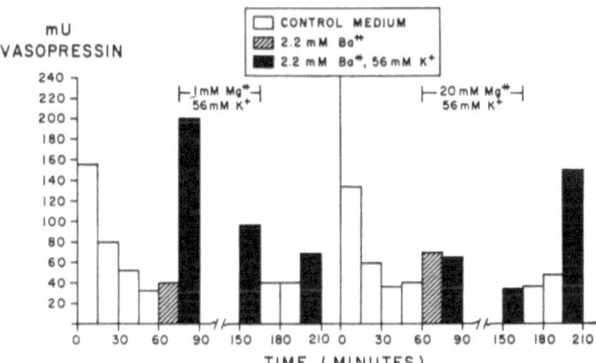

Fig. 4. Representative experiment of electrical stimulation of isolated posterior pituitaries of anesthetized dogs

Left hand portion: A male dog was anesthetized with nembutal and his mean arterial blood pressure was recorded; 30 minutes later the animal was sacrificed by means of an injection of 40 ml of saturated $MgSO_4$ solution; the posterior pituitary was removed, sliced in half and each half was incubated separately at 37 C in either 4 ml of normal Locke's solution (control medium) or Locke's solution which had Ca^{++} replaced by 2.2 mM Ba^{++}. The period of incubation was 15 minutes; electrical stimulation was carried out as previously described (17) in medium containing 2.2 mM Ba^{++}.

Right hand portion: An anesthetized dog was hemorrhaged and maintained at a blood pressure of 50 mm Hg for a period of 30 minutes prior to sacrifice. The isolated pituitary was then treated as described above; ordinate: milliunits vasopressin released over a 15 minute incubation period per half gland; abscissa: time in minutes.

The possibility that peripheral receptor mechanisms or central neurons could not maintain their activity under sustained hypotensive conditions was first examined. For example, the question was posed, "Could hormone secretion again occur at a high rate after a suitable recovery period following hemorrhage?" Fig. 3 shows the results of one of a series of such experiments. After 30 minutes of hemorrhage, reinfusion of blood restored the blood pressure and blood vasopressin (ADH) concentration to relatively normal values. However, a second hemorrhage one hour later failed to raise the concentration of hormone in the blood beyond the level observed just prior to blood infusion. Again, direct analysis showed that the attenuated release of vasopressin after 30 minutes of hemorrhage could not be attributed to exhaustion of the pituitary content of hormone. Nevertheless, this inhibition of vasopressin secretion appears to lie in part at the level of the pituitary. For example, pituitaries taken from hemorrhaged dogs released much less vasopressin in response to either electrical or K^+ ion stimulation, than pituitaries from nonhemorrhaged animals (Fig. 4, representative experiment). These experiments were done as follows. The stimulation of halved dog posterior pituitaries in vitro was carried out with minor modification of procedures previously described for preparations of isolated guinea pig glands (17). It had been shown in our own laboratory (17) and by Douglas et al. (18) that such preparations release vasopressin in response to either electrical stimulation or elevated concentrations of K^+ ions. Furthermore, Ba^{++} ions will increase the resting level of secretion and augment the release of hormone during either electrical or K^+ ion stimulation. In the case of the dog pituitaries incubated in vitro, the increments [mean $\pm$ SEM (no. expts.)] in hormone secretion upon electrical or K^+ ion stimulation were 61.3 ± 8.5 (4) and 156.2 ± 16.0 (6) milliunits per 15 minutes per half gland, respectively. Pituitaries taken from hemorrhaged animals, however, gave values for electrical or K^+ ion stimulation of 18.5 ± 12.5 (4) and 55.8 ± 25.4 (6) milliunits per 15 minutes per half gland, respectively.

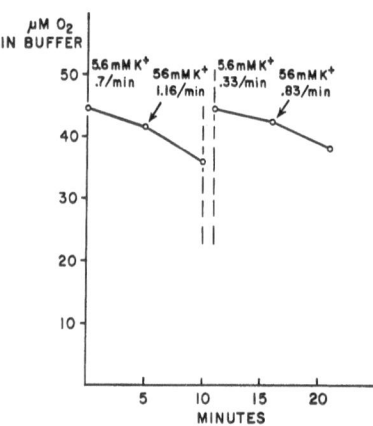

Fig. 5. Effect of K^+ on oxygen uptake by posterior pituitaries from dogs. 40.77 mg of tissue from two dogs sacrificed by i. v. injection of $MgSO_4$. Incubation medium was phosphate Ringer's at 37 C, equilibrated with air, pH 7.4, volume 2.0 ml. Incubation chamber was rinsed and buffer renewed during the time interval indicated by the dashed vertical lines. Oxygen uptake was measured by continuous recording with an oxygen electrode. Rates of O_2 uptake (in $\mu M\ O_2/min$) are given below the concentration of K^+ ions employed in the incubation media

A number of experiments indicated that the hypothalamo-neurohypophysial cells had not suffered irreversible damage due to decreased blood flow and hypoxia (or for other reasons) during hemorrhage (cf. 19, 20). These are:

1. EEG recordings from both surface and hypothalamic regions of the brain did not show any gross differences in electrical activity during 30 minutes of hemorrhage.

2. Isolated dog pituitaries were capable of O_2 uptake and showed a respiratory response to K^+ ions (Fig. 5). The rate of O_2 uptake and magnitude of the respiratory response to K^+ ions for pituitaries from hemorrhaged dogs were identical with that obtained with pituitaries from control animals.

3. Experiments carried out *in vitro* suggested that the secretory mechanisms are, in fact, quite resistant to extended periods of hypoxia. Although O_2 or an energy source is required for hormone release in response to K^+ ion stimulation [as reported by DOUGLAS et al. (*21*)], incubation of dog pituitaries for 1 to 2 hours in the absence of glucose and O_2 did not lead to irreversible damage of the secretory mechanisms. Transfer of pituitaries from the anoxic media to fresh buffer which contained glucose and O_2, resulted in a rapid restoration of responsivity.

The capacity of the neurohypophysis to release vasopressin in reponse to continued stimulation was studied further by means of the *in vitro* system. In analogy to the *in vivo* observations (i.e., hemorrhage) it was shown that stimulation of isolated dog pituitaries for extensive time periods *in vitro* also resulted in a progressive decline in hormone secretion; and this phenomenon was shown to occur in the absence of gland exhaustion. The question whether the attenuated release of vasopressin after prolonged stimulation *in vitro* was in fact due to the depletion of a readily releasable pool or was merely due to prolonged membrane depolarization was approached in the following way. Isolated dog pituitaries were divided in half; one half was incubated in the presence of a depolarizing concentration of K^+ for $1^1/_2$ hours while the other half was incubated in the presence of the same concentration of K^+ plus 20 mM Mg^{++} [which inhibits the release of hormone (*18*)]. In several such experiments it was shown that the pituitary halves incubated under the latter conditions (i.e., depolarization in the absence of a massive discharge of vasopressin), were capable of a much greater release of hormone in response to a subsequent stimulus under optimal conditions (increment $\pm$ SEM over prestimulation value, 79.5 $\pm$ 7.2 milliunits/15 minutes compared to 23.5 $\pm$ 4 milliunits/15 minutes for the corresponding pituitary halves which had been permitted to release vasopressin during the first stimulation period ($p < .01$).

Two experiments carried out *in vivo* have given essentially analogous results. For example, 2 dogs were hemorrhaged to a mean arterial blood pressure of 50 mm Hg under circumstances where both vagi were cut, and where the carotid sinuses were perfused at a high pulse pressure and at a normal mean arterial pressure. Under these conditions, hemorrhage does not lead to the expected discharge of vasopressin; indeed, the pituitaries taken from these animals after 30 minutes of hemorrhage released vasopressin in response to K^+ ion stimulation at an approximately normal rate (104 and 180 milliunits/15 minutes/half gland respectively).

The experiments described above are thus in accord with the view that the pool of neurohypophysial vasopressin is heterogeneous and that about 10—15% of the total pool of pituitary hormone may be discharged over a relatively short time interval (e.g. after hemorrhage, or K^+ ion stimulation *in vitro*). At present, the precise anatomical or intracellular location of this readily releasable pool is unknown. On the basis of many morphological studies (*1*) including those of BODIAN (*22*) the nerve endings would appear likely candidates as sites of storage of this pool.

References

1. Harris, G. W., and B. T. Donovan (Eds.): The Pituitary Gland, Vol. 3. Berkeley: University of California Press 1966.
2. Scharrer, E., and B. Scharrer: Hormones produced by neurosecretory cells. Rec. Progr. Hormone Res. **10**, 183 (1954).
3. Sachs, H.: Neurosecretion in the mammalien hypothalamo-neurohypophysial complex. In: H. Peeters (Ed.). Protides of the biological fluids, p. 181. Amsterdam: Elsevier 1965.
4. —, and Y. Takabatake: Evidence for a precursor in vasopressin biosynthesis. Endocrinology **75**, 943 (1964).
5. Galber, S., P. L. Campbell, G. E. Deibler, and L. Sokoloff: Effects of L-Thyroxine on amino acid incorporation into protein in mature and immature rat brain. J. Neurochem. **11**, 221 (1964).
6. Maggio, R., P. Siekevitz, and G. E. Palade: Studies on isolated nuclei. I. Isolation and chemical characterization of a nuclear fraction from guinea pig liver. J. Cell. Biol. **18**, 267 (1963).
7. Bondy, S. C., and H. Waelsch: Nuclear RNA polymerase in brain and liver. J. Neurochem. **12**, 751 (1965).
8. Sachs, H.: Vasopressin biosynthesis II. Incorporation of [^{35}S] Cysteine into vasopressin and protein associated with cell fractions. J. Neurochem. **10**, 299 (1963).
9. Takabatake, Y., and H. Sachs: Vasopressin biosynthesis III. In vitro studies. Endocrinology **75**, 934 (1964).
10. Edstrom, J. E., D. Eichner, and N. Schor: Quantitative ribonucleic acid measurements in functional studies of nucleus supraopticus. In: S. S. Kety, and J. Elkes (Eds.), Regional Neurochemistry, p. 274. Oxford: Pergamon Press 1960.
11. Weinstein, H., S. Malamed, and H. Sachs: Isolation of vasopressin-containing granules from the neurohypophysis of the dog. Biochim. Biophys. Acta **50**, 386 (1961).
12. Barer, R., H. Heller, and K. Lederis: The isolation, identification and properties of the hormonal granules of the neurohypophysis. Proc. Roy. Soc. B **158**, 388 (1963).
13. LaBella, F. S., G. Beaulieu, and R. J. Reiffenstein: Evidence for the existence of separate vasopressin and oxytocin-containing granules in the neurohypophysis. Nature (Lond.) **193**, 173 (1962).
14. Sachs, H.: Studies on the intracellular distribution of vasopressin. J. Neurochem. **10**, 289 (1963).
15. Weinstein, H., R. M. Berne, and H. Sachs: Vasopressin in blood: effect of hemorrhage. Endocrinology **66**, 712 (1960).
16. Share, L.: Acute reduction in extracellular fluid volume and the concentration of antidiuretic hormone in blood. Endocrinology **69**, 925 (1961).
17. Haller, E. W., H. Sachs, N. Sperelakis, and L. Share: Release of vasopressin from isolated guinea pig posterior pituitaries. Amer. J. Physiol. **209**, 79 (1965).
18. Douglas, W. W., and A. M. Poisner: Stimulus-secretion coupling in a neurosecretory organ: The role of calcium in the release of vasopressin from the neurohypophysis. J. Physiol. (Lond.) **172**, 1 (1964).
19. Rapela, L. E., and H. D. Green: Autoregulation of canine cerebral blood flow. Circulation Res. **14** (Suppl. 1): 205 (1964).
20. Kety, S. S.: Blood flow and metabolism of the human brain in health and disease. In: K. A. C. Elliott, I. H. Page, and J. H. Quastel (Eds.), p. 113. Springfield: Neurochemistry. Charles C. Thomas 1962.
21. Douglas, W. W., A. Ishida, and A. M. Poisner: The effect of metabolic inhibitors on the release of vasopressin from the isolated neurohypophysis. J. Physiol. (Lond.) **181** 753 (1965).
22. Bodian, D.: Herring bodies and neuro-apocrine secretion in the monkey. Bull. Johns Hopk. Hosp. **118**, 282 (1966).

Ultrastructural and Biological Evidence for the Presence and likely Functions of Acetylcholine in the Hypothalamo-neurohypophysial System

K. Lederis

M.R.C. Group for Research in Neurosecretion,
Department of Pharmacology, Medical School,
University of Bristol

Since the Bristol Symposium more information has become available on the mechanisms of storage, transport and release of the neurosecretory products in the hypothalamo-neurohypophysial system of vertebrates (Douglas and Poisner, 1964a, b; Lederis, 1964; Smith and Thorn, 1965; Daniel and Lederis, 1966; Ginsburg and Ireland, 1966; Ginsburg, Jayasena and Thomas, 1966). However, no evidence has been added to clarify the definition and the role of the so called synaptic vesicles in the neurohypophysis. It had been suggested that the definition synaptic be used with caution until evidence became available on whether or not these vesicles were indeed located in synaptic nerve endings and whether they contain a synaptic transmitter substance (Lederis, 1965).

Series of experiments were instigated in our laboratories to investigate the above problem. This report deals only with the examination of the neurohypophysis — firstly, for content of one synaptic transmitter agent — acetylcholine, secondly, effects of acetylcholine on hormone release from the posterior pituitary, and thirdly, ultrastructural considerations pertaining to synaptic or "synaptoid" nerve endings in the neurohypophysis.

Presence of Acetylcholine and of Cholinesterases in the Neurohypophysis

Homogenates of the rabbit neural lobe, anterior hypothalamus and of cerebral (temporal) cortex were tested for acetylcholine content as described by Lederis and Livingston, 1966. The leech muscle contracting activity (Szerb, 1961) found in the homogenates was shown to be due mainly to acetylcholine (Table 1). It was of interest to note that the tissue concentration of acetylcholine in the neural lobe was approximately comparable to that in the cerebral cortex; in both the above areas the acetylcholine content was somewhat lower than in the hypothalamus. Another observation made from over 20 experiments was that of a wide variation (several hundred-fold) in acetylcholine content in different batches of rabbits. The assumption seemed feasible that this variation may have a bearing on neurohypophysial hormone content in the corresponding neural lobes or, alternatively, on the physiological state of the animal in relation to the release of these hormones.

Table 1. *Inactivation of leech muscle-contracting activity of rabbit neural lobe and hypothalamus extracts by acetylcholinesterase (E.C. 3.1.1.7.). Extracts incubated for 1hr at 37° C in phosphate buffer, pH 7.4, containing 1 U/ml acetylcholinesterase. (from* Lederis *and* Livingston, *1966). Results of three experiments. N = neural lobe, H = hypothalamus extracts*

Tissue	Activity (g acetylcholine/g wet tissue × 10⁹)		% inactivation
	Before incubation	After incubation	
N	1531	67	96
H	239	61	74
N	23	<1.5	>90
H	31	9	71
N	237	54	77
H	259	33	87

In a number of experiments the rabbits were acutely stimulated to release neurohypophysial hormones at a high rate (ether anaesthesia and haemorrhage as described by Daniel and Lederis, 1966a). Such experiments failed to show significant differences in acetylcholine content between the stimulated animal neural lobes and controls (Lederis and Livingston, unpublished observations).

Cholinesterases in the Rabbit Neural Lobe

In view of histochemical observations that acetylcholinesterase can be demonstrated in the neural lobe of some mammals (cat, Koelle and Geesey, 1961; the hedgehog, Holmes, 1961) but not in others (Holmes, 1961), neural lobe homogenates of a number of mammalian species were tested for acetylcholine content. Broadly speaking, the amount of acetylcholine found was similar in the pituitaries of all the species examined, including the hedgehog (Table 2). It was then decided to test for the presence of acetylcholinesterase and other esterases in the neurohypophysis. Quantitative measurements (Livingston, 1966) were undertaken using the colourimetric procedure of Ellman, Courtney, Andres and Featherston, 1961. This method permits the estimation of true and pseudo-cholinesterases. The rabbit neural lobe was found to contain about half the concentration of cholinesterases as compared with the hypothalamus. Acetylcholinesterase accounted for more than 90 % of the total cholinesterase activity in both, the neural lobe and the hypothalamus. The remainder was found to be due mainly to butyrylcholinesterase. It thus becomes apparent that histochemical investigations on enzymes, especially negative findings, cannot be relied upon completely. Much more valuable information may be gained when histochemical and other morphological methods purporting to demonstrate presence or absence of biologically active substances are supported by direct measurements of the substances in question. Similar criteria have been shown to be necessary when considering quantitative aspects of hormone storage and release in the neurohypophysis (Moses, Leveque, Giambattista and Lloyd, 1963; Lederis, 1965; Daniel and Lederis, 1966a; Barer and Lederis, 1966).

Koelle and Geesey, 1961, and De Robertis, 1962, on the basis of histochemical and electron microscopical evidence respectively, advanced a hypothesis that acetylcholine acts as a local transmitter in the release of hormones from the neurohypophysial nerve terminals. Direct measurements of the effects of acetylcholine on hormone release from the neural lobe in several laboratories, have failed to confirm this contention (DOUGLAS and POISNER, 1964a, b; DANIEL and LEDERIS, 1966b; DICKER, 1966).

Table 2. *Acetylcholine content and ratios in the neural lobe (N), hypothalmus (H) and temporal cortex (C) of some mammalian species*

Species	Acetylcholine (g/g wet tissue × 10⁹)			Mean Ratio	
	N	H	C	N/H	N/C
Rabbit (19 expts)	76	127	51	0.57	1.06
Rat (6 expts)	72	171	196	0.58	0.88
Hedgehog (4 expts)	25	20	32	1.43	1.14
Cattle (2 expts)	146	142	—	1.03	—
Man (3 expts)	139	—	—	—	—

Table 3. *Cholinesterases in the rabbit neural lobe and hypothalamus, expressed as rates of hydrolysis of substrates (acetylthiocholine and butyrylthiocholine) in μ-moles of substrate hydrolysed/min/g wet tissue (means ± S.E.) (from* LIVINGSTON, *1966)*

Enzyme	Neural lobe (N)		Hypothalamus (H)		Ratio N/H
	No. of experiments	Rate	No. of experiments	Rate	
Acetylcholinesterease	15	$1.7^H \pm 0.11$	18	3.78 ± 0.60	0.63
Butyrylcholinesterase	14	0.16 ± 0.04	15	0.41 ± 0.08	0.29

Ultrastructural Considerations

If acetylcholine does not act as a synaptic transmitter on the neurohypophysial nerve endings, what is its role in the posterior pituitary ? Reappraisal of the electron microscopical appearance of the neurohypophysis permits the advancement of another hypothesis. When the immediate vicinity of blood vessels is examined, varying numbers of small nerve terminals can be seen which contain only the small ("synaptic") vesicles (Fig. 1, 2, 3). Such nerve terminals can be differentiated from the swellings and terminals of the hypothalamo-neurohypophysial nerve fibres as the latter contain either the elementary granules alone or, in some cases, varying numbers of the small vesicles, in addition to the hormonecontaining elementary granules. So far only the neural lobes of man, rabbit and rat have been re-examined. In many neural lobe sections of these species small nerve endings containing only the small vesicles can be found, usually near blood vessels (Fig. 4 and 5). Although it cannot be entirely excluded that such nerve endings may represent the extreme tips of hormone-containing nerve terminals, it is tempting to postulate that the small nerve terminals, found near the blood vessels, and containing only small vesicles, may be the terminals of cholinergic nerve fibres and that such nerve fibres — and therefore acetylcholine — may act directly on the capillary wall. Under conditions when large amounts of neurohypophysial hormones are required in the systemic circulation, acetylcholine may thus facilitate the

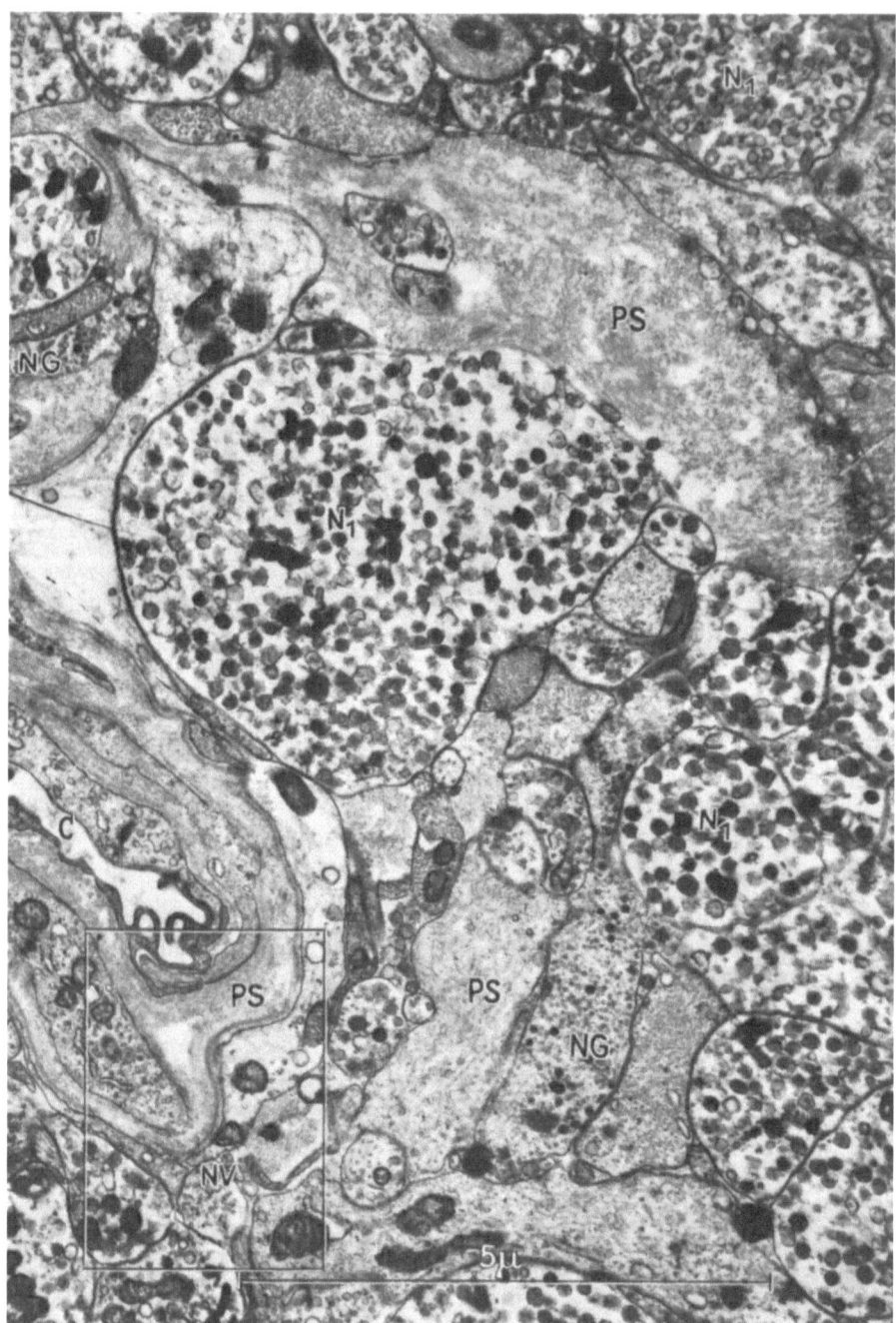

Fig. 1. Low power view of the human neurohypophysis showing the distribution of nerve terminals containing the hormone-containing elementary granules (N_1) and other, smaller, nerve terminals (NV, NG) close to the blood vessel (C) or abutting on the wide perivascular space (PS). NV = nerve terminals containing small electron lucent vesicles; NG = nerve terminals containing both, electron lucent vesicles and dense granules of similar size. Black square indicates area shown at higher magnification in Fig. 2. Mag. $\times$ 15000; $0{,}0_4$, Westopal, Uranylacetate. Siemens Elmiscope I

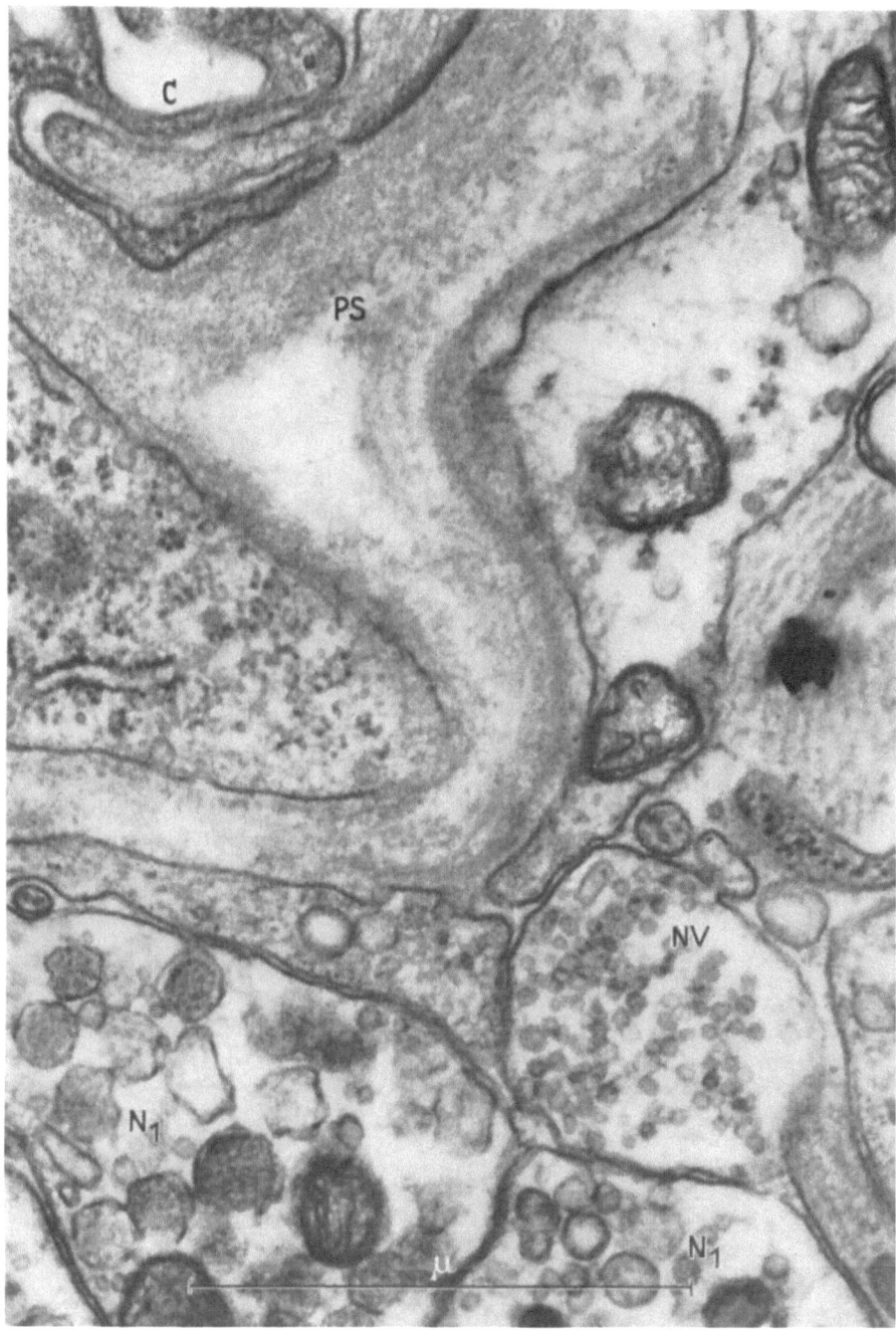

Fig. 2. Higher magnification of an area from Fig. 1 showing nerve swellings in which elementary granules and small vesicles occur (N_1). A small nerve terminal (NV) is seen near the perivascular space (PS) of a capillary (C). In this nerve terminal only small vesicles occur. Mag. $\times$ 71,000; O_sO_4, Westopal, Uranylacetate. Siemens Elmiscope I

160 K. Lederis:

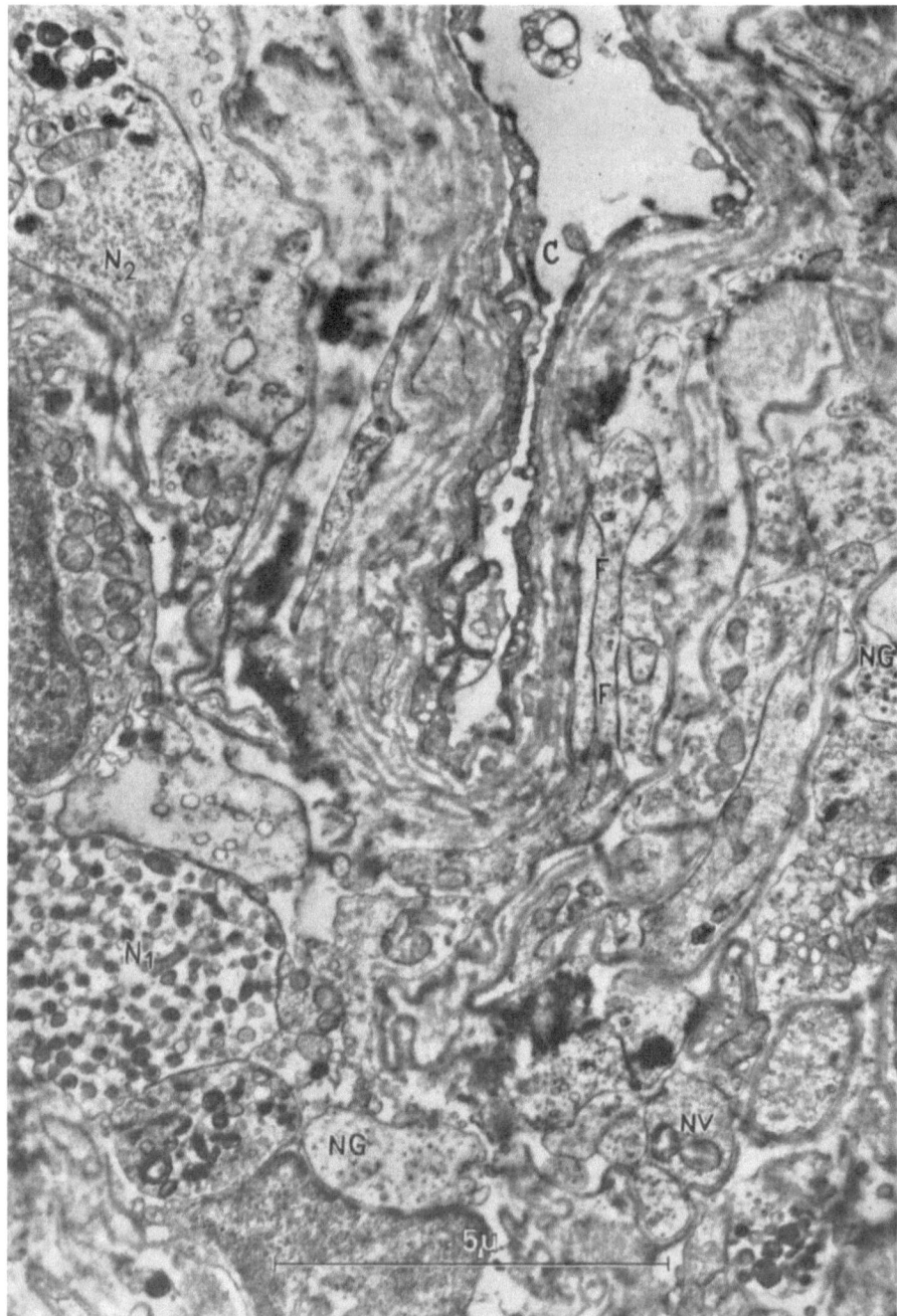

Fig. 3. Human neurohypophysis. Near the capillary (C) a narrow nerve fibre (F) is seen which dilates into a terminal. The latter contains only small vesicles. Other small nerve terminals containing only small vesicles (NV) or granules similar in size (NG). Swellings of the hypothalamo-neurohypophysial nerve fibres (N₁) contain elementary granules or the granules and small vesicles (N₂). Mag. × 11,200; O₄O₄, Vestopal, Uranylacetate. Hitachi Hs-7 S

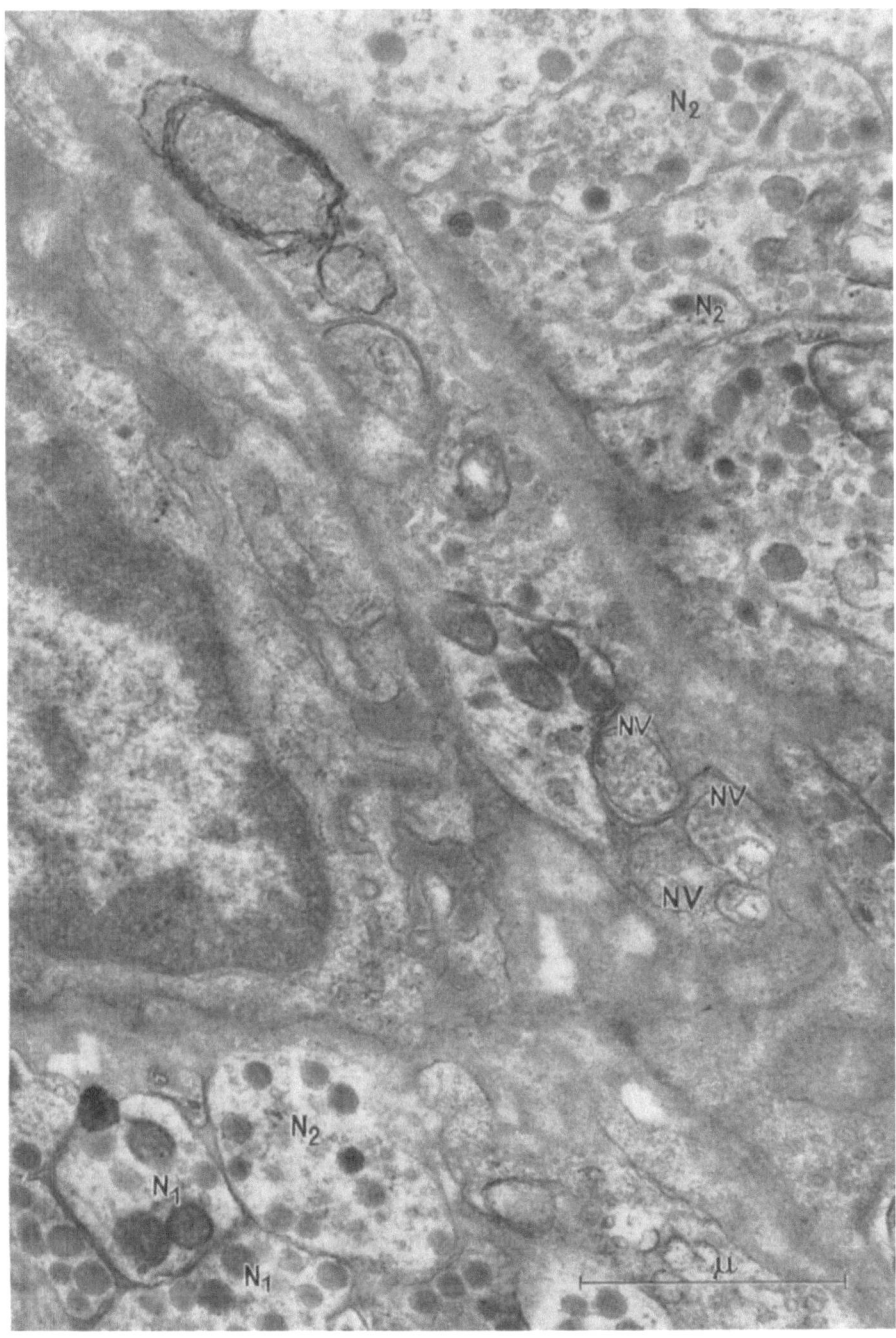

Fig. 4. Rabbit neural lobe. Nerve swellings containing elementary granules (N_1), others a mixture of the granules and small visicles (N_2). In the perivascular space several small nerve terminals are seen (NV) in which only the small vesicles occur. Mag. $\times$ 38,000; O_sO_4, Araldite, Uranylacetate; Siemens Elmiscope I

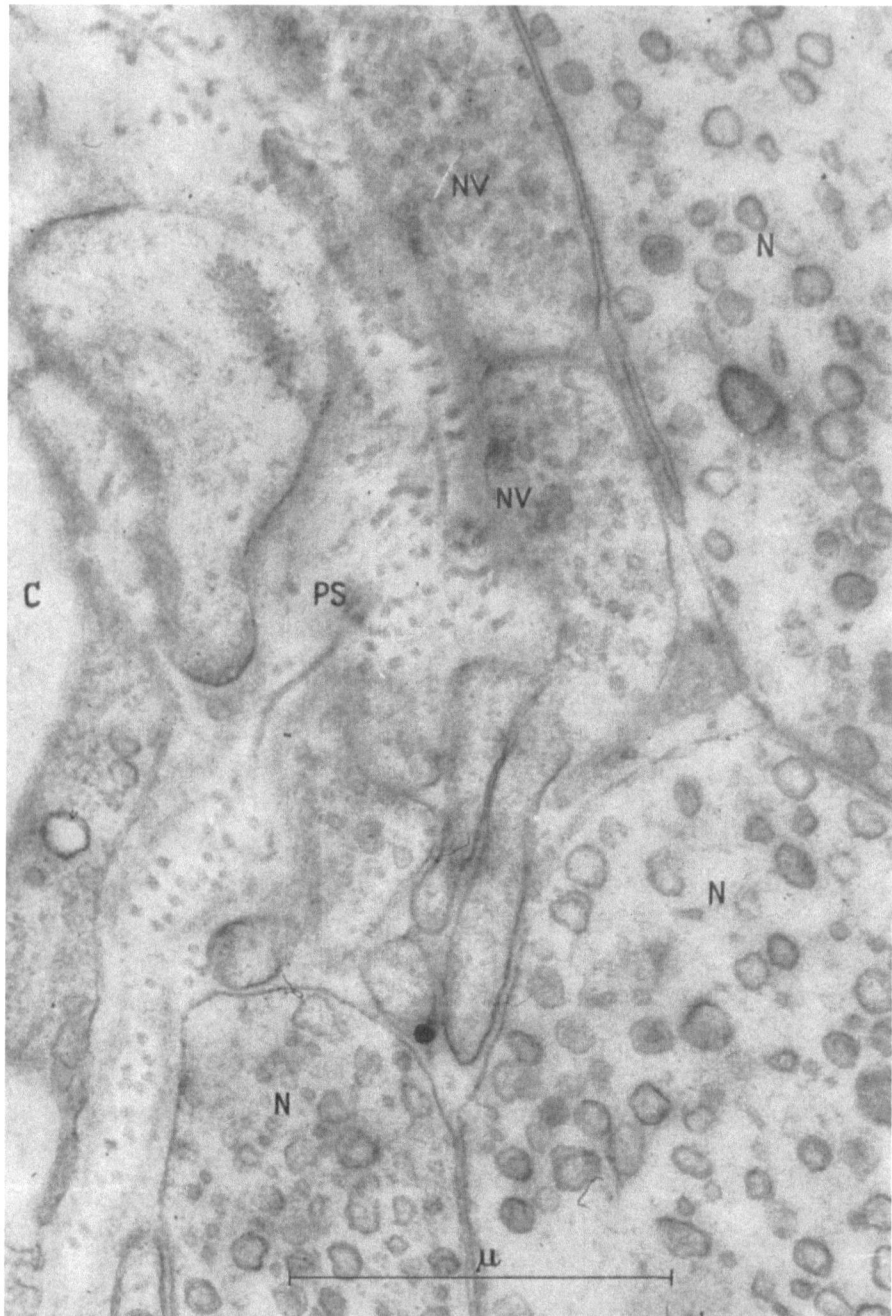

Fig. 5. Rat neural lobe showing a small area of the gland near a blood vessel. C = capillary lumen, PS = perivascular space. Abutting on the perivascular space are two small nerve terminals (NV) containing only the small vesicles. Parts of three larger nerve swellings are seen (N) in which elementary granules and small vesicles are present. Mag. $\times$ 54,700; O_sO_4, Araldite, Uranylacetate. Siemens Elmiscope I

transfer of hormones into the blood stream, possibly by causing vasodilatation. Such a speculation gains support from the occasional occurrence of nerve endings — also small, and also in the immediate vicinity of blood vessels — which contain small electron dense granules (Fig. 1 and 3). The nerve terminals, and the vesicles and dense granules contained within, conform to those which have been claimed to contain noradrenaline (DE ROBERTIS et al., 1961; RICHARDSON, 1966). It could thus be visualised that perhaps both components of the autonomic nervous system may be present in the neurohypophysis and that these may regulate the blood flow through the neural lobe in accord with changing rates of hormone release. The presence of autonomic nerve fibres in the neurohypophysis has been reported in the past (BARGMANN, 1962).

As already pointed out, speculations about function advanced on the basis of morphological observations require further investigation by other methods before they can be critically evaluated. Experiments are in hand to determine a) in which subcellular organelles of the neurohypophysis acetylcholine is lodged, b) whether it occurs in the same nerve endings in which vasopressin and oxytocin are stored, and c) whether catecholamines can also be found in the mammalian neurohypophysis.

References

BARER, R., and K. LEDERIS (1966): Ultrastructure of the rabbit neurohypophysis with special reference to hormone release. Z. Zellforsch. (in press).

BARGMANN, W. (1962): Histologie und mikroskopische Anatomie des Menschen, 5. Aufl., S. 354—358. Stuttgart: Georg Thieme.

DANIEL, A. R., and K. LEDERIS (1966a): Effects of ether anaesthesia and haemorrhage on hormone storage and ultrastructure of the rat neurohypophysis. J. Endocrin. 34, 91—104.

— — (1966b): Effects of acetylcholine on the release of neurohypophysial hormones in vitro. J. Endocrin. 34, 10—11.

DICKER, S. E. (1966): Release of vasopressin and oxytocin from isolated pituitary glands of adult and new-born rats. J. Physiol. 185, 429—444.

DOUGLAS, W. W., and A. M. POISNER (1964a): Stimulus-secretion coupling in a neurosecretory organ and the role of calcium in the release of vasopressin from the neurohypophysis. J. Physiol. 172, 1—18.

— — (1964b): Calcium movement in the neurohypophysis of the rat and its relation to release of vasopressin. J. Physiol. 172, 19—30.

ELLMAN, G. L., DIANE K. COURTNEY, V. JR. ANDRES, and R. M. FEATHERSTON (1961): A new and rapid colourimetric determination of acetyl-cholinesterase activity.

GINSBURG, M., and M. IRELAND (1966): The role of neurophysin in the transport and release of neurohypophysial hormones. J. Endocrin. 35, 289—298.

— K. JAYASENA, and P. J. THOMAS (1966): The preparation and properties of porcine neurophysine and the influence of calcium on the hormone-neurophysin complex. J. Physiol. 184, 387—401.

HOLMES, R. L. (1961): Esterases of the hypothalamo-hypophysial system. Proc. Anat. Soc. Gt. Brit. and Ireland, Nov. 1961. In: Cytology of Nervous Tissues. London: Taylor and Francis.

KOELLE, G. B., and C. N. GEESEY (1961): Localisation of acetylcholinesterase in the neurohypophysis and its functional implications. Proc. Soc. exp. Biol. Med. 106, 625—628.

LEDERIS, K. (1964): Fine structure and hormone content of the hypothalamo-neurohypophysial system of the rainbow trout (Salmo irideus) exposed to sea water. Gen. comp. Endocrin. 4, 638—661.

— (1965): An electron microscopical study of the human neurohypophysis. Z. Zellforsch. 65, 847—868.

—, and A. LIVINGSTON (1966): Acetylcholine content in the rabbit neurohypophysis. J. Physiol. 185, 37—38.

11*

LIVINGSTON, A. (1966): Acetylcholinesterase content in the rabbit neurohypophysis. J. Physiol. (in press).

MOSES, A. M., T. F. LEVEQUE, MARY GIAMBATTISTA, and C. W. LLOYD (1963): Dissociation between the content of vasopressin and neurosecretory material in the rat neurohypophysis. J. Endocrin. **26**, 273—278.

RICHARDSON, K. C. (1966): Electron microscopic identification of autonomic nerve endings. Nature (Lond.) **210**, 756.

DE ROBERTIS, E. (1962): Ultrastructure and function in some neurosecretory system. In: Neurosecretion. (H. HELLER, and R. B. CLARK, Eds.) pp. 3—20. London-New York: Academic Press.

— A. PELLEGRINO DE IRALDI, R. DE LORES ARNEIZ, and L. SALGANICOFF (1961): Electron microscope observations on nerve endings isolated from rat brain. Anat. Rec. **139**, 220.

SMITH, M. W., and N. A. THORN (1965): The effects of calcium on proteinbinding and metabolism of arginine vasopressin in rats. J. Endocrin. **32**, 141—151.

SZERB, J. C. (1961): The estimation of acetylcholine, using leech muscle in a microbath. J. Physiol. **158**, 8—9.

The Influence of Central Catecholamine Neurons on the Hormone Secretion from the Anterior and Posterior Pituitary*

K. FUXE and T. HÖKFELT

Department of Histology, Karolinska Institutet, Stockholm 60, Sweden

Thanks to the development of a highly specific and sensitive histochemical fluorescence method for the demonstration of dopamine (DA), noradrenaline (NA) and 5-hydroxytryptamine (5-HT) (FALCK, HILLARP, THIEME and TORP, 1962; HILLARP, FUXE and DAHLSTRÖM, 1966) it has been possible to demonstrate that the nuc. supraopticus and the nuc. paraventricularis are innervated by a dense plexus of NA nerve terminals (CARLSSON, FALCK and HILLARP, 1962; FUXE, 1965a). Furthermore, DA nerve terminals, which arise from axons originating from DA cell bodies present mainly in the nuc. arcuatus have been shown to surround the primary capillary plexus of the hypophyseal portal system (FUXE, 1963, 1964). Thus, central monoaminergic mechanisms in all probability participate in the regulation of hormone secretion from both the posterior and anterior pituitary. Experiments have now been performed to elucidate the neuroendocrinological role played by these NA and DA neuron systems.

The NA Innervation of the Magnocellular Neurosecretory Nuclei (Nuc. Supraopticus and Nuc. Paraventricularis)

Morphology. The terminals have the characteristic appearance of a monoamine nerve terminal (FUXE, 1965b) with abundant strongly fluorescent varicosities (around 1 μ in diameter) with high amine concentrations. The other parts of the monoamine neurons (cell body and non terminal axon) have much lower amine concentrations and the non-terminal axons are even difficult to identify in normal animals with the histochemical fluorescence technique. Some of the NA nerve terminals are localized in the immediate vicinity of the cell bodies (Fig. 2) but probably most of them lie close to the cell processes. This is particularly evident in the most ventral portion of the nuc. supraopticus, where the NA varicosities are most abundant, most of them lying without contact with nerve cell bodies. These findings are corroborated by electronmicroscopical studies (EICHNER, personal communication). With the help of lesions in the lateral midbrain tegmentum (ANDÉN, DAHLSTRÖM, FUXE, OLSEN and UNGERSTEDT, 1966) and large lesions in

* This study has been supported by grants (12 X-714-02) from the Swedish State Medical Research council and from Magnus Bergvall's Foundation. For generous supply of drugs we are indebted to Dr. CORRODI, AB Hässle, Göteborg (H 44/68) and Swedish Ciba, Stockholm (reserpine).

the medial ventral borderzone between the mesencephalon and the diencephalon (Andén, Fuxe and Larson, 1966) it has been shown that these terminals arise from axons, which originate from NA cell bodies situated in the pons and the medulla oblongata. Thus, we are dealing at least mainly with rhombencephalic afferents. At least the NA nerve fibres giving axon branches to the paraventricular nucleus (Fig. 2) run in the lateral hypothalamic area, since electrolytic lesions in this part will cause marked anterograde degenerative changes in most of the NA nerve terminals of the paraventricular nucleus (Andén, Dahlström, Fuxe and

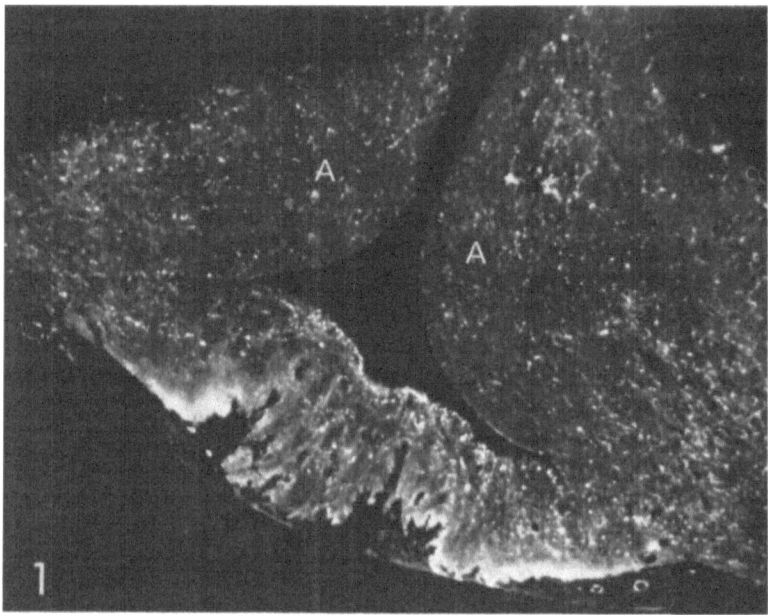

Fig. 1. The median eminence of normal rat. Cross-section. The high density of DA nerve terminals in the external layer of the median eminence give a high fluorescence intensity to this part of the median eminence. The strongly fluorescent varicosities of the NA nerve terminals in the nuc. arcuatus (A) and internal layers of the median eminence are also observed. × 110

Larsson, 1965). — So far no yellow-fluorescent 5-HT nerve terminals have been discovered innervating the magnocellular nuclei, not even after monoamineoxidase inhibition, which is known to increase very markedly the intraneuronal amine levels of the 5-HT neurons (Dahlström and Fuxe, 1965). Direct 5-hydroxytryptamin-ergic mechanisms therefore do not seem to be involved in the regulation of oxytocin and antidiuretic hormone (ADH) secretion.

Function. It is known that an increased impulse-flow affect the amine levels of the central and peripheral CA neurons only to a small degree, probably due to an increased resynthesis of neurotransmitter in the terminal parts of the neuron to compensate for the increased release (Andén, Carlsson, Hillarp and Magnus-son, 1965; Andén, Corrodi, Dahlström, Fuxe, and Hökfelt, 1966). Therefore changes in activity cannot be detected by measuring the intraneuronal amine levels. Thanks to the development of potent inhibitors of the first rate-limiting step in the CA biosynthesis (for references see ANDÉN, CORRODI, DAHLSTRÖM, FUXE, and HÖKFELT, 1966), however, the increased and decreased amine release existing in connection with high and low neuronal activity respectively, can be revealed, since after synthesis-inhibition no compensatory resynthesis can occur. Under these conditions the result will be an increased and decreased rate of depletion of the CA stores respectively as compared to controls, which can be observed histochemically and biochemically. We have now used this method to

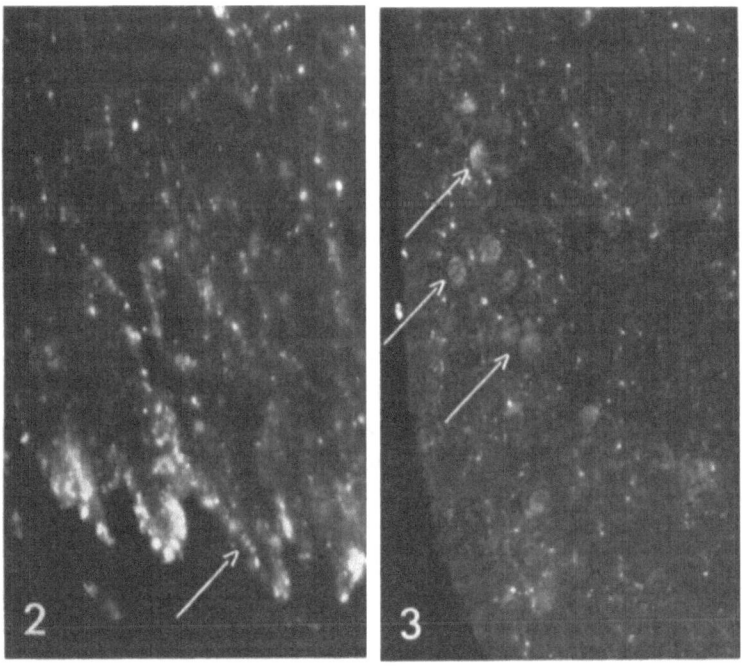

Fig. 2   Fig. 3

Fig. 2. Median eminence of normal rat. Cross-section of an araldite-embedded specimen (HÖKFELT, 1965). Thanks to the thinness of the section (1—2 μ) the individual varicosities (→) of the DA nerve terminals can now be observed as they lie on the outer surface of the median eminence. × 660

Fig. 3. Nuc. arcuatus of normal rat. Cross-section. Small, round to oval DA nerve cell bodies with a very weak to weak green fluorescence (→) are observed just below the ependyma. × 270

study the activity of NA nerve terminals of the supraoptic and paraventricular nuclei during stimulation of osmoregulation, resulting in ADH release (rat, 4—21 days with 1.5—2.5% sodium chloride as drinking water). As inhibitor the α-methyl-p-tyrosine methylester (H 44/68) was chosen. Preliminary results indicate that 8 hours after treatment with the inhibitor (250 mg/kg, i.p.) more NA nerve terminals remain in the supraoptic nuclei of the experimental rats than in those of the control rats. These preliminary findings indicate that there is a decreased impulse flow in the supraoptic NA nerve terminals during ADH secretion, which imply that the synapses formed by the NA terminals on the processes and cell bodies of the supraoptic cells are inhibitory in function. This is supported by many

workers who have observed stimulation of ADH secretion after reserpine treatment (Gaunt, Renzi, Antonchak, Miller, and Gilman, 1954; Gabe, Tuchmann-Duplessis, and Mercier-Parot, 1961; Miline, Stern, Serstenev, and
Muhibic, 1957) which causes a blockade of the monoamine neurotransmission
(cf. Carlsson, 1966). Thus, after reserpine treatment an increase in neurosecretory products is observed in the supraoptic neuroglandular cells and an
increased depletion rate of ADH occurs during osmostimulation from the neural
lobe under the influence of reserpine.

These studies will be continued by water load experiments (cf. Olivecrona,
1957). If the present interpretation is correct the NA nerve terminals should in
this case show an increased depletion rate after synthesis inhibition, since under
these conditions a decrease in ADH secretion will occur. — The inhibitory effect
of ethanol on the release of oxytocin during parturition, which probably is due to
central inhibition of the reflex release of oxytocin (Fuchs, 1966) can very well be
explained if it is assumed that also the NA nerve terminals innervating the nuc.
paraventricularis has an inhibitory function. Thus, ethanol has recently been
shown to cause an increase in the activity of the NA nerve terminals of the hypothalamus (Corrodi, Fuxe, and Hökfelt, 1966).

The Tubero-infundibular DA Neuron System

Morphology (Figs. 1, 2, 3). Small, oval DA cell bodies giving rise to this system
are situated mainly in the nuc. arcuatus and in the ventral part of the anterior
periventricular nucleus. Some cells are found also in the caudal midline part of the
retrochiasmatic area. The cells are normally only weakly green-fluorescent and in
order to describe their distribution in detail it has been necessary to inject pharmacological drugs which increase their amine level. E.g. after treatment with a
monoamine oxidase inhibitor (e.g. nialamide) in combination with the precursor
3,4-dihydroxypehnylalanine (L-DOPA) a marked increase is observed in the
amine levels of the entire neuron. The number of cell bodies are considerably increased and their processes can be observed as well as the axons, which in some
cases can be traced down to the external layer of the median eminence (Duxe, and
Hökfelt, 1966). Similar findings have also been obtained in mice after intraperitoneal injection of very high doses of NA (Lichtensteiger, and Langemann,
1966). Recently, also intraventricular injections of α-methyl-NA have been made
in our laboratory (Fuxe, and Ungerstedt, 1966), and a marked uptake and
concentration of the amine was observed in cell bodies in the arcuate nuclei, the
anterior periventricular nuclei and the retrochiasmatic area, which in all probability were identical with the DA cell bodies. These data are corroborated by auto-
radiographic studies (Fuxe, Ritzén, and Ungerstedt, unpublished data). All
this evidence together with the fact that after lesion of the median eminence
(Fuxe, and Hökfelt, 1966), there is an accumulation of fluorescence in the DA
cell bodies, which in all probality represent a retrograde cell body reaction (cf.
Dahlström, and Fuxe, 1965), leave no doubt that there exists a tubero-infundibular DA neuron system.

This system seems at least partly to be identical with the tubero-infundibular
fibre system detected in Golgi preparations by several workers (cf. Szenthágothai, Flerkó, Mess, and Halász, 1962). This is *inter alia* supported by the fact

that most of the DA nerve terminals are not in close contact with the capillary loops but lie on the outer surface of the external layer adjacent to the rich "Mantelplexus" (Figs. 1, 2, 4), which drains into the portal vessels in the same way as does the capillary loops. Furthermore, practically no DA nerve terminals traverse the external layer to enter the pars tuberalis, which are empty of mono-amine nerve terminals except for the adrenergic nerve terminals surrounding the superior hypophyseal arteries. Similar results have been obtained in Golgi studies.

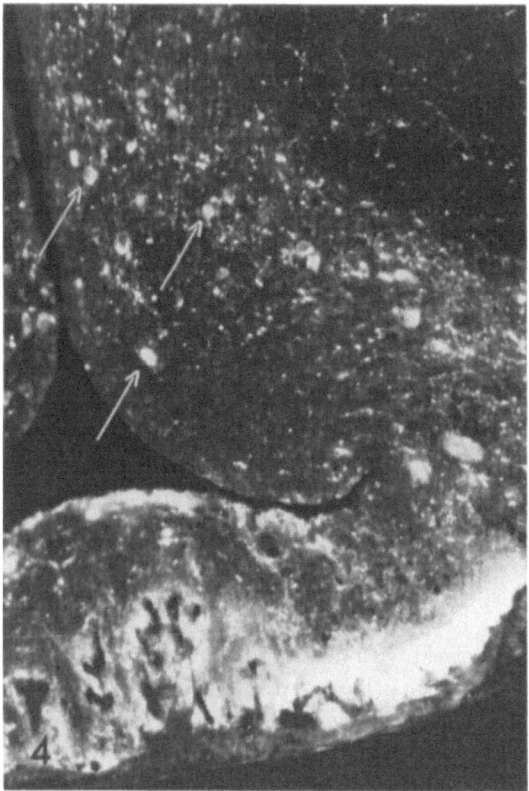

Fig. 4. Nuc. arcuatus and median eminence of rat on day 4 of pregnancy. Cross-section. Clear increases are observed in the number and intensity of DA cell bodies (→) in the nuc. arcuatus. The external layer is strongly green-fluorescent due to the presence of a dense plexus of DA nerve terminals. × 180. (FUXE, HÖKFELT, and NILSSON, unpublished material)

It must be pointed out that the DA neurons only constitute a minor proportion of the neuron population in the nuc. arcuatus. Thus, there may well exist other systems projecting onto the primary capillary plexus of the hypophyseal portal system, and which may be of importance for the regulation of the anterior pituitary secretion.

It has been shown that the DA tubero-infundibular neuron system contains two uptake mechanisms; one is the reserpine-sensitive uptake-storage mechanism of the amine granules, which are produced in the DA cell bodies and transported down to the terminals via the axons; the other is a reserpine-resistent amine uptake-concentration mechanism for CA which is present in the entire neuron and probably localized at the level of the nerve cell membrane (FUXE, and HILLARP, 1964; FUXE, and UNGERSTEDT, 1966). This uptake mechanism for CA has been possible to demonstrate thanks to the fact that the DA nerve terminals and non-terminal axons lie outside the blood-brain barrier, which is impermeable to CA. It has been possible to block this reserpine resistent accumulation of amine with amphetamine but not with desimipramine (FUXE, HAMBERGER, and MALMFORS, 1966). The effect of other drugs on this mechanism, especially those with known endocrinological effects (chlorpromazine, guanethidine, morphine, cocaine) are tested at the present time.

It has hitherto not been possible to identify with certainty the perivascular DA nerve terminal at the ultrastructural level. The most common nerve terminal in the perivascular zone of the median eminence of guinea pig (MAZZUCA, 1965) and rat (RINNE, 1966) seems to be one containing small agranular vesicles, so called synaptic vesicles (diameter about 500 Å) and in addition varying number of large granular vesicles (diameter about 700—1500 Å). In previous studies a similar type of nerve terminal has been found in other brain regions rich in monoamine nerve terminals (FUXE, HÖKFELT, and NILSSON, 1965). However, evidence was obtained for the view that a considerable part of the CA are stored in those structures which appear as small agranular vesicles. This probably is due to technical difficulties in fixation procedure, during which the amines may be dissolved, thus causing the dense core of small granular vesicles to disappear. Support for this view has recently been obtained by using potassium permanganate fixation (RICHARDSON, 1966). In the locus coeruleus area of rat, a region rich in monoamine nerve terminals, small granular vesicles have been demonstrated in certain nerve endings (HÖKFELT, 1967a). Furthermore, after incubation of brain slices from the hypothalamus including the median eminence in an α-m-NA containing medium it has been possible to show small granular vesicles in certain perivascular nerve endings, which probably are identical with dopamine containing varicosities demonstrated in the fluorescence microscope (HÖKFELT, 1967b).

Function. Purely on morphological grounds it seems probable that the DA which is highly concentrated in the varicosities of the DA nerve terminals is released into the primary capillary plexus of the hypophysial portal system to influence the hormone secretion of the cells in the anterior pituitary. If this is so, the tubero-infundibular DA neuron system possesses the property of participating in the control of an endocrine organ, although indirectly by way of a short special vessel pathway. In view of this the DA neuron system can probably be classified as a neurosecretory neuron system (KNOWLES, and BERN, 1966) and thus represent the final common pathway for the specific neuroendocrine function it regulates. The trophic releasing factors for thyroid stimulating hormone (TSH) and luteinizing hormone (LH) release has recently been shown by GUILLEMIN et al., 1966, to be simple molecules with a molecular weight probably below 500. The prolactin inhibitory factor (PIF) also seems to be a simple molecule (MEITES, and NICOLL, unpublished data). Since the molecular weight of DA is below 200, it is not improbable that DA or possibly a DA derivative or conjugate may, in fact, be one of the trophic releasing or inhibitory factors. At the present time, however, it cannot be in any way excluded that the DA released by the nerve impulse instead may release another substance which in this case would be one of the adenohypo-physeal releasing or inhibitory factors. This factor is probably stored in another type of terminal in the median eminence.

The endocrinological effects of reserpine which cause a blockade of monoamine neurotransmission by blocking the uptake-storage mechanism of the amine storage granules (CARLSSON, HILLARP, and WALDECK, 1963; DAHLSTRÖM, FUXE, and HILLARP, 1965) clearly indicate that monoaminergic mechanisms participate in controlling the gonadotrophin [follicle stimulating hormone (FSH) and luteinizing hormone (LH) and prolactin], in rats and mice identical with luteotrophic hormone (LTH) secretion from the anterior pituitary (cf. FLERKO, 1963; MEITES, NICOL, and TALWALKER, 1963; MEITES, and NICOLL, 1966). It has been shown that reserpine blocks e.g. spontaneous ovulation in rats (BARRACLOUGH, and SAWYER, 1957) as does chlorpromazine and completely suppresses ovulation (no LH release) in the immature rat (COPPOLA, LEONARDI, and LIPPMANN, 1966) as does other mono-amine depletors such as tetrabenazine. The studies of COPPOLA et al., 1966, and those of BROWN, 1966, strongly support the view that these effects are central in origin. Furthermore, reserpine and chlorpromazine induce pseudopregnancy (increase in LTH secretion) in rats (BARRACLOUGH, and SAWYER, 1959) as does other drugs which reduce brain CA levels (COPPOLA, LEONARDI, LIPPMANN, PERRINE, and RINGLER, 1965). The most striking effect of reserpine is, however, its ability to stimulate prolactin secretion hereby inducing lactation and mammary growth (cf. MEITES, NICOLL, and TALWALKER, 1963). Furthermore, investigations by MAYER, 1963, indicate that the blockade of implantation obtained with reserpine is due to interference with a central mechanism.

So far we have only studied the tubero-infundibular DA neurons during pregnancy, especially during the implantation period in rats and to a certain extent also during lactation with or without pretreatment with a potent inhibitor of the DA and NA biosynthesis (H 44/68).

The studies performed on the DA neurons during the gestation period have been done in close cooperation with Doctor OVE NILSSON, Department of Anatomy, University of Uppsala (FUXE, HÖKFELT, and NILSSON, 1966).

The day following the night of mating has been defined as day one of pregnancy. There was observed marked increase in the number and intensity of DA nerve cell bodies in the arcuate and anterior periventricular nuclei on day 4 to 6 (Fig. 4). This increase in amine levels had started on day 3 but was not present on day 1 and 2. The increase was still present on day 7 to 10. Otherwise no changes were observed in the DA neurons as compared to normal animals.

The increase of fluorescence intensity observed in many of the DA cell bodies may reflect an increased formation of amine storage granules since there is no reason to believe that a decreased transport of these amine granules should occur. Nor is it likely that an increased formation of DA is responsible for the observed increases in fluorescence, since inhibition of monoamine oxidase, which breaks down DA intraneuronally does not result in any considerable increases in fluorescence intensity. The increased formation of amine granules is probably induced by an increased neuronal activity since increases in amine levels in CA cell bodies in the medulla oblongata are found after haloperidol treatment (ANDÉN, DAHL-STRÖM, FUXE, and HÖKFELT, 1966), a central adrenergic blocking agent, which is

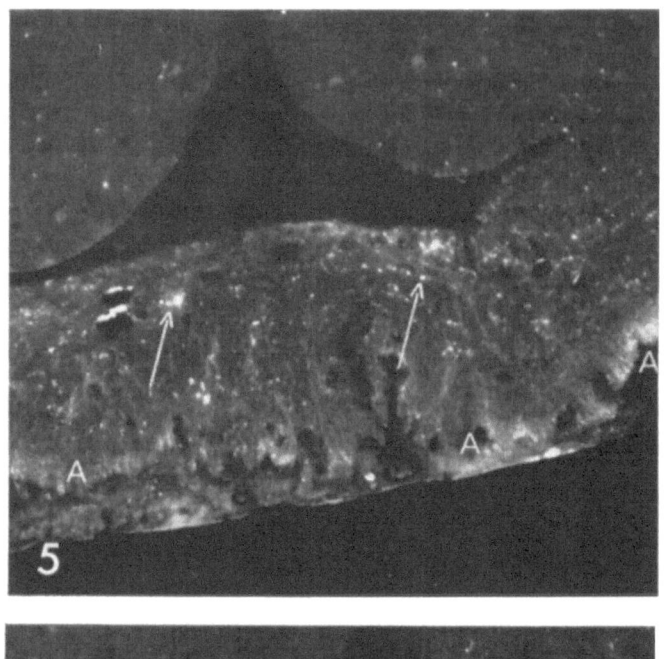

Fig. 5

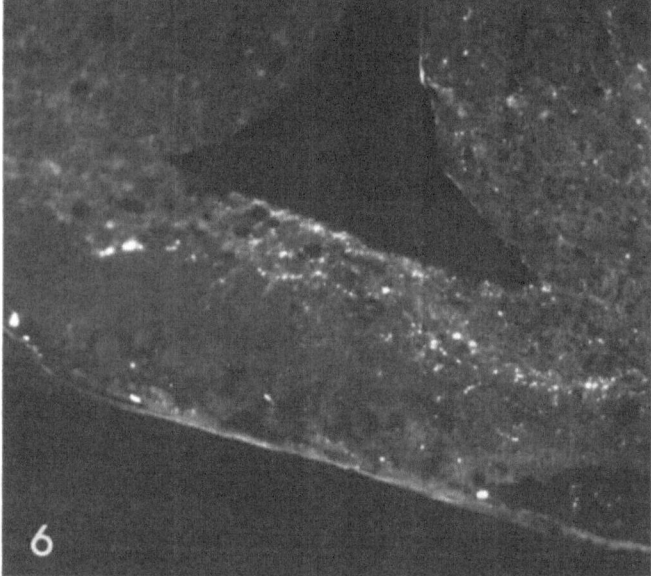

Fig. 6

Fig. 5. Median eminence of rat treated with H 44/68 (250 mg/kg, i. p., 6 hours before killing). Cross-section. A weak green fluorescence (A) remains in the external layer and the NA nerve terminals (→) in the innermost layers are strongly green-fluorescent. × 180. (Fuxe, Hökfelt, and Nilsson, unpublished material)

Fig. 6. The median eminence of rat on day 4 of pregnancy after H 44/68 treatment in the same way as in the control rat (see text to Fig. 5). No green fluorescence remains in the external layer but the NA nerve terminals of the innermost layers are still strongly green-fluorescent as in the control rat. × 180. (Fuxe, Hökfelt, and Nilsson, unpublished material)

known to increase the activity in central CA neurons (CORRODI, FUXE, and HÖK-FELT, 1967). With the help of synthesis inhibition, using H 44/68, direct evidence has been obtained that the tubero-infundibular DA neurons are activated on day 4 and 6 of pregnancy. It could be shown in the experimental animals that the external layer was completely empty of DA nerve terminals, whereas in the control rats weakly fluorescent DA terminals still remained (Figs. 5, 6). It seems likely from these data that the tubero-infundibular DA neuron system participate in the regulation of gonadotrophin and/or prolactin secretion. It is e.g. known that pregnancy is associated with a suppression of gonadotrophin secretion from the anterior pituitary and a moderate release of prolactin (see *inter alia* DOMINIC, 1966).

Fairly high daily doses (1 mg/kg) of reserpine have to be used to block the implantation effectively (MAYER, 1963). Histochemical fluorescence studies with daily doses between 0.5—1.5 mg/kg show that this is necessary, since the DA neuron system recover fluorescence in their terminals rapidly and before the other central CA neuron systems. This may be due to the fact that the neurons are very short and newly formed intact amine granules in the cell bodies can therefore reach the terminals rapidly. Guanethidine has also been tried in high daily doses (75 mg/kg, twice daily) in order to block implantation. The reason for using guanethidine, which is known to block peripheral adrenergic transmission, is that it does not penetrate the blood-brain barrier and thus the only central monoamine nerve terminals to be affected are the DA and NA nerve terminale of the median eminence. Guanethidine also causes a partial depletion of the peripheral NA stores. The results with this drug were negative, however. In no instance was guanethidine able to block implantation and there were never observed any detectable decreases in the amine levels of the DA nerve terminals of the median eminence. Decreases in amine levels were present, however, in the adrenergic vasomotor terminals and in the NA terminals of the median eminence. Thus, DA nerve terminals are probably not affected by guanethidine in the same way as NA nerve terminals.

Studies are now in progress to test the implantation blocking ability of other drugs (e.g. metaraminol, H 44/68, tetrabenazine) which interfere with the CA metabolism.

So far the tubero-infundibular DA neuron system has been studied during lactation (increased prolaction secretion) only in some rats. On the 5th day after parturition there was a slight increase in the amine levels of the DA cell bodies, whereas on day ten and especially day 15 the DA cell bodies had clearly increased amine levels although not as pronounced as during pregnancy. These preliminary results indicate that the tubero-infundibular DA neuron may increase their activity above normal in the later part of the lactation period. These results will be checked by the use of H 44/68.

The effect of stress (5% sodiumchloride, i.p., 10 ml, 30—60 min before killing or insulin-induced hypoglycemia), hydrocortisone treatment (25 mg/kg given i.p. for 14—21 days) and bilateral adrenalectomy (1, 2 and 14 days before killing) on the tubero-infundibular DA neurons has also been studied. So far no certain changes have been observed in the amine levels of the DA neurons after these treatments. Furthermore, hydrocortisone treatment or adrenalectomy did not accelerate or retard the depletion of DA from the DA neurons after synthesis inhibition. Thus, the activity of these neurons does not seem to be changed to any significant degree during hydrocortisone treatment or after adrenalectomy. Further experiments, however, are necessary to elucidate this point. These results are opposed by those of Akmayev and Donath, 1965, who found marked increases and decreases of the amine contents of the tubero-infundibular DA neurons following adrenalectomy and hydrocotisone treatment, respectively.

The present findings clearly indicate that the tubero-infundibular DA neurons are concerned with the regulation of gonadotrophin and/or prolactin secretion from the anterior pituitary and probably not with the regulation of adrenocortico-trophic hormone (ACTH) secretion.

It is interesting to note that the DA neurons are absent in the avian brain, where the neural mechanisms which regulate prolactin secretion probably are fundamentally different from those of the mammalian brain. In the mammalian brain regulation is probably established by means of secretion of a prolactin inhibitory factor (PIF), whereas the bird brain probably uses a prolactin secretory factor (cf. Meites, and Nicoll, 1966). After e.g. reserpine administration no increase in prolactin secretion is observed in birds. Furthermore, studies on the neurosecretory structure of the median eminence in the white-crowned sparrow (Oksche, 1962) have shown that unlike in mammals fibres from the nuc. supra-opticus contribute to a considerable degree to the nerve plexus in the external layer of the median eminence. In this connection it should be pointed out that CA probably are stored in the periodic acid-Schiff (PAS)-positive cells of the anterior pituitary, especially in those of the cat and that these cells also can take up and decarboxylate L-DOPA to a high degree (Dahlström, and Fuxe, 1966). DA is also taken up but in considerably lesser amounts. Thus, there seem to exist possibilities for DA to reach and to be taken up by PAS-positive cells to influence *inter alia* gonadotrophin secretion. Too few data exist, however, to be able to explain adequately the functional role of the DA tubero-infundibular neuron system played in the regulation of prolactin and FSH-LH release.

Although the central CA neuron systems discussed in the present paper are those directly concerned with the regulation of hormone release from the anterior and posterior pituitary, is has to be remembered that there exist other central CA and 5-HT neuron systems which may be of some importance for the neuroendo-crinological effects observed after injection of drugs interfering with the mono-amine metabolism e.g. reserpine and chlorpromazine. Especially the possible endocrinological role played by the NA nerve terminals of the arcuate nuclei and the anterior periventricular nuclei and by those in the inner layer of the median eminence has not been considered. Nor has the possible function of the rich plexus of CA nerve terminals of central origin present in the intermediate lobe of mammals (Fuxe, 1964; Dahlström, and Fuxe, 1966). The CA released from these terminals probably produce inhibition of melanocyte stimulating hormone release (Iturriza, 1966).

References

Akmayev, I. G., u. T. Donáth (1966): Die Katecholamine der Zona palisadica der Eminentia mediana des Hypothalamus bei Adrenalektomie, Hydrocortisonverabreichung und Stress. Z. mikr.-anat. Forsch. 74, 84—91.

Andén, N.-E., A. Carlsson, N.-Å. Hillarp, and T. Magnusson (1965): Noradrenaline release by stimulation of the spinal cord. Life Sci. 4, 129—132.

ANDÉN, N.-E. H., CORRODI, A. DAHLSTRÖM, K. FUXE, and T. HÖKFELT (1966): Effects of tyrosine hydroxylase inhibition on the intraneuronal amine levels of the central monoamine neurons. Life Sci. 5, 561—568.
— A. DAHLSTRÖM, K. FUXE, and K. LARSSON (1965): Mapping out of catecholamine and 5-hydroxytryptamine neurons innervating the telencephalon and diencephalon. Life Sci. 4, 1275—1279.
— — —, and T. HÖKFELT (1966): The effect of haloperidol and chlorpromazine on the amine levels of central monoamine neurons. Acta physiol. scand. in press.
— — — L. OLSON, and U. UNGERSTEDT (1966): Ascending monoamine neurons to the telencephalon and diencephalon. Acta physiol. scand. (in press).
— K. FUXE, and K. LARSSON (1966): Effect of large mesencephalic-diencephalic lesions on the noradrenaline, dopamine and 5-hydroxytryptamine neurons of the central nervous system. Experientia (Basel) (in press).
BARRACLOUGH, C. A., and C. H. SAWYER (1957): Blockade of the release of pituitary ovulating hormone in the rat by chlorpromazine and reserpine: Possible mechanisms of action. Endocrinology 61, 341—351.
— — (1959): Induction of pseudopregnancy in the rat by reserpine and chlorpromazine. Endocrinology 65, 563—571.
BROWN, P. S. (1966): The effect of reserpine, 5-hydroxytryptamine and other drugs on induced ovulation in immature mice. J. Endocr. 35, 161—168.
CARLSSON, A. (1966): Drugs which block the storage of 5-hydroxytryptamine and related amines. In: Handbuch der exp. Pharmak. Ergänzungswerk (Ed. V. ERSPAMER) pp. 529—592. Berlin-Göttingen-Heidelberg: Springer.
— B. FALCK, and N.-Å. HILLARP (1962): Cellular localization of brain monoamines. Acta physiol. scand. 56, Suppl. 196, 1—28.
— N.-Å. HILLARP, and B. WALDECK (1963): Analysis of the Mg^{**}-ATP dependant storage mechanism on the amine granules of the adrenal medulla. Acta physiol. scand. 59, Suppl. 215, 1—38.
COPPOLA, J. A., R. G. LEONARDI, and W. LIPPMANN (1966): Ovulatory failure in rats after treatment with brain norepinephrine depletors. Endocrinology 78, 225—228.
— — — J. W. PERRINE, and I. RINGLER (1965): Induction of pseudopregnancy in rats by depletors of endogenous catecholamines. Endocrinology 77, 485—490.
CORRODI, H., K. FUXE, and T. HÖKFELT (1966): The effect of ethanol on the activity of central catecholamine neurons in rat brain. J. pharm. pharmacol. 18, 821—823.
— — — (1967): The effect of neuroleptics on the activity of central catecholamine neurons. Life Sci. (in press).
DAHLSTRÖM, A., and K. FUXE (1964): Evidence for the existence of monoamine neurons in the central nervous system. I. Demonstration of monoamine on the cell bodies of brain stem neurons. Acta physiol. scand. 62, Suppl. 232, 1—55.
— — (1965): Evidence for the existence of monoamine neurons in the central nervous system. II. Experimentally induced changes in the intraneuronal amine levels of bulbospinal neuron systems. Acta physiol. scand. 64, Suppl. 247, 1—36.
— — (1966): Monoamines and the pituitary gland. Acta Endocrinol. 51, 301—314.
— —, and N.-Å. HILLARP (1965): Site of action of reserpine. Acta pharmacol. toxicol. 22, 277—292.
FALCK, B., N.-Å. HILLARP, G. THIEME, and A. TORP (1962): Fluorescence of catechol amines and related compounds condensed with formaldehyde. J. Histochem. Cytochem. 10, 348—354.
FLERKÓ, B. (1963): The central nervous system and the secretion and release of luteinizing hormone and follicle stimulating hormone. In: Advances in Neuroendocrinology. (Ed. A. V. NALBANDOV) pp. 211—224. Urbana: University of Illinois Press.
FUCHS, A.-R. (1966): The inhibitory effect of ethanol on the release of oxytocin during parturition in the rabbit. J. Endocrin. 35, 125—134.
FUXE, K. (1963): Cellular localization of monoamine in the median eminence and infundibular stem of some mammals. Acta physiol. scand. 58, 383—384.
— (1964): Cellular localization of monoamines in the median eminence and infundibular stem of some mammals. Z. Zellforsch. 61, 710—724.

FUXE, K. (1965a): Evidence for the existence of monoamine neurons in the central nervous system. IV. The distribution of monoamine nerve terminals in the central nervous system. Acta physiol. scand. **64**, Suppl. 247, 39—85.

— (1965b): Evidence for the existence of monoamine neurons in the central nervous system. III. The monoamine nerve terminal. Z. Zellforsch. **65**, 573—596.

— B. HAMBERGER, and T. MALMFORS (1966): Inhibition of amine uptake in tubero-infundibular dopamine neurons and in catecholamine cell bodies of the area postrema. J. Pharm. Pharmacol. **18**, 543—544.

—, N.-Å. HILLARP (1964): Uptake of L-dopa and noradrenaline by central catecholamine neurons. Life Sci. **3**, 1403—1406.

—, and T. HÖKFELT (1966): Further evidence for the existence of tubero-infundibular dopamine neurons. Acta physiol. scand. **66**, 243—244.

— T. HÖKFELT, and O. NILSSON (1965): A fluorescence and electron microscopic study on certain brain regions rich in monoamine nerve terminals. Amer. J. Anat. **117**, 33—46.

— — — (1966): Changes in amine levels of the tubero-infundibular dopamine neuron system during implantation in rats. In: Proc. V. World Congress on Fertility and Sterility. (Eds. A. INGELMAN-SUNDBERG, and B. WESTIN) in press. Amsterdam-New York-London-Milan-Tokyo-Buenos Aires: Excerpta Medica Foundation.

—, and U. UNGERSTEDT (1966): Localization of catecholamine uptake in rat brain after intraventricular injection. Life Sci. **5**, 1817—1824.

GABE, M., H. TUCHMANN-DUPLESSIS, and L. MERCIER-PAROT (1961): Influence de la reserpine sur la neurosécrétion hypothalamo-hypophysaire du rat albinos. C. R. Acad. Sci. (Paris) **252**, 1857—1859.

GAUNT, R., A. A. RENZI, N. ANTONCHAK, G. J. MILLER, and M. GILMAN (1954): Endocrine aspects of the pharmacology of reserpine. Ann. N. Y. Acad. Sci. **59**, 22—35.

GUILLEMIN, R., R. BURGUS, E. SAKIZ, and D. N. WARD (1966): Nouvelles données sur la purification de l'hormone hypothalamique TSH-hypophysiotrope, TRF. C. R. Acad. Sci. (Paris) **262**, 2278—2280.

HILLARP, N.-Å., K. FUXE, and A. DAHLSTRÖM (1966): Central monoamine neurons. In: Mechanisms of release of biogenic amines. (Eds. U. S. VON EULER, S. ROSELL, and B. UVNÄS) pp. 31—56. Stockholm: Pergamon Press.

HÖKFELT, T. (1965): A modification of the histochemical fluorescence method for catecholamines and 5-hydroxytryptamine using araldite as embedding medium. J. Histochem. Cytochem. **13**, 518—519.

— (1967a): On the ultrastructural localization of noradrenaline in the central nervous system of rat. Z. Zellforsch. (in press).

— (1967b): The possible ultrastructural identification of tubero-infundibular dopamine-containing nerve endings in the median eminence of the rat. Brain Res. (in press).

ITURRIZA, F. C. (1966): Monoamines and control of the pars intermedia of the toad pituitary. General and comparative Endocrinology **6**, 19—25.

KNOWLES, F., and H. A. BERN (1966): Function of neurosecretion in endocrine regulation. Nature (Lond.) **210**, 271—272.

LICHTENSTEIGER, W., and H. LANGEMANN (1966): Uptake of exogenous catecholamines by monoamine-containing neurons of the central nervous system: Uptake of catecholamine by arcuato-infundibular neurons. J. Pharm. exptl. Ther. **151**, 400—408.

MAYER, G. (1963): The experimental control of oval implantation. In: Techniques on endocrine researches. (Eds. P. ECKSTEIN, and F. KNOWLES) pp. 245. New York: Academic Press.

MAZZUCA, M. (1965): Structure fine de l'eminence médiane du cobaye. J. microscopie **4**, 225—238.

MEITES, J., and C. NICOLL (1966): Adenohypophysis. Prolactin. Ann. Rev. Physiol. **28**, 57—88.

— C. S. NICOLL, and P. K. TALWALKER (1963): The central nervous system and the secretion and release of prolactin. In: Advances in Neuroendocrinology. (Ed. A. V. NALBANDOV) pp. 238—277. Urbana: University of Illinois Press.

MILINE, R., P. STERN, E. SERSTENEV et M. MUHIBIC (1957): Effet de la réserpine et de la réserpine associée au luminal sur le complex hypothalamo-hypophysaire. In: Psychotropic Drugs. (Eds. S. GARATTINI, and V. GHETTI) pp. 332—349. Amsterdam: Elsevier Publ. Co.

OKSCHE, A. (1961): The fine nervous neurosecretory and glial structure of the median eminence in the white-crowned sparrow. Proc. III. int. Symp. Neurosecretion. (Eds. H. HELLER, and R. B. CLARK) pp. 199—206. London-New York: Academic Press.

OLIVECRONA, H. (1957): Paraventricular nucleus and pituitary gland. Acta physiol. scand. 40, Suppl. 136, 1—178.

RICHARDSON, K. C. (1966): Electron microscopic identification of autonomic nerve endings. Nature (Lond.) 210, 756.

RINNE, U. K. (1966): Ultrastructure of the median eminence of the rat. Z. Zellforsch. 74, 98—122.

SZENTHÁGOTHAI, J., B. FLERKÓ, B. MESS, and B. HALÁSZ (1962): Hypothalamic control of the anterior pituitary. Budapest: Académiai Kiadó.

Stimulus-Secretion Coupling in the Adrenal Medulla and the Neurohypophysis: Cellular Mechanisms of Release of Catecholamines and Posterior Pituitary Hormones

W. W. DOUGLAS

Department of Pharmacology, Albert Einstein College of Medicine, Bronx 10461, New York

One of the most fascinating problems in the field of secretion concerns the nature of regulation of release of the secretory products. How, it may be asked, is a particular cell made to secrete at the appropriate time ? What, indeed, are the cellular events that are initiated on stimulation, and how do these lead to the extrusion of the secretory product ? To these questions, which may be embraced by the term "Stimulus-Secretion Coupling" (DOUGLAS, and RUBIN, 1961a), only partial answers can be given. We know, of course, that most secreting cells are under chemical control. Where the cells receive a secretomotor supply the chemical stimulant (secretagogue) is a neurohumor. Where such nerves are absent, the chemical stimulant is a hormone or "releasing factor". This much is clear; and we have even a fair amount of information on the chemical identity of the various secretagogues. Very little information, however, is available to tell us how these chemical stimuli act at the cellular level. Moreover, the secretory process itself which these stimuli initiate, is usually ill-defined. Most evidence we possess on this particular point derives from histological studies on fixed material which, all too often, allows for a variety of interpretations.

In the last few years my colleagues and I have been attempting to unravel some of the factors involved in stimulus-secretion coupling in various systems with the use of a variety of physiological, pharmacological, biophysical, and biochemical techniques, and my purpose today will be to review for you our principal findings. Our experiments have not been confined to neurosecretory systems, but it so happens that the bulk of evidence we have obtained derives from the mammalian adrenal medulla and neurohypophysis, secretory systems that fall within the province of the present meeting. The neurohypophysis — or, more properly, the hypothalamo-hypophyseal system — is, of course, the classical mammalian neurosecretory system. But the developmental origins of the medullary chromaffin cells certainly entitle them to consideration by those interested in neurosecretion, and because we have much more extensive evidence on events involved in stimulus-secretion coupling in medullary chromaffin cells I intend to describe our findings with this system first, and defer discussion of the more classical (dare I say banal ?) hypothalamo-hypophyseal system.

The Adrenal Medullary Chromaffin Cell

The chromaffin cells of the adrenal meduall have long been known to be supplied by secretomotor nerves in the splanchnic branches of the sympathetic system, and it is now more than 30 years since FELDBERG, MINZ, and TSUDZIMURA, 1934, provided evidence that these nerves are cholinergic, and that acetylcholine is thus the immediate physiological stimulus causing the chromaffin cells to release their hormones (the catecholamines: adrenaline and noradrenaline). The problem with which we are here concerned is how acetylcholine stimulates the chromaffin cells; and how this stimulation leads up to the release of the stored hormones. When Dr. RUBIN and I took up this problem some years ago, we thought that a useful approach might be to explore the possibility that acetylcholine stimulated by some action on the plasma membrane of the chromaffin cell influencing its permeability to the common species of inorganic ions. This seemed to be mechanism of action of acetylcholine at other sites in the body where it acted as the chemical transmitter of nervous activity, i.e. at neuromuscular junctions and nervous synapses. By studying the effects of varying the extracellular concentration of commonly occurring cations we accumulated considerable evidence in favor of this possibility (DOUGLAS and RUBIN, 1961a), but I shall begin by describing recent experiments, involving intracellular recording techniques, that provide more direct evidence that acetylcholine does indeed act on the plasma membrane of the chromaffin cell.

Intracellular recording from chromaffin cells. Intracellular recording has proved to be one of the most valuable techniques for the analysis of mechanisms involved in neurohumoral transmission at a variety of synapses, and it seemed likely that its application to the chromaffin cell would help to define the actions of the transmitter there. It soon became evident, however, that we were unlikely to obtain useful information by applying conventional microelectrode techniques to the whole adrenal gland. In the first place, the medullary cells *in situ* were difficult to impale: not only were the cells very small but they were only loosely suspended in the spongy structure of the medulla and offered a poor target for impalement. Moreover, even when we succeeded in recording from cells in the medullary region of the intact gland, we were left in doubt about whether the potentials recorded came from chromaffin cells. Although it seemed likely that they did, we could not be certain about this for the medulla contains other elements. A means of overcoming these difficulties was found when we succeeded in isolating and maintaining medullary chromaffin cells *in vitro* by techniques adopted from the field of tissue culture. In essence, the successful method involved the dispersal of adrenal medullary cells (from the gerbil, Meriones Unguiculatus) by tissue dissociation techniques, and the subsequent incubation of the free cells in culture chambers containing a "feeder culture" of hamster lung cells to provide essential nutrient factors. After about 10 hours or so, when the cells had become firmly attached to the culture chamber, chromaffin cells were identified by their characteristic size and content of fine granules under high power phase-contrast microcsopy. Control experiments showed that cells identified in this way gave the classical chromaffin reaction when treated with fixatives containing potassium dichromate. The cells we have studied are thus, by definition, medullary chromaffin cells. When chromaffin cells had been identified, they were impaled with glass microelectrodes under direct visual control.

With this method (DOUGLAS, KANNO, and SAMPSON, 1966 and 1967), it was found that the chromaffin cells had a resting potential of about 30 mV inside negative. The potential fell as the potassium concentration of the medium was

12*

raised, indicating that the ratio $[K]_i : [K]_0$ was an important factor contributing to the potential; but sodium also played a part, for there was a clear rise in resting potential when all sodium was removed from the extracellular environment (DOUGLAS, KANNO, and SAMPSON, unpublished). The effect of reducing sodium suggests that permeability may be higher in the chromaffin cell than in, for example, nerves and muscles; and this might account for the somewhat lower value of resting potential found in the chromaffin cell. But more evidence is needed to establish the ionic basis of the transmembrane potential in chromaffin cells. For the present purposes it suffices that the experiment showed the plasma membrane of the chromaffin cell to be polarized with the inside considerably more negative than the outside. The principal finding relevant to stimulus-secretion coupling was that the addition of acetylcholine to the extracellular environment caused a sharp fall in this potential. This depolarizing effect provides unequivocal evidence of an action of acetylcholine on the plasma membrane of the chromaffin cell. Depolarization appears to be mainly the result of an increased permeability to sodium for the effect waned as the sodium in the extracellular environment was replaced with osmotically equivalent amounts of sucrose. But even when $[Na]_0$ was reduced to zero some depolarization in response to acetylcholine persisted. This depolarization increased with increasing concentrations of extracellular calcium, and it can therefore be concluded that acetylcholine also increases the permeability of the plasma membrane to calcium. This corroborates an earlier conclusion drawn from the finding that acetylcholine increases the rate of Ca^{45} uptake in the adrenal medulla (DOUGLAS, and POISNER, 1962a). The microelectrode studies thus provide direct evidence that acetylcholine is acting on the medullary chromaffin cell in much the same way as it acts at other synapses where the innervated structure is a nerve or a muscle, that is to say on the plasma membrane to increase its permeability to commonly occurring species of ions.

The question now is how far these effects go to explaining the stimulant effect of acetylcholine on medullary secretion. It is commonplace that changes in membrane potential are instrumental in regulating activity at other sites of cholinergic transmission. For example, ACh-induced depolarization is the factor initiating impulses in skeletal muscles and sympathetic neurones (the latter are developmental homologues of the chromaffin cell) and impulse formation is the critical link in mediating the functional response of the receptive cells. This prompts the suspicion that the fall in membrane potential observed at the chromaffin cell exposed to acetylcholine may be instrumental in inducing secretion. In harmony with this possibility is the evidence that the chromaffin cells are depolarized by each of a wide variety of medullary stimulants other than acetylcholine (DOUGLAS, KANNO, and SAMPSON, 1967). This group of secretagogues includes not only substances pharmacologically related to acetylcholine, such as nicotine and muscarine (medullary chromaffin cells in the species we have studied contain muscarinic as well as receptors as shown by FELDBERG, MINZ, and TSUDZIMURA, 1934, and by DOUGLAS, and POISNER, 1965a), but also the biogenic amines, histamine and 5-hydroxytryptamine and the polypeptides, bradykinin and angiotensin. The suspicion is further strengthened by the following observations: 1) that drugs (hexamethonium and atropine) known to block the stimulant effect of acetylcholine and related agents on secretion, also block the depolarizing effect of these secretagogues; and, 2) that depolarization increases with increasing concentrations of acetylcholine over a range 3×10^{-6} g/ml to 10^{-3} g/ml, a range where secretion also increases from threshold to near maximal levels (DOUGLAS, KANNO, and SAMPSON, 1966, 1967). However, there are grounds for questioning the functional importance of the fall in membrane potential in the chromaffin cell exposed cell to ACh. Thus, I have mentioned that a reduction in extracellular sodium *reduces* the depolarizing effect of acetylcholine. Yet, from other experiments that I will shortly mention (DOUGLAS, and RUBIN, 1963) we know that such reduction in extracellular sodium *augments* the secretory response. Certainly depolarization is not in itself sufficient to induce secretion, for depolarization in response to acetylcholine (or excess K) persists in Ca-free media (DOUGLAS, KANNO, and SAMPSON, unpublished) where, as we shall see, secretion does not occur. Perhaps, then, we should regard the change in membrane potential on exposure to acetylcholine as being simply the electrical sign of an increased permeability of the plasma membrane, and enquire whether this permeability change may be the critical event. One simple conjecture would then be that the plasma membrane rendered "leaky" by acetylcholine's action allows the escape of catecholamines that are free in the cell sap. But I believe we can dismiss this possibility, for ACh continues to depolarize (i.e. produce the increase in membrane permeability) in a calcium-free environment (DOUGLAS, KANNO, and SAMPSON, unpublished) where, as will be described later, no secretion occurs. Furthermore, there is no escape of catecholamines even on prolonged exposure to calcium-free solutions which, as would be expected on general grounds, render the plasma membrane unduly permeable as evidenced by a progressive fall in membrane potential (DOUGLAS, KANNO, and SAMPSON, unpublished) and by an increased rate of efflux of potassium (DOUGLAS, and POISNER, unpublished). Indeed, the fact that no catecholamines escape in such circumstances calls into question the view of HILLARP, 1960, and others that a significant pool of "free" catecholamines exists within the cell sap (DOUGLAS, 1965b). In seeking an alternative explanation we might next consider whether it is the movement of the commonly occurring cations in response to acetylcholine that is the critical event initiating secretion. Our evidence has indicated that permeability increases to both sodium and calcium when the cell is exposed to acetylcholine, and that these ions then penetrate the plasma membrane by running down their electrochemical gradients from the outside of the cell to the inside. The possibility, then, is that entry of these ions (or one of them) is the factor evoking catecholamine secretion.

Experiments on perfused adrenal glands. Precisely such a conjecture was advanced by DOUGLAS, and RUBIN, 1961a, b, as a result of experiments made on cats' adrenal glands perfused with solutions of different ionic composition. From evidence that acetylcholine failed to evoke secretion in the absence of calcium, and on other grounds, they concluded that acetylcholine might stimulate the chromaffin cell to secrete by causing an influx of calcium ions, and that the appearance of an excess of free calcium ions somewhere in the cell was the factor leading to extrusion of the hormones. Before reviewing the findings relevant to calcium however, I should point out that the experiments offered no evidence that extracellular sodium was needed: acetylcholine continued to act when all sodium in the perfusion medium had been replaced with osmotically equivalent amounts of sucrose. Thus, although the electrophysiological experiments show that the inward (depolarizing) current is mainly carried by sodium ions, with calcium ions contributing less, the movement of sodium ions — and, indeed, the consequent depolarization — does not seem to be contributing to the secretory response. In fact sodium ions exert a depressant effect: in their absence the response to ACh is increased, possibly because (1) there is competition between sodium and calcium for channels of entry, (2) the ionic strength of the medium is critical, (3) hyperpolarization favors secretion (DOUGLAS, and RUBIN, 1963).

What now is the other evidence supporting the possibility that calcium entry initiates secretion? This evidence may be summarized as follows:

1. The effect of the extracellular concentration of calcium is graded: as the concentration of calcium is increased there is a progressive increase in the secretory response to acetylcholine (DOUGLAS, and RUBIN, 1961a).

2. Acetylcholine increases the rate of Ca^{45} uptake in the medulla and the effect increases with the calcium concentration of the perfusion medium (DOUGLAS, and POISNER, 1962a). Evidence that calcium entry in response to ACh increases with increasing $[Ca]_0$ has also been obtained from intracellular recordings showing that depolarization in response to acetylcholine increases as $[Ca]_0$ is increased: in these experiments Ca^{++} was the only extracellular cation (DOUGLAS, KANNO, and SAMPSON, unpublished).

3. Calcium is required, not only for the stimulant effect of acetylcholine, but also for the stimulant effect of each of a number of adrenal secretagogues of widely different chemical structure. These include not only other ACh-like drugs such as nicotine, DMPP and carbachol (DOUGLAS, and RUBIN, 1961b), but also the biogenic amines, histamine and 5-hydroxytryptamine, and the polypeptides, bradykinin and angiotensin (POISNER, and DOUGLAS, 1966). These different classes of drugs are known to be able to promote calcium entry into various tissues, such as smooth muscle (DANIEL, 1964). There is no doubt that these various secretagogues increase membrane permeability of the chromaffin cell to common cations, for they all depolarize chromaffin cells (DOUGLAS, KANNO, and SAMPSON, 1967).

4. Calcium is required when stimulation is evoked by raising the potassium concentration of the extracellular environment (DOUGLAS, and RUBIN, 1961a). Excess K is effective in concentrations far below that required to depolarize the cell completely (DOUGLAS, KANNO, and SAMPSON, 1966) indicating that stimulation occurs when the concentration of extracellular potassium is lower than that within the cell. This makes it unlikely that the rise in extracellular potassium stimulates by altering the internal environment of the cell. It seems more probable that the effect is due to the fall in membrane potential produced by the change in the ratio $[K]_i : [K]_0$ with a consequent increase in membrane permeability leading to calcium influx. An increased influx of Ca^{45} in response to a rise in $[K]_0$ has been demonstrated in the medulla (DOUGLAS, and POISNER, 1961).

The ability to act on the plasma membrane of the chromaffin cell, to depolarize it and induce calcium entry is the only property, as far as we can discern, that is shared by potassium and the chemically diverse secretagogues we have studied.

5. Calcium itself, in the absence of any of the familiar secretagogues, (such as acetylcholine) can be shown to be an effective medullary secretagogue in conditions where the permeability of the plasma membrane of the chromaffin cell is

increased, and where calcium may be supposed to have relatively easy access to the cell interior. The stimulant effect of calcium can be shown by simply withdrawing calcium from the extracellular environment for a sufficient period of time and then reintroducing it. As would be expected on general grounds (HEILBRUNN, 1956; MORRILL, KABACK, and ROBBINS, 1964), the adrenal cells become leaky after prolonged calcium deprivation as witnessed by increased K efflux (DOUGLAS, and POISNER, unpublished) and by progressive depolarization (DOUGLAS, KANNO, and SAMPSON, unpublished). When calcium is reintroduced under such conditions there is a violent secretory response that passes off within a few minutes as the cell recovers its normal relative impermeability to calcium. A diagram depicting the supposed sequence of events will be found elsewhere (DOUGLAS, 1965a). I would emphasize that there is no leakage of catecholamines from the calcium deprived cell even although it is leaky to the common cations.

6. The simple addition of barium to the perfusion fluid is sufficient to evoke catecholamine secretion. The effect is a direct one on the chromaffin cells and, unlike the stimulant effect of calcium, can be shown readily in the normal cell without recourse to calcium deprivation. It has been suggested that barium owes its stimulant effect to the relative ease with which it penetrates cell membranes; and the phenomenon thus supports the idea that secretion is normally induced by the activation of some sensitive to alkaline earth metals, normally, of course, calcium. Barium, I should point out, evokes intense secretion even in calcium-free media. It is the only secretagogue we have studied that does so (DOUGLAS, and RUBIN, 1964).

7. Secretion in response to acetylcholine, or the other medullary secretagogues we have tested, is powerfully inhibited by magnesium; and this alkaline earth metal can be shown to be an antagonist of calcium-induced secretion in the chromaffin cell (DOUGLAS, and RUBIN, 1963).

In conclusion then, the evidence obtained from the perfused adrenal glands and the isolated chromaffin cells provides strong grounds for the view (DOUGLAS, and RUBIN, 1961a, b) that acetylcholine owes its stimulant effect on the chromaffin cell to some action exerted on the plasma membrane that increases the permeability of the membrane to calcium, and that calcium, running down its electrochemical gradient to some strategic site in the cell, *(which need be no further than the inner surface of the plasma membrane)*, then initiates the process that leads to catecholamine release.

If the above conclusion is correct, then the next step would be to identify this calcium-dependent link. In any event, it is clear that we can make no significant progress until the cellular mechanism for extrusion of catecholamines has been identified. The theories of morphologists, physiologists, pharmacologists, biochemists, and others, on the mechanism of release of the adrenal medullary hormones present an awesome variety of alternatives. The suggestions have ranges all the way from a holocrine type of secretion to simple leakage of free amines a cross the plasma membrane (for references see DOUGLAS, 1965a). In recent years it has come to be accepted that extrusion of amines occurs without disruption of the cell, and conjecture has centered on the newer evidence concerning the mechanisms of intracellular storage of amines where, from the results of cell fractionation and differential centrifugation on the one hand, and electron microscopy on the other, it has become evident that the bulk of catecholamines in chromaffin cell is lodged in membrane-limited granules distributed throughout the cytoplasm. These "chromaffin granules" appear to be limited by a lipid membrane of the commonly occurring type. Just how much of the catecholamines within the chromaffin cell is lodged in such granules is uncertain. On cell fractionation and differential centrifugation about 75% of the catecholamines may be recovered in the granule fraction and the rest is extragranular. While it seems likely that some at least of the extragranular catecholamines ("free" catecholamine) is an artefact of the fractionation procedure and represents material that has escaped from granules, it has been argued that a significant amount of catecholamines is free normally in the cytoplasm of the cell (HILLARP, 1960). A further complexity is introduced by evidence that the granules themselves are of different types. The most common type is characterized by its extremely high content of adenine nucleotides, principally ATP. The molar ratio of nucleotide to catecholamines is about 1 : 4, a value at which the opposing charges on the two substances balance one another and which therefore suggests that the function of the nucleotide is to combine with the catecholamine and retain it within the granule as acomplex (BLASCHKO, 1958). According to HILLARP, 1960, however, some of the chromaffin granules are devoid of ATP and the catecholamines must be held in some other form there. The problem that confronts us then is to find out which of these three "pools" of catecholamines is immediately involved (i.e. drawn on) when the chromaffin cell is exposed to acetylcholine; and, hopefully, once that has been done, to learn just how this pool is tapped.

In casting around for an approach to this problem it seemed to us that a search for substances escaping along with the catecholamines might be rewarding. Particularly it seemed worthwhile seeking adenine nucleotides. In the first place, as I have mentioned, these substances are present in enormous concentration in the principal amine pool, the so-called "heavy" chromaffin granule, secondly, there was already evidence that the level of adenine nucleotide in adrenal glands subjected to stimulation was low (CARLSSON, HILLARP, and HÖKFELT, 1957) — and the fate of the adenine nucleotide was unknown and, third, there were available highly sensitive methods for the measurement of ATP and related substances based on the use of firefly luciferase. When we examined the venous effluent from cats' adrenal glands perfused with Locke's solution we soon found that massive amounts of AMP appeared along with the catecholamines on exposure to acetylcholine, and that the efflux of AMP was highly correlated with that of the catecholamines. This suggested that the classical nucleotide-rich chromaffin granules were immediately involved in the acute secretory response and encouraged us (DOUGLAS, and POISNER, 1966a) to perform another series of experiments where we measured other nucleotides. We found, in addition to AMP, considerable amounts of adenosine, smaller amounts of ADP and traces of ATP; and when the balance sheet was drawn up, the molar ratio of catecholamines to ATP plus metabolites turned out to be 4 : 1, i.e. a ratio corresponding closely with that found in the "heavy" chromaffin granules of the cat (HILLARP, and THIEME, 1959). Furthermore, when measurements were made on successive drops of venous effluent escaping in the few seconds before and after beginning stimulation, it became evident that the time courses of efflux of the nucleotides and the catecholamines were similar. We were led to conclude that the nucleotide-rich chromaffin granules are the pool of amines that the cell draws uppon when it is stimulated. It may yet turn out that granules of this sort are the only significant repository of amines in the normal intact cell. There is no convincing evidence that the "light" (ATP-free) granules or the "free" cytoplasmic amines have any existence other than in the homogenizer and ultracentrifuge.

Although the main purpose of the experiments just described was to identify the intracellular source of catecholamines that is tapped by stimulation, the findings also offered us a possible approach to the second of the two questions confronting us, namely "How does acetylcholine draw on the pool involved?" Thus, the nucleotide we had found in the venous effluent from the stimulated gland, while equivalent in *amount* to that present in the chromaffin granules with a corresponding amount of catecholamine, was different in *composition*. Although most of the nucleotide in the chromaffin granules is ATP (HILLARP, and THIEME, 1959), only very small amounts of ATP were present in the adrenal venous effluent — there was much more AMP, adenosine and ATP. The presence of these breakdown products of ADP at once raises the question whether hydrolysis of the ATP within the granules may occur on stimulation and, by breaking down the catecholamine-ATP complex, lead to the release of these substances. Just such a hypothesis was advanced by HILLARP, 1958, some years ago. He had then made the discovery of an ATPase associated with the chromaffin granules (seemingly in their membranes) — a finding recently corroborated by BANKS, 1965 — and he proposed that during stimulation this ATPase might somehow be activated, hydrolyse the intracellular ATP and thus free the granule amines to diffuse out of the granule and through the cytoplasm and plasma membrane to the outside of the cell. HILLARP's proposal was, to us, a most exciting one, for we possessed two additional pieces of evidence consistent with it: first, we had found metabolites of ATP in the effluent from the secreting adrenal gland; and, second, our evidence indicated that ACh acted by promoting calcium influx into the cell and calcium was known to activate various ATPases. All at once, it seemed that that the pieces of the puzzle were falling together and that we had in our grasp the molecular basis of catecholamine secretion. Unfortunately, it was not long before the cold winds of contrary evidence chilled our enthusisam for this attractive biochemical scheme, for we soon found (as we should have suspected on general grounds) that if we added ATP to the perfusion medium it was almost all broken down of passage through the adrenal blood vessels; indeed, the pattern of metabolites resembled closely that escaping from the glands stimulated with ACh (DOUGLAS, POISNER, and RUBIN, 1965; DOUGLAS, and POISNER, 1966a). Clearly then, the presence of ATP metabolites in the effluent from the ACh-stimulated gland could not be taken as evidence that ATP splitting occurred within the chromaffin cells. These metabolites could equally well have resulted from breakdown of ATP after its release, presumably by phosphatases known to be present in blood vessels. Our colleague, Dr. ALEX B. NOVI-KOFF (personal communication) kindly demonstrated for us such enzymes in the adrenal vasculature by histochemical techniques. The next line of experiment was obvious: we should contrive somehow to inhibit the vascular phosphatases and repeat the experiments with ACh. None of the enzyme inhibitors we tried, however, was satisfactory. All caused a violent discharge of catecholamines. We had thus to abandon this approach. A simple, although not entirely satisfactory, alternative presented itself when we found that we could inhibited the responsible vascular enzymes by omitting calcium and magnesium from the perfusion medium and adding to it a small amount of EDTA. Under such conditions ATP largely survived perfusion through the adrenal glands, Since ACh is ineffective in evoking catecholamine secretion when calcium is absent from the extracellular environment we set up secretion with barium. In these experiments the pattern of nucleotides recovered along with the amines in the venous effluent on stimulation was quite different. Massive amounts of ATP, unhydrolysed, appeared along with the catecholamines and there was relatively little of the ATP metabolites. If we are correct in our view that barium stimulates by activating the normally calcium-receptive link and thus sets in motion the same mechanism as does acetylcholine, then it may be concluded that splitting of ATP within the chromaffin granules is not a key event in the normal release mechanism (DOUGLAS, and POISNER (1966 b). It seems curious that the chromaffin cell amasses extraordinary high amounts of ATP only to discard it intact, as a byproduct of catecholamine secretion: but nature is frequently prodigal in the means deployed to achieve particular ends.

Although these experiments have failed to explain *how* the ATP-rich chromaffin granules are made to release their contents when the cell is stimulated, they do suggest *where* release occurs. Thus it seems improbable that release is from the granule to the cytoplasm. If it were, then one would surely expect that much of the ATP released would be hydrolysed by the several sources of ATPase (BANKS, 1965) that are present there; and the remaining ATP would not be expected to traverse the plasma membrane so readily as to maintain the observed ratio of ATP : catecholamines found in the venous effluent. Rather it would seem more plausible that release from the granules occurs at the cell surface in such a way that the secreted substances are delivered directly to the cell exterior by some process such as reverse micropinocytosis (exocytosis), as hinted at in the electron micrographs of DE ROBERTIS and VAZ FERREIRA, 1957; DE ROBERTIS, and SABATINI, 1960, and COUPLAND, 1965. This conclusion (DOUGLAS, and POISNER, 1966 b) has been reinforced by recent elegant experiments in which protein characteristic of the catecholamine granules has been demonstrated in the effluent from stimulated adrenal glands by immuno assay techniques (BANKS, and HELLE, 1966). Using a less sensitive methode for protein measurement, Dr. POISNER and I (DOUGLAS, and POISNER, 1965 b) had noted that protein efflux from the adrenal gland during acetylcholine's action was sufficiently low that we could exclude some of the grosser forms of secretion favored in some light microscope studies (see DOUGLAS, 1965 a), but the method was not sensitive enough, nor specific enough, to give a satisfactory answer about extrusion of "granule" protein. A further insight into the cellular events involved in catecholamine extrusion may well come from examination of the effluent from secreting glands for other substances. Already an unsaturated hydroxy-carboxylic acid, prostaglandin $F_{1\alpha}$, has been detected there (RAMWELL, SHAW, DOUGLAS, and POISNER, 1966) and this raises a number of questions about lipid metabolism related to secretion. It is of interest that the adrenal medulla is exceptionally rich in lysolecithin (HAJDU, WEISS, and TITUS, 1957; DOUGLAS, POISNER, and TRIFARO, 1966) and that much of this seems to be associated with the chromaffin granules (BLASCHKO, FIREMARK, SMITH, and WINK-

LER, 1966). It is conceivable that phospholipase activation may be involved in catecholamine secretion (RAMWELL, SHAW, DOUGLAS, and POISNER, 1966), but the evidence at present is no more than to hint at such a possibility. It must be concluded that we have no satisfactory explanation of the biochemical events responsible for amine extrusion. The evidence I have reviewed, however, suggests that the following factors are involved in stimulus-secretion coupling: (1) an action of acetylcholine on the plasma membrane of the cell that results in entry of calcium ions. (2) The activation of some calcium-dependent process which (3) leads to the release of amines from the ATP-rich granules at the surface of the cell by some process akin to reverse micropinocytosis.

The Neurohypophysis

I need not remind this audience that the hypothalamo-hypophyseal system shares a common (although, admittedly, remote) developmental heritage with the adrenal medulla. And, further, that the pituitary hormones are stored (at least in large part) in membrane-limited granules, the so-called elementary granules, not unlike the chromaffin granules. It was these considerations that suggested the possibility that stimulus-secretion coupling in the hypothalamo-hypophyseal system, might involve links similar to those that were them emerging from the work on the adrenal gland. At first sight the hypothalamo-hypophyseal system seemed to be much less favorable than the adrenal gland for studies of the sort needed to explore this possibility: the system seemed so inaccessible. However, this notion was rapidly dispelled when it was found that the neurohypophysis could be extirpated (from rats) to yield a preparation responsive to stimulation *in vitro*. When, in the very first experiments, it became evident that secretion (as indicated by vasopressin release into the incubation medium) was calcium-dependent, it seemed likely that calcium entry might again be the factor responsible for releasing the stored hormones (DOUGLAS, 1963). In the experiments just referred to, secretion was evoked by raising the extracellular potassium concentration ten-fold, a procedure adopted with the purpose of mimicking the depolarizing effect of impulses discharged down the hypothalamo-hypophyseal tract. Although it was not then established that such impulses did occur or did normally provide the immediate physiological stimulus for release of the posterior pituitary hormones, evidence existed that at least some neurosecretory cells were capable of generating impulses, and impulse conduction along other neurosecretory axons had been demonstrated (see BERN, 1962). That impulses did provide the stimulus for secretion thus seemed likely on general grounds (see HARRIS, 1960). The scheme seemed still more probable when it was found that the isolated neurohypophysis secreted briskly when stimulated electrically (DOUGLAS, and POISNER, 1964a). Further support for the "calcium-entry" hypothesis came from experiments showing that depolarization (by excess K) caused an increased uptake of Ca[45] into the neurohypophysis (DOUGLAS, and POISNER, 1964b); that secretion in response to a rise in extracellular K (DOUGLAS, and POISNER, 1964a) or electrical impulses (MIKITEN, and DOUGLAS, 1966) varies with the calcium concentration of the extracellular environment over a wide range and is inhibited by magnesium; and that calcium has a stimulant effect on secretion when introduced during incubation with calcium-free media rich in potassium (DOUGLAS, and POISNER, 1964a).

By way of emphasizing the importance of calcium and providing some evidence of the specificity of its action, I should like now to contrast its effects with those of sodium. It may be reasonably supposed that impulse propagation in the hypo-thalamo-hypophyseal tract is mediated by currents carried principally by sodium, as is true in other axons. Hence a massive influx of sodium ions may be expected to occur at the neurosecretory terminals with the arrival of each impulse. However, secretion in response to excess K persists when all sodium is omitted from the extracellular environment. Indeed, the secretory response to potassium is then strikingly potentiated (DOUGLAS, and POISNER, 1964a) just as it is in the adrenal gland — and possibly for one or other of the reasons I have already advanced. Thus it is evident that sodium entry is not directly linked to extrusion of the pituitary hormones, and it seems likely that the role of sodium in the system is to assure the propagation of impulses from the perikarya to the neurosecretory terminals and the depolarization of these terminals. Depolarization, to judge from the experiments with high $[K]_0$ would then suffice to drive calcium into the terminals and initiate secretion.

Since there are close parallels between the results yielded by the neurohypophysis and those yielded by the adrenal medulla, a particular interest attaches to the suggestion that acetylcholine may be involved in the release of posterior pituitary hormones *at the level of the neurosecretory terminals*. According to this conjecture (ABRAHAM, KOELLE, and SMART, 1957; KOELLE, 1962; KOELLE, and GEESE, 1961) the wave of excitation reaching the neurosecretory terminals would first liberate acetylcholine which would then, in turn, liberate the posterior pituitary hormones much as acetylcholine liberates catecholamines from the chromaffin cells — with the important difference that the secretagogue (ACh) and the hormones (the pituitary hormones) are in this instance both supposed to derive from the same cell. A similar suggestion has also been put forward by GERSCHENFELD, TRAMEZZANI, and DE ROBERTIS, 1960. However, it is apparent that these conjectures are based on rather slender evidence: namely, that some cholinesterase activity is present in the hypothalamo-hypophyseal tract, and that the neurosecretory terminals contain clear vesicles reminiscent of those found in cholinergic nerves. Pharmacological tests performed on the isolated neurohypophysis have provided no evidence to support the scheme: ACh and related drugs failed to stimulate secretion of hormones; the anticholinesterase, eserine, had no discernible effect, and acetylcholine-blocking drugs — with the exception of atropine in high dose — did not inhibit release evoked by potassium or electrical stimulation (DOUGLAS, and POISNER, 1964a; MIKITEN, 1966). Unless more convincing evidence is advanced to support the conjecture that acetylcholine is involved at the terminals, it seems preferable to favor the simpler hypothesis that the steps involved in release of the posterior pituitary hormones are as follows: (1) arrival of impulses down the hypothalamo-hypophyseal tract, (2) depolarization of the neurosecretory terminals by these impulses, (3) influx of calcium ions across the plasma membrane as a result of depolarization, (4) activation of some calcium-dependent process leading to hormone extrusion.

Although this "calcium-dependent" process could be associated with the peculiarity of storage of the posterior pituitary hormones (evidence has recently been provided to show that calcium can lead to dissociation of these hormones from neurophysin (SMITH, M. W., and N. A. THORN, 1965); it seems more likely that the role of calcium in the intact neurohypophysis (and in the adrenal medulla) is concerned with some more general phenomenon common to secreting cells that "package" their secretions in membrane-limited granules. The fact that calcium is also required for extrusion of proteins from exocrine glands (e.g. the salivary glands) favours this hypothesis and offers an additional hint that this phenomenon may be reverse micropinocytosis (Douglas, and Poisner, 1962b, 1963). Since measurement of substances released along with the catecholamines has helped to define the mechanism of hormone release from the chromaffin cell, a similar approach to the neurohypophysis may prove rewarding: if, for example, it is found that neurophysin (a very bulky substance) escapes on stimulation, this would provide strong grounds for supposing that secretion involves reverse micropinocytosis or some similar process.

References

ABRAHAMS, V. C., G. B. KOELLE, and P. SMART (1957): Histochemical demonstration of cholinesterases in the hypothalamus of the dog. J. Physiol. 139, 137—144.

BANKS, P. (1965): The adenosine triphosphatase activity of adrenal chromaffin granules. Biochem. J. 95, 490—496.

BLASCHKO, H. (1958): The development of current concepts of catecholamine formation. In: Symp. on Catecholamines; held October 16—18, 1958. Pharmacol. Rev. 11, (1959), pp. 307—316.

— H. FIREMARK, A. D. SMITH, and H. WINKLER (1966): Phospholipids and cholesterol in particulate fractions of adrenal medulla. Biochem. J. 98, 24 P.

BERN, H. A. (1962): The properties of neurosecretory cells. Gen. comp. Endocr. Suppl. 1, 117—132.

CARLSSON, A., N.-Å. HILLARP, and B. HÖKFELT (1957): The concomitant release of adenosine triphosphate and catechol amines from the adrenal medulla. J. biol. Chem. 227, 243—252.

COUPLAND, R. E. (1965): Electron microscopic observations on the structure of the rat adrenal medulla. I. Ultrastructure and organization of chromaffin cells in the normal medulla. J. Anat. (Lond.) 99, 231—254.

DANIEL, E. E. (1964): Effect of drugs on contractions of vertebrate smooth muscle. Ann. Rev. Pharmacol. 4, 189—222.

DE ROBERTIS, E. D. P., and D. D. SABATINI (1950): Submicroscopic analysis of the secretory process in the adrenal medulla. Fed. Proc. 19, 70—78.

—, and A. VAZ FERREIRA (1957): Electron microscope study of the excretion of catechol-containing droplets in the adrenal medulla. Exp. Cell Res. 12, 568—574.

DOUGLAS, W. W. (1963): A possible mechanism of neurosecretion: release of vasopressin by depolarization and its dependence on calcium. Nature (Lond.) 197, 81—82.

— (1965a): Calcium-dependent links in stimulus-secretion coupling in the adrenal medulla and neurohypophysis. In: Mechanisms of release of Biogenic Amines. A symposium held in Stockholm, Feb. 21—24, 1965, pp. 267—290. Oxford: Pergamon Press 1966.

— (1965b): The mechanism of release of catecholamines from the adrenal medulla. Symp. on Catecholamines, Milano, 1965. Pharmacol. Rev. 18 (1966), pp. 471—480.

— T. KANNO, and S. R. SAMPSON (1966): Intracellular recording from adrenal chromaffin cells: effects of acetylcholine, hexamethonium and potassium on membrane potentials. Proc. Physiol. Soc., July 15, 1966, p. 57—58.

— — — (1967): Effects of acetylcholine and other medullary secretagogues and antagonists on the membrane potential of adrenal chromaffin cells: an analysis employing techniques of tissue culture. J. Physiol. (in press).

—, and A. M. POISNER (1961): Stimulation of uptake of ^{45}Ca in the adrenal gland by acetylcholine. Nature (Lond.) 192, 1299.

— — (1962a): On the mode of action of acetylcholine in evoking adrenal medullary secretion: increased uptake of calcium during the secretory response. J. Physiol. 162, 385—392.

— — (1962b): Importance of calcium for acetylcholine evoked salivary secretion. Nature (Lond.) 196, 379—380.

Douglas, W. W. (1963): The influence of calcium on the secretory response of the submaxillary gland to acetylcholine or to noradrenaline. J. Physiol. **165**, 528—541.
— — (1964a): Stimulus-secretion coupling in a neurosecretory organ: the role of calcium in the release of vasopressin from the neurohypophysis. J. Physiol. **172**, 1—18.
— — (1964b): Calcium movement in the neurohypophysis of the rat and its relation to the release of vasopressin. J. Physiol. **172**, 19—30.
— — (1965a): Preferential release of adrenaline from the adrenal medulla by muscarine and pilocarpine. Nature (Lond.) **208**, 1102—1103.
— — (1965b): Efflux of adenine nucleotides and their derivatives and of protein from adrenal glands during stimulation of the splanchnic nerve or exposure to acetylcholine. XXIII International Congress of Physiological Sciences, Tokyo, September, 1965. Abstracts: p. 484.
— — (1966a): Evidence that the secreting adrenal medullary chromaffin cell releases catecholamines directly from ATP-rich granules. J. Physiol. **183**, 236—248.
— — (1966b): On the relation between ATP splitting and secretion in the adrenal chromaffin cell: extrusion of ATP (unhydrolyzed) during release of catecholamines. J. Physiol. **183**, 249—256.
— —, and R. P. Rubin (1965): Efflux of adenine nucleotides from perfused adrenal glands exposed to nicotine and other chromaffin cell stimulants. J. Physiol. **179**, 130—137.
— —, and J. M. Trifaro (1966): Lysolecithin and other phospholipids in the adrenal medulla of various species. Life Sci. **5**, 809—815.
—, and R. P. Rubin (1961a): The role of calcium in the secretory response of the adrenal medulla to acetylcholine. J. Physiol. **159**, 40—57.
— — (1961b): Mechanism of nicotinic action at the adrenal medulla: calcium as a link in stimulus-secretion coupling. Nature (Lond.) **192**, 1087—1089.
— — (1963): The mechanism of catecholamine release from the adrenal medulla and the role of calcium in stimulus-secretion coupling. J. Physiol. **167**, 288—310.
— — (1964): Stimulant action of barium on the adrenal medulla. Nature (Lond.) **203**, 305—307.
Feldberg, W., B. Minz, and H. Tsudzimura (1934): The mechanism of the nervous discharge of adrenaline. J. Physiol. **81**, 286—304.
Harris, G. W. (1960): Central control of pituitary secretion. In: Handbook of Physiology. Section I. Neurophysiology, vol. II. Chapter XXXIX. pp. 1007—1038. Washington: Amer. Phys. Soc.
Hajdu, S., H. Weiss, and E. Titus (1957): The isolation of cardiac active principle from mammalian tissue. J. Pharmacol. **120**, 99—113.
Heilbrunn, L. V. (1956): The Dynamics of Living Protoplasm. 1st ed., pp. 32 etc. New York: Academic Press.
Hillarp, N.-Å. (1958): Enzymic systems involving adenosinephosphates in the adrenaline and noradrenaline containing granules of the adrenal medulla. Acta physiol. scand. **42** 144—165.
— (1960): Different pools of catecholamines stored in the adrenal medulla. Acta physiol. scand. **50**, 8—22.
—, and G. Thieme (1959): Nucleotides in the catecholamine granules of the adrenal medulla. Acta physiol. scand. **45**, 328—338.
Koelle, G. B. (1962): A new general concept of the neurohumoral functions of acetylcholine and acetylcholinesterase. J. Pharm. (Lond.) **14**, 65—90.
—, and C. N. Geesey (1961): Localization of acetylcholinesterase in the neurohypophysis and its functional implications. Proc. Soc. exp. Biol. (N. Y.) **106**, 625—628.
Mikiten, T. M. (1966): The effect of acetylcholine antagonists and eserine on the release of vasopressin from isolated neurohypophysis. Fed. Proc. **25**, 2 part 1., 253.
—, and W. W. Douglas (1965): Effect of calcium and other ions on vasopressin release from rat neurohypophysis stimulated electrically in vitro. Nature (Lond.) **207**, 302.
Morrill, G. E., H. R. Kaback, and E. Robbins (1964): Effect of calcium on intracellular sodium and potassium concentrations in plant and animal cells. Nature (Lond.) **204**, 641—642.
Ramwell, P. W., J. E. Shaw, W. W. Douglas, and A. M. Poisner (1966): Efflux of prostaglandin from adrenal glands stimulated with acetylcholine. Nature (Lond.) **210**, 273—274.
Smith, M. W., and N. A. Thorn (1965): The effects of calcium on protein-binding and metabolism of arginine-vasopressin in rats. J. Endocr. **32**, 141—151.

Localisation d'amines biogènes dans le système neurovégétatif périphérique. (Etude radioautographique en microscopie électronique après injection de noradrénaline-^{3}H et de 5-hydroxytryptophane-^{3}H.)

J. Taxi et B. Droz

Laboratoire de Cytologie, Faculté des Sciences, Paris, Centre de Microscopie électronique appliquée à la Biologie, C. N. R. S., Paris, et Département de Biologie, C. E. A., Saclay

La détection histochimique des amines biogènes par la microscopie de fluorescence a fait récemment des progrès remarquables, tant dans le système nerveux central que périphérique, grâce à la méthode de Falck, 1962.

Cette technique donne des résultats remarquables pour l'étude de la distribution topographique des catécholamines dans les organes, mais elle ne permet pas de connaitre les caractères structuraux des cellules ou parties de cellules repérées, dont on ne voit qu'une silhouette fluorescente.

Par contre, la radioautographie combinée à la microscopie électronique offre la possibilité d'étudier la localisation et le renouvellement de ces substances dans les ultrastructures cellulaires intactes, permettant de traduire en termes de structure la masse impressionnante de données établies par les études de fractionnements biochimiques (voir en particulier les revues récentes d'Axelrod, 1965; et de Wurtman, 1965).

La détection radioautographique des amines biogènes peut être pratiquée de deux façons:

— soit après l'injection d'un *précurseur* marqué du médiateur, dont on décèle ensuite les *produits* auxquels il a donné naissance. Ainsi, après injection de 5-hydroxytryptophane-^{3}H comme précurseur, la 5-hydroxytryptamine (sérotonine) peut être décelée par radioautographie (Gershon et coll., 1965).

— soit l'injection directe du médiateur marqué. Whitby, Axelrod et Weil-Malherbe, 1961, ont en effet montré l'aptitude des fibres adrénergiques à capter et stocker la noradrenaline du milieu intérieur.

Sur la base des données de Wolfe, Potter, Richardson et Axelrod, 1962, nous avons repris l'étude des modalités du captage et du stockage de la noradrénaline-^{3}H dans les fibres les nerveuses de l'épiphyse, puis nous avons étendu ces observations au canal déférent, au ganglion cervical supérieur, à l'intestin.

Matériel et méthodes

Des rats mâles de 120 g ont reçu une injection dans la veine cave supérieure de 5-mCi de DL-noradrénaline-7^{3}H (ac. spécif. 10,1 Ci/mM.). Les animaux ont été sacrifiés 2 min, 30 min et 5 heures après l'injection. Une autre expérience a été faite avec le 5-HTP-³H (ac. spécif. 2,45 Ci/mM.) injecté dans les mêmes conditions.

Sur un rat traité par la noradrénaline-³H, on a fait agir la réserpine dans les conditions suivantes: 30 min après l'injection de noradrénaline-³H, un canal déférent a été prélevé comme témoin, puis immédiatement après on a injecté 5 mg/kg de réserpine; l'animal a été sacrifié 3 heures après.

Les pièces prélevées ont été fixées soit par le tétroxyde d'osmium à 2%, tamponné selon Palade au véronal-acétate de sodium, soit par le glutaraldéhyde à 5% selon Miller, 1962, suivi de tétroxide d'osmium.

Les pièces ont été incluses dans l'araldite ou dans l'épon. Les coupes, recueillies sur un film de collodion porté par une lame de verre, sont contrastées à l'acétate d'uranyle (20 min), suivi ou non de citrate de plomb (10 min); puis on les recouvre d'une pellicule de carbone. Elles sont enfin recouvertes d'émulsion Ilford L4 ou Gevaert NUC 307, selon la technique de Granboulan, 1965.

Résultats

A) Noradrénaline-³H.

a) Epiphyse. Deux minutes après l'injection, le marquage des faisceaux nerveux est remarquablement intense. Il est nettement moindre au bout de 30 min, puis n'apparait plus modifié de façon nette entre 30 min et 5 heures après l'injection.

Les grains d'argent sont localisés sur les faisceaux nerveux, nombreux dans les lacunes de l'épiphyse. Ils sont situés aussi bien sur des fibres associées à une cellule de Schwann que sur des fibres nues (dépourvues de satellite schwannien) abondantes à ce niveau (fig. 1). Un nombre important des ces dernières se rencontre également au sein même du parenchyme épiphysaire, représentant selon toute vraisemblance les «terminaisons» (au sens physiologique du terme), bien qu'aucune différenciation ne permette de reconnaître des zones synaptiques sur la base des critères connus pour d'autres tissus. Le seul dispositif rencontré suggérant des rapports fonctionnels est une gouttière déprimant la surface de certaines cellules pinéales, dans laquelle est logée une fibre nerveuse, les deux membranes plasmiques étant séparées par un espace de l'ordre de 200 Å.

Les fibres marquées contiennent des vésicules de 300 à 600 Å de diamètre dont une proportion variable, mais toujours importante, contient un granule dense Après injection de réserpine, les vésicules apparaissent vides dans la plupart des fibres, comme l'avaient observé Pellegrino de Iraldi et de Robertis, 1961. Quelques fibres cependant présentent encore quelques vésicules à granules dense, marquées de un ou deux grains d'argent. Il faut signaler pour finir que quelques rares fibres ne paraissent avoir été affectées ni dans leur contenu vésiculaire ni dans leur marquage.

b) Canal déférent. Sur les fibres nerveuses du canal déférent, tant dans les faisceaux que dans les fibres isolées (fig. 3A), un marquage tout à fait comparable à celui de l'épiphyse a été observé.

c) Ganglion cervical supérieur. On sait depuis le travail de Kappers, 1960, que c'est dans le ganglion cervical supérieur que siègent les périkaryons des fibres nerveuses de l'épiphyse. Nous avons nous-même constaté la disparition ou l'

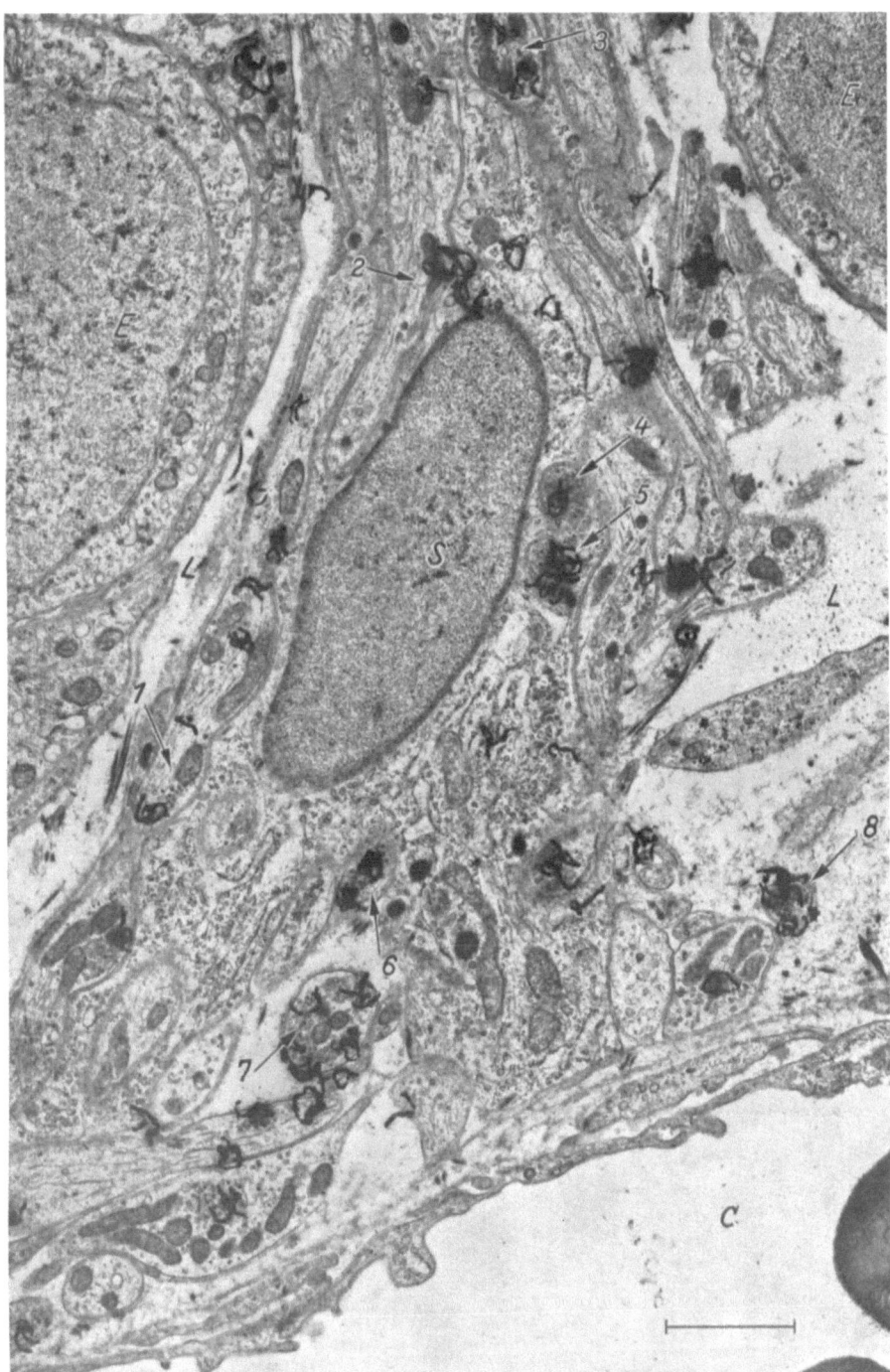

Fig. 1. ($\times$ 20.000) Epiphyse de Rat. Deux minutes après injection de noradrénaline [3]H. De nombreuses fibres sont marquées. Les fibres *1, 2, 3, 4, 5, 6*, entre autres, appartiennent à une «fibre amyélinique composée» centrée sur la cellule schwannienne de noyau (*S*). La fibre *7* est partiellement indépendante. La fibre *8* est totalement nue, entourée seulement d'une membrane basale. *E* = cellules épiphysaires. *L* = lacunes, toujours très développées dans l'épiphyse après fixation osmiée. *C* = capillaire sanguin

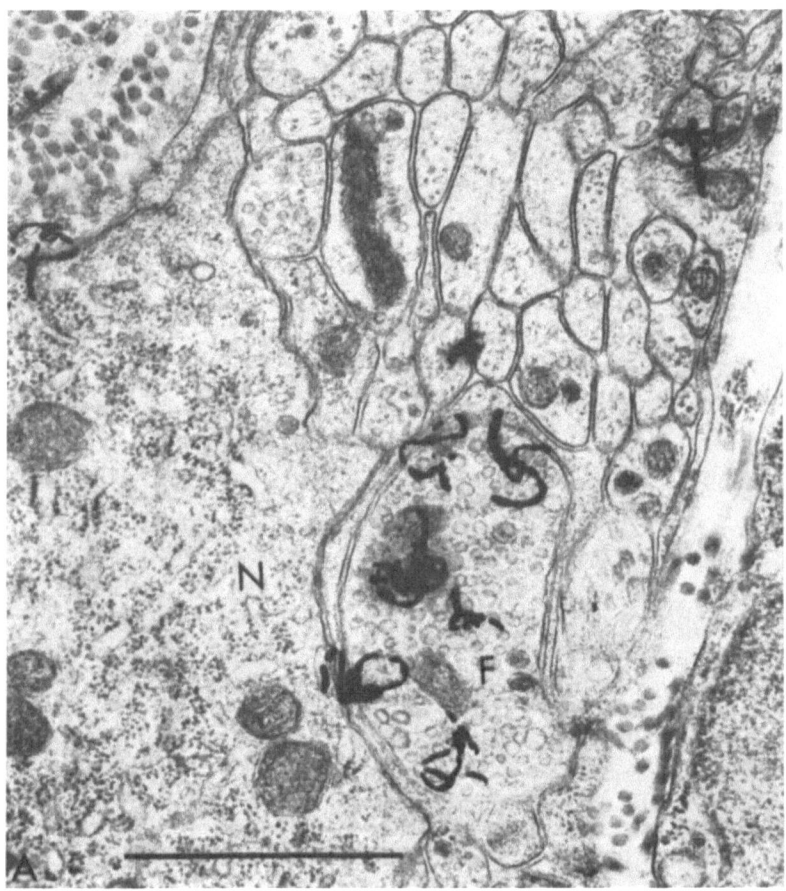# 194 J. TAXI et B. DROZ:

altération des fibres nerveuses dans l'épiphyse huit jours après la section bilatérale des nerfs postganglionnaires issus du ganglion cervical supérieur.

Cependant le marquage des périkaryons est ici extrêmement pauvre et probablement dénué de signification. Les rares localisations qui ont pu être observées concernaient des fibres contenant quelques vésicules à granule dense, probablement des dendrites.

d) Intestin. Dans la musculeuse circulaire, la seule qui chez le Rat possède une innervation intramusculaire (TAXI, 1965), les fibres nerveuses se montrent dépourvues de tout marquage.

Les seules fibres nerveuses marquées dans l'intestin sont situées d'une part dans la sous-muqueuse, d'autre part dans les plexus d'AUERBACH et de MEISSNER.

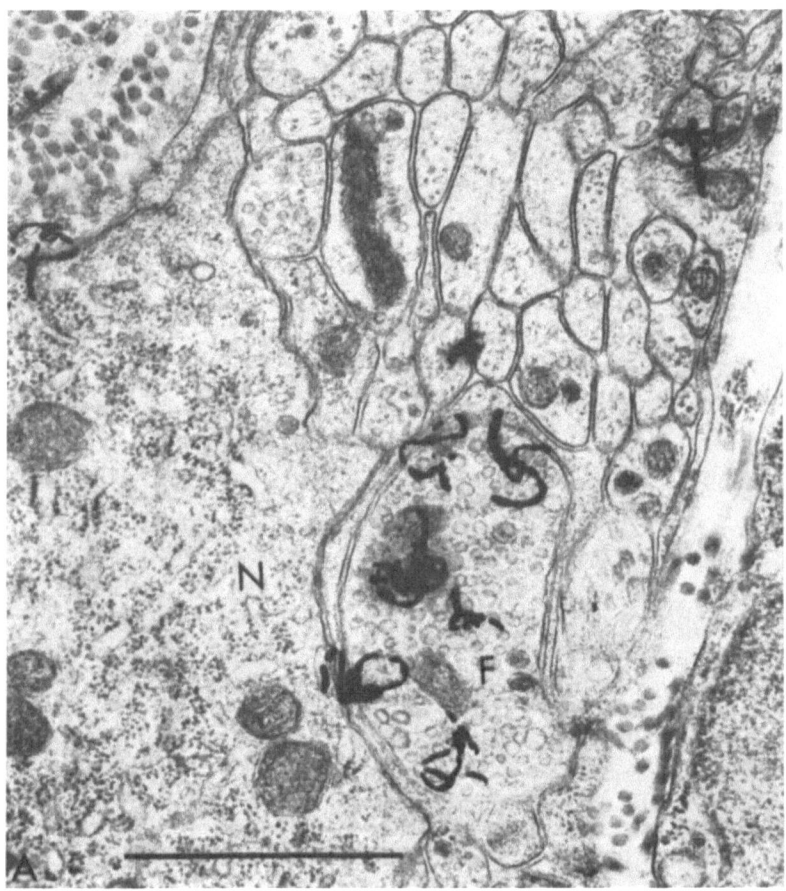

Fig. 2 A

Fig. 2 A et B. A = (× 44.000). B = (× 33.750). Intestin de Rat — 30 minutes après injection de noradrénaline-³H. Les deux figures sont relatives à deux sections très proches l'une de l'autre du plexus de MEISSNER. N = neurone. F = fibre richement marquée, ayant les caractères d'une fibre proche d'un contact synaptique (notamment l'abondance des vésicules). On remarquera que, à la différence de celles des fig. 1 et 4 notamment, aucune de ces vésicules ne contient de granule dense. Certaines par contre, notamment figure 3 B (flèche), semblent plus grandes que normalement

Dans la sous-muqueuse, le marquage intéresse des petits faisceaux, souvent situés à proximité d'un vaisseau ou de la muscularis mucosae.

Dans les plexus, le marquage concerne un nombre restreint de fibres nerveuses; caractérisées par leur taille supérieure à la moyenne (environ 1 µ) et l'intensité de la réaction radioautographique qu'elles produisent. Le caractère vraiment significatif de ce marquage est attesté par l'existence de grains d'argent sur des sections successives de la même fibre (fig. 2). Il convient en outre de souligner que les nombreuses vésicules contenues dans ces fibres ne contiennent pas l'inclusion dense rencontrée jusqu'ici dans tous les autres organes étudiés (épiphyse, canal déférent, innervation périvasculaire).

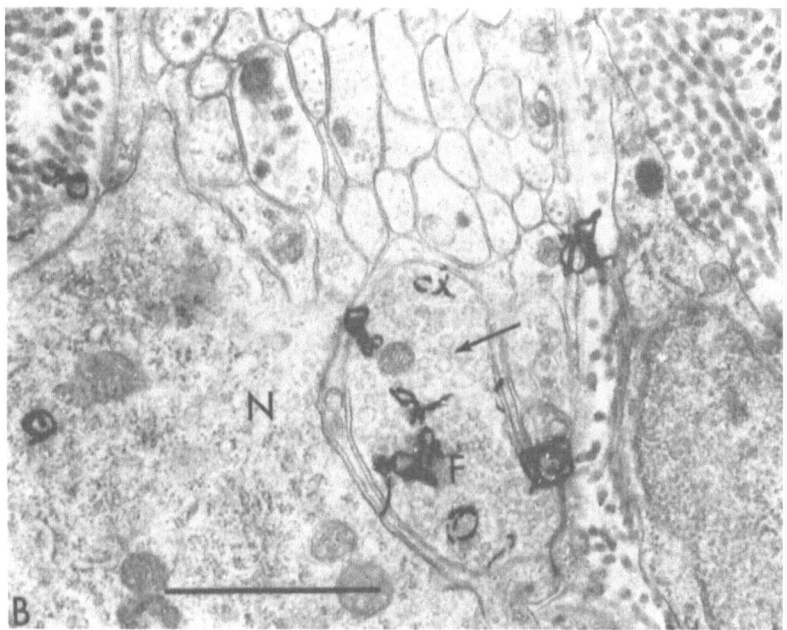

Fig. 2 B

B) 5-Hydroxytryptophane-³H

Dans l'épiphyse, 35 min après l'injection, un assez grand nombre de fibres nerveuses sont marquées (fig. 4). La radioactivité est toutefois moins intense qu' après administration de noradrenaline-³H.

Dans le canal déférent, un nombre limité de fibres se montrent marquées (fig. 3 B). Cependant le fait que la concentration de la radioactivité est environ 20 fois plus forte sur les fibres nerveuses que sur le reste du tissu montre que ce marquage est tout à fait significatif.

Par contre, aucun marquage significatif n'a été observe dans cette expérience sur le ganglion cervical supérieur ou sur l'intestin.

Discussion

Noradrénaline-³H. Epiphyse. Canal déférent.

La morphologie permet de reconnaître dans les axones du système nerveux périphérique, et tout spécialement dans les régions présynaptiques, au moins trois types de vésicules, ceci en particulier sur la foi des observations de DE ROBERTIS et PELLEGRINO DE IRALDI, 1961; GRILLO et PALAY, 1962; RICHARDSON, 1962, et TAXI, 1965. Ces trois types sont:

1. Vésicules synaptiques, apparemment vides, d'un diamètre compris entre 300 et 600 Å, contenant probablement de l'acétylcholine (voir sur ce point la revue de WHITTAKER, 1965).

2. Vésicules de même taille que les précédentes, mais contenant une inclusion très dense. Les travaux biochimiques (VON EULER et LISHAJKO, 1961), pharmacologiques (en particulier, action de la réserpine, PELLEGRINO de IRALDI et DE ROBERTIS, 1961), et radioautographique (WOLFE et al., 1962, TAXI et DROZ, 1966), ont apporté un faisceau d'arguments convergents en faveur du fait que ces vésicules contiendraient de la noradrenaline.

3. Vésicules plus grandes (diamètre compris entre 800 et 1600 Å), contenant également une inclusion dense. Ces vésicules, qui ne sont pas sensibles à l'action de la réserpine, sont présentes dans les terminaison cholinergiques et adrénergiques, en quantité largement variable selon le matériel. Il n'est nullement prouvé qu'elles aient partout la même signification chimique. Dans les terminaisons préganglionnaires, CLEMENTI et al., 1966, ont montré récemment quer leur nombre augmente après injection de DOPA plus iproniazide.

Sur la nature du produit mis en évidence par la présence de grains d'argent, la vidange obtenue par action de la réserpine tend bien à montrer qu'il s'agit d'une catécholamine. Le fait que la déplétion n'ait pas été totale dans notre expérience, contrairement à ce qui a été observé par CLEMENTI, 1965, est peut être en rapport avec la faible intervalle de temps (3 heures au lieu de 24) entre l'injection et le prélèvement. Enfin, d'après les travaux biochimiques (WHITBY et al., 1961) une partie importante au moins de la radioactivité décelée dans les divers tissus serait due à la présence de noradrenaline.

En accord avec les résultats de WOLFE et al., 1962, on peut déduire que les fibres contenant des vésicules de type 2 sont les fibres adrénergiques du système nerveux autonome périphérique. Nos observations montrent de plus que le captage de la noradrénaline par les fibres nerveuses se fait probablement sans intermédiaire, puisque le marquage le plus intense est observé pour les temps les plus courts (2 min) après l'injection. Il y a une chute importante du taux de radioactivité dans les premières minutes, puis le taux se stabilise, ce qui parait en accord avec les données biochimiques (WHITBY et al., 1961; IVERSEN, GLOWINSKI et AXELROD, 1965).

Ganglion cervical supérieur.

Le marquage observé sur les fibres nerveuses de l'épiphyse contraste de façon frappante avec la rareté des grains situés sur les périkaryons d'origine de ces fibres, situés dans le ganglion cervical supérieur. Ceci peut traduire l'incapacité des périkaryons soit à capter la noradrénaline, soit plus probablement à la retenir sous une forme capable de se maintenir en place au cours de la fixation et de la déshydratation des tissus. L'utilisation de techniques différentes pour la préparation des pièces pourra peut être modifier profondément ce résultat. On ne peut pas manquer de rapprocher l'absence presque totale de radioactivité sur les périkaryons de la rareté des petites vésicules à coeur dense (type 2) à ce niveau (TAXI, 1965);

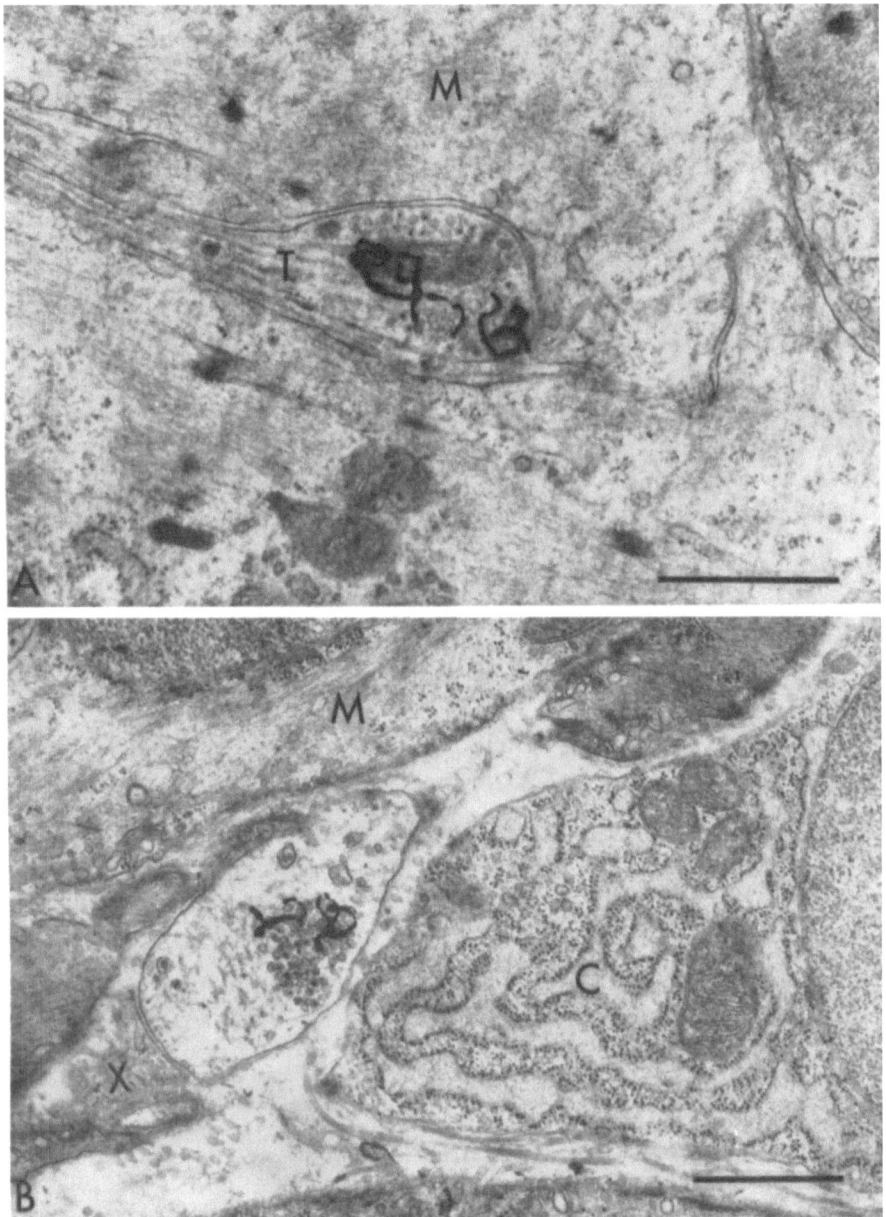

Fig. 3 A et B. Tunique musculaire du canal déférent de Rat. A = (× 25.500) — 30 minutes après injection de noradrénaline-^{3}H. B = (× 22.000) — 35 minutes après injection de 5-hydroxytryptophane-^{3}H. Dans les deux cas, une fibre nerveuse est marquée au niveau ou se trouvent des vésicules contenant un granule dense. Dans la fig. A, la partie gauche de fibre nerveuse contient des tubules (T). La partie droite, dilatée, déprime la surface de la cellule musculaire (M), l'espace entre les deux membranes plasmiques étant d'environ 250 Å à ce niveau. Dans la fig. B, la fibre nerveuse est associée à une plage de cytoplasme (x), de nature indéterminé. C = cellule conjonctive de type plasmocyte. M = cellule musculaire lisse

ces vésicules sont peut être le support nécessaire à une liaison suffisamment solide de la noradrénaline aux structures pour résister aux traitements de la technique usuelle pour la microscopic électronique.

Intestin.

L'absence totale, dans les faisceaux nerveux situés au sein de la musculeuse, de fibres marquées est à mettre en parallèle avec les données purement morphologi-

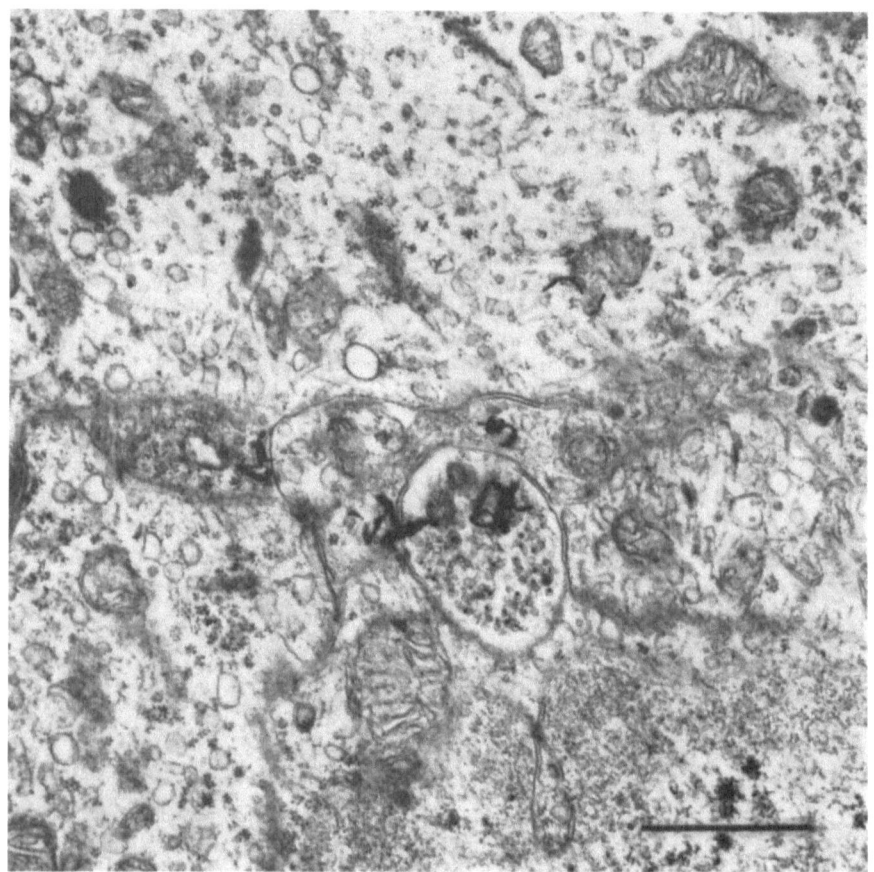

Fig. 4. (× 25.000) Epiphyse de Rat — 35 minutes après injection de 5-hydroxytryptophane-[3]H. Une fibre nerveuse située au sein du parenchyme épiphysaire est marquée de deux grains (flèche)

ques sur l'absence de vésicules de type 2 dans ces fibres (Taxi, 1964, 1965). Ce fait impose l'abandon de la conception de Langley sur l'antagonisme sympathique-parasympathique dans l'intestin, puisqu'il parait exclus que les fibres adrénergiques agissent directement sur les cellules musculaires.

Les seules fibres marquées, en dehors de celles de la sous-muqueuse, sont situées au sein du plexus d'Auerbach et surtout de Meissner. Il paraît logique de penser que ces fibres, situées au voisinage immédiat des neurones des plexus, exercent directement sur eux leur action inhibitrice. D'ailleurs les fibres marquées rencontrées ont nettement par leur dimensions et leur contenu le caractère de fibres proches d'un contact synaptique. Si l'on admet que les neurones (du plexus d'AUERBACH notamment) donnent naissance aux fibres cholinergiques susceptibles de stimuler des contractions intestinales, il semble que l'action modératrice du système orthosympathique sor la motricité intéstinale pourrait s'expliquer par une action inhibitrice des fibres adrénergiques sur des périkaryons des neurones du plexus.

Rappelons que c'est à une conclusion semblable que sont parvenus NORBERG, 1964, et JACOBOWITZ, 1965, sur la base d'observations faites par la méthode de fluorescence. Par contre, utilisant également la méthode de fluorescence des catécholamines, HOLLANDS et VANOV, 1965, signalent l'existence de nombreuses fibres adrénergiques à l'intérieur du muscle, dont nous n'avons pas trouvé trace avec notre méthode.

Un autre problème est posé par le fait que, à la différence de ce qui a été rapporté pour les autres matériels, le marquage intéresse des fibres dont le contenu vésiculaire apparaît du type «vésicule synaptique«, sans inclusion dense à l'intérieur (type 1). Ce fait inattendu est susceptible de plusieurs interprétations. La première est qu'il s'agit d'un simple artefact, le contenu dense de la vésicule ayant disparu au cours de la fixation. En effet, RICHARDSON, 1966, a récemment montré que la fixation par le permanganate de potassium à forte concentration pouvait mettre en évidence un contenu dense dans des vésicules qui en sont souvent dépourvues, par exemple dans le canal déférent de la Souris. Mais, dans ce matériel, que nous avons nous-même étudié, il y a toujours des endroits où le contenu dense des vésicules se trouve conservé, ce qui n'est pas du tout le cas de l'intestin, où de très nombreuses observations ne nous ont jamais permis d'observer de vésicules de type 2.

On remarquera d'ailleurs que la vidange totale des vésicules serait peu compatible avec la rétention des produits radioactifs au niveau de vésicules de même type que celles de l'épiphyse, puisque l'action de la réserpine montre que le marquage disparaît avec les granules denses. On est ainsi plutôt amené à admettre que l'on se trouve ici devant une nouvelle catégorie de vésicules, qui ne se distinguent pas par la simple morphologie des vésicules des terminations cholinergiques.

Il se pourrait d'ailleurs que le contenu des fibres en question ne soient pas de même nature que celles de l'épiphyse et du vas deferens, où il y a toute chance qu'il s'agisse de noradrenaline (v; plus haut).

On remarquera encore que les fibres riches en vésicules de type 3, présentes dans les plexus (HAGER et TAFURI, 1959, HONJIN et al., 1965; TAXI, 1965) ne semblent pas avoir de propriétés particulières vis - à - vis de la noradrenaline.

5-hydroxytryptophane tritié.

Les résultats obtenus mettent en évidence la capacité des fibres adrénergiques, définies par la présence des vésicules de type 2, de fixer également le 5-HTP-^{3}H. D'après les résultats des dosages obtenus après injection de 5-HTP marqués au ^{14}C par UDENFRIEND, WEISSBACH et BOGDANSKI, 1957, et après injection de 5-HTP-^{3}H par GERSHON, DRAKONTIDES et ROSS, 1965, il y a lieu de penser que le produit visualisé est de la sérotonine. Les vésicules de type 2 ont donc la propriété d'emmagasiner et probablement de synthétiser la sérotonine. C'est un argument en faveur de l'hypothèse selon laquelle la sérotonine pourrait suppléer le mécanisme adrénergique normal lorsqu'il est défaillant.

Résumé

La méthode radioautographique a été employée pour étudier la localisation, dans les axones du système neurovégétatif, des médiateurs chimiques de l'excitation nerveuse. Les observations ont été faites après injection soit d'un médiateur tritié, soit de son précurseur marqué au tritium, lorsqu'on sait que ce dernier peut être prompé et stocké par certaines fibres nerveuses.

Après injection de noradrénaline tritiée, l'examen de l'épiphyse a permis de confirmer que le médiateur se fixe au niveau d'axones contenant des vésicules à grain dense, (300—600 Å de diamètre), dans lesquels il semble qu'on puisse reconnaître les fibres adrénergiques. La dynamique du phénomène a éte précisée grâce à des prélèvements faits à des temps variés après l'injection; ces observations ont été étendues à plusieurs autres matériels (canal déférent, artères, . . .). Dans les conditions où nous nous sommes placés, il y a une opposition très nette entre le marquage toujours très intense des axones postganglionnaires et l'absence presque totale de marquage des périkaryons correspondants, qui siègent dans le ganglion cervical supérieur. La portée de cette observation est discutée.

Dans l'intestin, cette technique permet de conclure à l'absence à peu près complète de fibres adrénergiques au sein de la musculeuse intestinale. Les seules fibres marquées, servant en quelque sorte de témoin au résultat négatif précédent, se rencontrent d'une part dans la sous-muqueuse, d'autre part dans les plexus d'Auerbach et de Meissner; ce marquage n'est pas associé ici à des vésicules à grain dense, mais à des vésicules de même taille apparemment vides. Ce résultat amène à remettre en question le schéma classique de Langley sur le mécanisme de l'antagonisme sympathique-parasympathique dans l'intestin. Il semble maintenant probable que les fibres adrénergiques exercent leur action inhibitrice directement sur les neurones moteurs des plexus entériques.

Après injection de 5-hydroxytryptophane tritié, certaines fibres contenant des vésicules à grain dense, et donc capables de fixer la noradrenaliné, sont marquées; ceci a été constaté dans l'épiphyse et le canal déférent. Ces observations suggèrent que les fibres adrénergiques sont probablement en outre capables de former de la sérotonine à partir du 5-THP.

Summary

Radioautography combined with electron microscopy allows to study, in the axons of the autonomic nervous system, the localization of neurotransmitters. Our observations were made after injection of a labeled transmitter or its precursor.

After injection of norepinephrine-^{3}H, the label is localized within nerve fibres containing dense-core vesicles, about 300—600 Å in diameter. Such labeled fibres were found in the pineal gland, was deferens and around blood vessels. The label disappears from nerve fibres at a very high rate within the first minutes, then more slowly. Under the conditions we worked, the large amount of label in the nerve fibers of the pineal gland contrasts with the rare silver grains seen over the perikaryons in the superior cervical ganglion. In the intestine, no labeled nerve fibers was observed within the muscular layers. Labeled nerve fibers are confined to the submucosa and to the AUERBACH's and MEISSNER's plexuses. Here the labeled fibers are filled with vesicles which do not contain a dense core.

The distribution of adrenergic nerve fibres in the intestine wall call in question the classical Langley's schema on the sympathetic-parasympathetic antagonism. It seems now probable that adrenergic (sympathetic) fibers exert their inhibitory action directly on the motor neurons of the enteric plexuses.

After injection of 5-hydroxytryptophane-³H, most of the nervous fibers containing dense core vesicles, i.e. adrenergic fibers, are labelled, in the pineal gland and to a lesser extent in the vas deferens. This observation suggests that adrenergic fibers are also capable to synthetize serotonin from 5-HTP and store it.

Bibliographie

AXELROD, J. (1965): The metabolism, storage and release of catecholamines. Rec. Prog. Horm. Res. 21, 597—619.

CLEMENTI, F. (1965): Modifications ultrastructurelles provoquées par quelques médicaments sur les terminaisons nerveuses adrénergiques et sur la médullaire surrénale. Experientia (Basel) 21, 171—187.

— P. MANTEGAZZA, and M. BOTTURI (1966): A pharmacologic and morphologic study on the nature of the dense-core granules present in the presynaptic endings of sympathic ganglia. Inv. J. Neuropharmacol. 5, 281—285.

EULER, U. S. VON, and F. LISHAJKO (1961): Noradrenalin release from isolated nerve granules. Acta physiol. scand. 51, 193—203.

FALCK, B. (1962): Observations on the possibilities for the cellular localization of monoamines by a fluorescence method. Acta physiol. scand. 56, suppl. 197, 1—25.

GERSHON, P. M., A. B. DRAKONTIDES, and L. I. ROSS (1965): Serotonin: synthesis and release from the myenteric plexus of the mouse intestine. Science 149, 197—199.

GRANBOULAN, P. (1965): The use of radioautography in investigating protein synthesis (ed. by C. P. LEBLOND et K. B. WARREN) p. 43. London-New York: Academic Press.

GRILLO, M. A., and S. L. PALAY (1962): Granule containing vesicles in the autonomie nervous system. Vth Int. Congr. Electron Microscop., Philadelphia 2, p. U. 1. London-New York: Academic Press.

HAGER, H., u. W. L. TAFURI (1959): Elektronenoptischer Nachweis sog. neurosekretorischer Elementargranula in marklosen Nervenfasern des Plexus myentericus (Auerbach) des Meerschweinchens. Naturwissenschaften 46, 332—333.

HOLLANDS, B. C. S., and S. VANOV (1965): Localization of catécholamines in visceral organs and ganglia of the rat, guinea-pig and rabbit. Brit. J. Pharmacol. 25, 307—316.

HONJIN, R., A. TAKAHASHI, and H. MARNYAMA (1965): Two types of synaptic nerve processes in the ganglia of Auerbach's plexus of mice, as revealed by electron microscopy. J. Electr. Micr. 14, 43—49.

IVERSEN, L. L., J. GLOWINSKI, and J. AXELROD (1965): The uptake and storage of ³H-norepinephrine in the reserpine pretreated rat heart. J. Pharm. exp. Ther. 150, 173—183.

JACOBOWITZ, D. (1965): Histochemical studies of the autonomic innervation of the gut. J. Pharm. exp. Ther. 149, 358—364.

KAPPERS, J. ARIENS (1960): The development, topographical relations and innervation of the epiphysis cerebri in the albinos rat. Z. Zellforsch. 52, 163—215.

MILLER, F. (1962): Acid phosphatase localization in neural protein absorption droplets. Vth Int. Congr. Electron Microscop. Philadelphia. 2, p. Q 2. London-New York: Academic Press.

NORBERG, K. (1964): Adrenergic innervation of the intestinal wall studied by fluorescence microscopy. Int. J. Neuropharmacol. 3, 379—382.

PELLEGRINO DE IRALDI, A., and E. ROBERTIS (1961): Action of reserpine on submicroscopic morphology of the pineal gland. Experientia (Basel) 17, 122—123.

Richardson, K. G. (1962): The fine structure of autonomic nerve endings in smooth muscle of the rat vas deferens. J. Anat. **96**, 427—442.
— (1966): Electron microscopic identification of autonomic nerve endings. Nature (Lond.) **210**, 756.
Robertis, E. de, and A. Pellegrino de Iraldi (1961): Plurivesicular secretory processes and nerve endings in the pineal gland. J. biophys. biochem. Cytol. **10**, 361—372.
Taxi, J. (1964): Etude au microscope électronique de l'innervation du muscle lisse intestinal, comparée à celle de quelques autres muscles lisses de Mammifères. Arch. Biol. (Liège), **75**, 301—328; Contribution à l'étude des connexions des neurones moteurs du système nerveux autonome. Ann. Sci. Nat. (Zool.), 12e série, **7**, 413—674.
—, et B. Droz (1966): Etude de l'incorporation de noradrénaline-^{3}H (NA-^{3}H) et de 5-hydroxytryptophane-^{3}H (5-HTP-^{3}H) dans l'épiphyse et dans le ganglion cervical supérieur. C. R. Acad. Sci. (Paris) **263**, sous-presse.
Udenfriend, S., H. Weissbach, and D. F. Bogdanski (1957): Increase in tissue serotonin following administration of its precurssor 5-hydroxytryptophan. J. biol. Chem. **224**, 803—810.
Whittaker, V. P. (1965): The application of subcellular fractionation techniques to the study of brain function. Progr. Biophys. molec. Biol. **15**, 39—96.
Whitby, L. G., J. Axelrod, and H. Weil-Malherbe (1961): The fate of H^3-norepinephrine in animals. J. Pharm. exp. Ther. **132**, 193—201.
Wolfe, E. D., L. T. Potter, K. C. Richardson, and J. Axelrod (1962): Localizing tritiated norepinephrine in sympathetic axons by electron microscopic autoradiography. Science **138**, 440—442.
Wurtman, R. J. (1965): Catecholamines. New Engl. J. Med. **273**, 637—646; 693—700; 746—753.

Phénomèns neurosécrétoires au niveau de la chaîne nerveuse chez les Invertébrés

H. Herlant-Meewis, J. Naisse et J. Mouton

Laboratoire de Biologie animale et d'Histologie comparée Université de Bruxelles

C'est vraisemblablement par analogie avec la localisation au sein du cerveau des cellules neurosécrétrices des Vertébrés que, chez les Invertébrés, les ganglions cérébroïdes furent les premiers explorés et sont actuellement les mieux connus.

Les neurosécrétions issues de ces ganglions semblent jouer un rôle important dans la physiologie des Invertébrés.

Néanmoins, les expériences destinées à mettre ce rôle en évidence aboutirent parfois à des résultats incohérents ou même à des échecs. C'est pourquoi, les investigations se sont étendues aux autres ganglions nerveux dans lesquels des cellules neurosécrétrices avaient été mises en évidence par l'hématoxyline de Gomori et la fuchsine paraldéhyde ou par la technique à l'azocarmin. L'application de la méthode au bleu alcian oxyde d'Adams et Sloper modifiée par M. Herlant a permis de distinguer aisément plusieurs types de cellules et d'observer les variations d'aspect qu'elles subissent au cours de cycle sécrétoires.

On sait actuellement qu'il existe des cellules neurosécrétrices dans les ganglions infra-oesophagiens et dans les autres ganglions de la chaîne nerveuse chez la plupart des Invertébrés et le rôle de certaines d'entre elles a déjà été envisagé.

Nous résumerons ici quelques observations faites chez les Annélides, les Mollusques, les Crustacés et les Insectes en nous attachant plus spécialement aux Annélides et aux Insectes.

I. Annélides

1. Polychètes. Chez *Nereis diversicolor*, Polychète errante, nous avons observé (Herlant-Meewis et van Damme, 1962) la présence, à l'avant de chaque ganglion de la chaîne nerveuse de une ou deux cellules neurosécrétrices latérales et de deux petits massifs symétriques composés de 6 à 7 cellules ventrales.

Chez diverses Polychètes sédentaires, Arvy, 1954, signale la présence, dans tous les ganglions, de cellules différentes par l'aspect du produit de sécrétion qui peut se présenter sous la forme de flaques denses ou de fines granulations et se colorer, soit par l'hématoxyline de Gomori, soit par la phloxine. L'auteur observe dans certains cas, et notamment, chez les Terebellides, le cheminement de la sécrétion le long de l'axone mais elle ne nie pas la possibilité d'élimination du produit élaboré à travers la membrane du péricaryon.

2. Oligochètes. Chez les Oligochètes terrestres, on connaît l'existence de cellules neurosécrétrices dans les ganglions ventraux de *Lumbricus* depuis les travaux de B. Scharrer, 1937.

Ces observations ont été confirmées plus récemment par Harms, 1948, par Brandenburg, 1956, qui signale le cheminement de la sécrétion tout le long de la chaîne nerveuse, par Hubl, 1956, par Michon et Alaphilippe, 1959, et par Aros et Vigh, 1961.

Hubl, 1956, signale l'apparition de cellules neurosécrétrices qu'il appelle ,,u-Zellen", dans le ganglion infra-oesophagien de *Lumbricus terrestris*, à la suite d'une section dans la région postérieure du corps. Lorsque le ver est intact, il ne distingue aucun élément sécréteur dans ce ganglion. De telles cellules ont cependant été décrites depuis par Otremba, 1961, vers l'avant du ganglion infra-oesophagien, à proximité des connectifs péri-oesophagiens. L'auteur signale leur

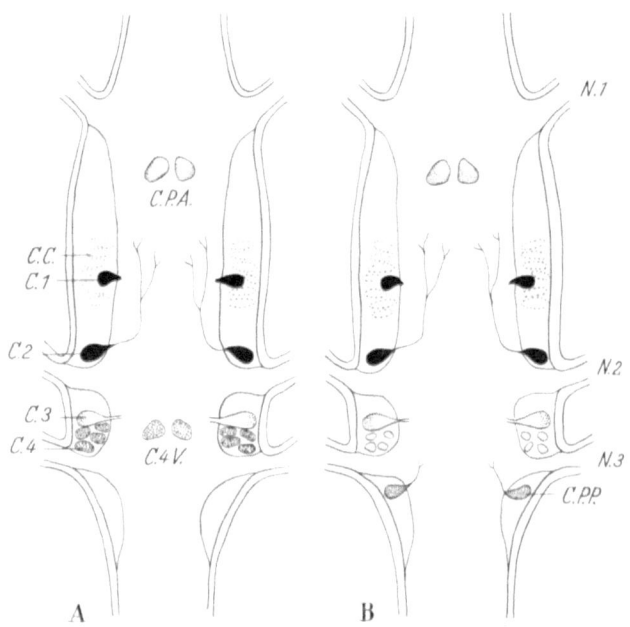

Fig. 1 A et B. Localisation des cellules neurosécrétrices de la chaîne nerveuse ventrale d'*Eisenia foetida*. A: au niveau du segment 13. B: au niveau du segment 40. *C.C.*: cellules chromophiles; *C.P.A.*: cellules phloxinophiles antérieures; *C.P.P.*: cellules phloxinophiles postérieures; C_4V.: cellules C_4 ventrales; N_1, N_2, N_3: nerfs

ressemblance avec les cellules «a» du cerveau, elles se colorent par l'hématoxyline de Gomori.

D'après Takeuchi, 1965, elles existent au même endroit chez *Pheretima communissima* et *hilgendorfi*.

Michon, Maissiat et Angevain, 1964, observent, chez *Eiseniella tetraedra*, le présence de deux types de cellules, les unes permanentes, les autres apparaissant lors de la régénération.

Deux types de cellules ont également été observés par Juberthie et Mestrov, 1962, chez *Pelodrilus leruthi*, les unes ressemblent aux cellules «a» du cerveau, les autres présentent des plages colorées par la phloxine.

De notre côté (Herlant-Meewis et van Damme, 1962), nous avons observé, dans tous les ganglions ventraux d'*Eisenia foetida*, la présence de différents types de cellules neurosécrétrices, que nous avons appelées, en raison de leur localisation antéro-postérieure, C_1, C_2, C_3, C_4. Elles sont caractérisées par leur taille, l'aspect et la colorabilité de leurs inclusions, nous les avons décrites en détail dans un article récent (HERLANT-MEEWIS, 1966). De plus, en avant du ganglion, existe un groupe de cellules que nous avons appelées chromophiles (fig. 1).

Les ganglions infra-oesophagiens constitués en fait par la fusion des deux premiers ganglions ventraux, renferment, vers l'arrière, toutes les cellules neuro-sécrétrices d'un ganglion ventral et vers l'avant, les cellules de type «a» décrites par les auteurs précédents.

En 1965, JUBERTHIE et MESTROV décrivent 4 groupes de cellules neurosécrétri-ces dans chacun des ganglions ventraux d'*Eophile pyrenaica*, soit, de chaque côté, un groupe antérieur, situé entre le 1 er et le 2 ème nerf, colorées en bleu ciel parle bleu alcian, une volumineuse cellule colorée enbleu foncé, à l'avant du nerf 2, une cellule phloxinophile près de la racine du nerf 3 et deux cellules ventrales se colorant en bleu clair au niveau des nerfs postérieurs. Nous croyons pouvoir homologuer le groupe antérieur à nos cellules chromophiles, la cellule bleu foncé à C_2 et les cellules bleu clair aux C_4.

Reprenant récemment l'étude de ces ganglions (HERLANT-MEEWIS et RAMU, inédit), nous avons également observé des éléments phloxinophiles sous la forme de 2 cellules antérieures ventrales (fig. 1, 3 a), et 2 cellules postérieures, une de chaque côté à l'arrière du point d'origine du nerf 3 (fig. 1 B, 3 b). Ces dernières cellules ne sont visibles que dans les ganglions postérieurs à la région génitale (fig. 1 B).

Par contre, c'est uniquement dans la région sexuelle, que les cellules C_4 sont actives. De plus, les segments mâles (10 et 11) et femelles (12 et 13) renferment une paire ventrale de cellules C_4 particulièrement volumineuses dans les segments femelles (fig. 1 A).

Chez les Oligochètes limicoles, DEUSE-ZIMMERMANN, 1960, décrit 2 cellules neurosécrétrices disposées symétriquement dans les ganglions infra-oesophagiens d'*Enchytraeus albidus*; leurs axones chargés de flaques de sécrétion se distinguent tout le long de la chaîne nerveuse. Elle trouve aussi de très nombreuses cellules neurosécrétrices (22 à 32), différentes par la grosseur de leurs sécrétats, dans les ganglions ventraux de *Tubifex tubifex*, leurs axones empruntent la voie du nerf 2 pour rejoindre des cellules sensorielles dans l'épiderme.

Chez *Naïs communis*, espèce où aucune cellule neurosécrétrice n'a été mise en évidence dans le cerveau, il existe 2 à 8 cellules neurosécrétrices dans chaque ganglion, elles sont également en rapport avec l'épiderme.

3. Hirudinées. Chez *Theromyzon*, étudié par HAGADORN, 1958, les ganglions supra- et infra-oesophagiens ne sont pas isolés, ils forment un anneau autour du tube digestif, ils contiennent des cellules neurosécrétrices α colorables par la fuchsine paraldéhyde et des cellules β, acidophiles. Ces deux types de cellules existent dans la partie correspondant aux ganglions infra-oesophagiens.

De l'ensemble de ces observations, on peut conclure que les ganglions de la chaîne nerveuses ventrale des Annélides renferment des cellules orientées dans le sens sécrétoire. Quant à leur rôle, il est encore fort hypothétique.

Chez *Eisenia foetida*, le fait que les cellules C_4 deviennent actives au moment de la puberté, que cette activité est particulièrement intense lors de la maturité génitale et que ces éléments sont localisées dans les segments sexuels, suggère qu'ils pourraient sécréter une substance intervenant dans la reproduction.

Par contre, les cellules C_1 et C_2 sont actives dès la naissance et pendant toute la croissance du ver; au moment de la maturité sexuelle, elles paraissent bloquées, elles se bourrent de sécrétion et les ramifications de leur axone renferment également d'importantes flaques de matériel sécrété qui stagne sans être éliminé.

Les produits élaborés par ces cellules pourraient intervenir dans la croissance.

Depuis les expériences de Morgan, 1902, l'influence du système nerveux dans la régénération fut maintes fois discutée tant chez les Vertébrés que chez les Invertébrés et l'intervention de phénomènes neurosécrétoires a été envisagée.

On sait actuellement que chez les Polychètes, le cerveau est indispensable à la régénération postérieure, il semble que les cellules neurosécrétrices cérébrales interviennent au moment de la cicatrisation et lors des premières phases de la régénération (voir bibliographie dans Herlant-Meewis, 1965).

Chez les Oligochètes, au contraire, la régénération caudale peut s'effectuer en l'absence des ganglions cérébroïdes (voir bibliographie dans Saussey, 1966), aussi a-t-on mis en cause des phénomènes neurosécrétoires prenant naissance dans la chaîne nerveuse. En 1965, Gersch et Wohlrabe ont observé des transformations au niveau des deux cellules décrites par Deuse-Zimmermann dans le ganglion infra-oesophagien d'*Enchytraeus albidus*: 30 min après l'amputation des 10 derniers segments du ver, ces cellules sont complètement déchargées, elles se rechargent très fortement dans les heures qui suivent, les deux types de cellules neurosécrétrices du cerveau suivent le même cycle. Les auteurs ont réussi la suppression sélective de ces différentes cellules et montré qu'elles sont indispensables à la cicatrisation et à la formation du blastème de régénération; en leur absence, l'accumulation des coelomocytes nécessaires à l'obturation de la plaie est insuffisante et la croissance de la chaîne nerveuse dans le blastème indispensable au développement de celui-ci ne se produit pas.

Après l'ablation d'un certain nombre de segments postérieurs chez *Eophila pyrenaica*, Juberthie et Mestrov remarquent des modifications dans l'aspect des cellules neurosécrétrices des ganglions voisins de la section et notamment une vidange des cellules phloxinophiles.

Nous avons sectionné des *Eisenia foetida* jeunes et adultes au niveau du 40e segment.

Chez les jeunes (Herlant-Meewis et Gallardo, 1965), nous avons observé que les cellules C_1 et C_2 sont particulièrement actives immédiatement après la section. Chez les adultes (en collaboration avec Pillart et Ramu), tandis que se forme le bouchon cicatriciel de coelomocytes, les cellules C_1 et C_2 de l'ensemble des ganglions subissent un déblocage, les granules de sécrétions redeviennent visibles dans le péricaryon et dans l'axone.

Cette activité ne se manifeste que pendant les processus de cicatrisation et de formation du blastème. Les cellules phloxinophiles postérieures semblent également subir des modifications. Immédiatement après la section, leur volume s'accroît, des plages plus colorées apparaissent à la périphérie du péricaryon, l'axone se colore en rouge (fig. 3 b) et des fibrilles peuvent devenir apparentes dans la cellule et dans l'axone ramifié. Après deux jours, ces cellules ont repris leur aspect habituel.

Comme Juberthie et Mestrov, nous avons donc observé des transformations dans les éléments phloxinophiles, mais il semble qu'il existe des différences spécifiques dans l'allure de leur activité. Quoi qu'il en soit, tous les auteurs qui ont abordé cette question s'accordent pour admettre que chez les Oligochètes, différents types de cellules neurosécrétrices appartenant aux ganglions ventraux, subissent des transformations à la suite d'une section et qu'elles pourraient intervenir dans la régénération. Leur activité serait liée à la cicatrisation et à la formation du blastème mais on ignore encore le rôle exact des substances qui seraient libérées à ce moment.

Toutes ces cellules sont-elles neurosécrétrices ?

L'examen histologique ne laisse, à notre avis, aucun doute pour certaines d'entre elles, telles chez *Eisenia*, les cellules C_1 et C_2 qui renferment un produit figuré cheminant le long de l'axone et qui peut être déversé dans les capillaires sillonannt le neuropile. Lorsque la cellule est en activité, les dictyosomes sont bien visibles parmi les granules de sécrétion. Lors du blocage, les granules se tassent les uns contre les autres et l'appareil de Golgi ne se voit plus; au cours du déblocage, il réapparaît en même temps que des vésicules plus volumineuses qui paraissent de nature lysosomiale.

Les cellules C_4 semblent plus sujettes à caution quant à leur qualification de cellules neurosécrétrices, leur axone est peu visible. Le sécrétat dense occupe une région bien limitée de la cellule, entre une plage juxta-nucléaire renfermant les dictyosomes et une bordure péripherique basophile.

Les cellules phloxinophiles ont le même aspect cytologique, péricaryon et axone semblent dépourvus de produits de sécrétion sous la forme de granules.

Nous avons abordé l'étude de ces cellules en microscopie électronique. Les premiers résultats que nous avons obtenus confirment nos observations cytologiques concernant l'association de l'appareil de Golgi et des granules de sécrétion (NAISSE, 1961; HERLANT-MEEWIS et VAN DAMME, 1962) et la démonstration ultrastructurale qui en a été faite simultanément par BERN, NISHIOKA et HAGADORN, 1961, chez *Theromyzon* et par STIENNON et DROCHMANS, 1961, chez *Carausius* et retrouvée par E. SCHARRER et BROWN, 1961, chez *Lumbricus*.

Nos images confirment également l'existence de plusieurs types de cellules neurosécrétrices, différentes par la taille des granules et par l'aspect des mitochondries semblables à celles qui ont été décrites dans les ganglions cérébroïdes par DE ROBERTIS et BENNETT, 1954, chez *Lumbricus* et par HAGADORN, BERN et NISHIOKA, 1963, chez *Theromyzon*.

II. Mollusques

Chez les Mollusques, le système nerveux ventral est représenté par les ganglions pleuraux, pédieux, palléaux et viscéraux. Des cellules neurosécrétrices de différents types ont été décrites dans ces ganglions. GABE, 1965, en a fait le relevé dans un rapport récent, nous ne le reprendrons pas ici. Leur classification est peu claire, car dès le début. leur étude s'est heurtée à un écueil. En effet, les cellules nerveuses de beaucoup de Mollusques, et tout particulièrement celles d'*Helix*, renferment de nombreuses inclusions chromolipoïdes qui se colorent par les techniques de mise en évidence des produits de neurosécrétion. Par ailleurs, le plus souvent, les neurosécrétats ne se colorent ni par l'hématoxyline de Gomori, ni par la fuchsine paraldéhyde, ils sont acidophiles et sont mis en évidence notamment par l'azocarmin.

Enfin, des auteurs ont admis la possibilité d'une elimination des produits élaborés au travers de la membrane du péricaryon pour expliquer l'absence de cheminement le long de l'axone.

Pour ces raisons conjuguées, de nombreuses «fausses cellules neurosécrétrices» ont été décrites et il est vraisemblable que certaines «vraies» aient échappé jusqu'à présent, aux investigations. La microscopie électronique a déjà permis de relever un certain nombre d'erreurs (Simpson, Nishioka et Bern, 1963; Nolte, Brencker et Kuhlmann, 1965) et d'ores et déjà on peut admettre qu'il existe dans les ganglions ventraux des Mollusques comme dans ceux des Vers, des cellules neuro-sécrétrices authentiques, les unes Gomori-positives et les autres phloxinophiles excrètant leur produit de sécrétion par voie axonale (voir Gabe, 1965).

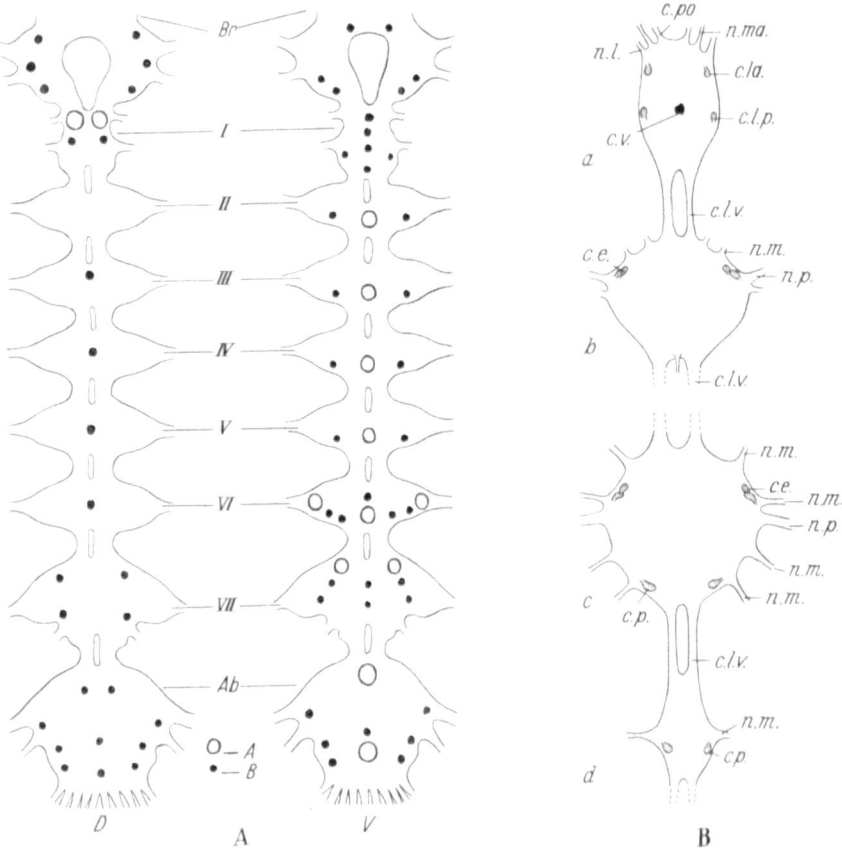

Fig. 2 A et B. Localisation des cellules neurosécrétrices de la chaîne nerveuse ventrale des Crustacés et des Insectes. A: *Armadillidium vulgare* (Isopode). D: vue dorsale; V: vue ventrale; *Ab*: ganglions abdominaux; *Br*: cerveau; *I—VII*: ler ganglion — 7e. ganglion (Matsumoto, 1959). B: *Carausius morosus* (Phasmide-Orthoptère). a: ganglion infra-oesophagien; b: ganglions thoraciques I et II; c: ganglion thoracique III; d: ganglions abdominaux 1, 2, 3, 4. *C.a.*: cellules antérieures des ganglions thoraciques; *C.l.a.*: cellule latérale antérieure; *c.l.p.*: cellule latérale postérieure; *c.l.v.*: connectif longitudinal ventral; *c.p.*: cellules postérieures des ganglions abdominaux; *c.p.o.*: collier péri-oesophagien; *c.v.*: cellules ventrales; *n.l.*: nerf labial; *n.m.*: nerf innervant la musculature; *n.ma.*: nerf mandibulaire; *n.p.*: nerf innervant les pattes

Néanmoins, la plupart de ces observations ont été faites au niveau des ganglion-cérébroïdes: dans cette région, la libération des produits au niveau d'organes neuros hémaux a été décrite chez les Pulmonés par VAN MOL, 1960, par ROHNISH, 1964, et par NOLTE, 1965.

VAN MOL (inédit) a pu montrer des phénomènes semblables au niveau des ganglions viscéraux de *Succinea putris*: les produits de neurosécrétion qui se colorent par l'azocarmin et qui sont particulièrement abondants au moment de la maturation sexuelle cheminent le long des axones qui se ramifient dans la paroi de l'aorte antérieure à la hauteur des ganglions de la chaîne viscérale.

Quant au rôle des sécrétats issus des ganglions ventraux, il est encore fort peu connu. Néanmoins, quelques données histophysiologiques suggèrent leur inter-vention dans la reproduction chez les Gastéropodes (GABE, 1951; KRAUSE, 1960; GORF, 1961) et chez les Lamellibranches (LUBET, 1956—1965; NAGABUSHANAM, 1963). D'après LEVER et ses collaborateurs (1961), des phénomènes neuro-endo-crines issus des ganglions pleuraux interviendraient dans la balance hydrique chez *Limnaea stagnalis*.

III. Crustacés

Le système neurosécréteur ventral des Crustacés présente également une grande complexité; il est constitué de différents types d'éléments répartis dans toute la chaîne nerveuse. C'est ainsi que chez les Malacostracés, où il fut le plus étudié, on observe des cellules neurosécrétrices dans tous les ganglions (fig. 2 A).

Ces cellules neurosécrétrices se groupent suivant leurs caractères morphologi-ques et leurs affinités tinctoriales (MATSUMOTO, 1954—1959). Le produit de sécré-tion se décharge soit à travers la membrane du péricaryon soit le long de l'axone (MATSUMOTO, 1958). Dans ce dernier cas, il peut gagner le cerveau et les pédoncules oculaires, ou les nerfs des pattes ou bien encore se déverser dans le neuropile (MATSUMOTO, 1958). On ne possède à l'heure actuelle, que peu de données sur le rôle de ces cellules. Certaines d'entre elles interviendraient dans les processus de mue en général (MATSUMOTO, 1962) ou dans les phénomènes de pigmentation (MATSUMOTO, 1954B), ou de reproduction (OTSU, 1960).

IV. Insectes

Un des premiers auteurs qui s'intéressa à la chaîne nerveuse des Insectes fut DAY ,1940, qui décrivit dans les ganglions infra-oesophagiens et thoraciques des Lépidoptères des cellules semblables à celles de la pars intercerebralis.

Par la suite, sur la base d'observations cytologiques, des cellules neurosécré-trices furent signalées dans tous les ganglions de la chaîne nerveuse des Insectes étudiés: chez les Aptérygotes Thysanoures (BART, 1963,) chez les Ephéméroptères et Odonatoptères (ARVY et GABE, 1952), chez les Dictyoptères (B. SCHARRER, 1941; GELDIAY, 1959), chez les Isoptères (NOIROT, 1957), chez les Chéleutoptères (RAABE, 1965a; NAISSE et MOUTON, 1965; PASTEELS, 1965), chez les Orthoptères (BAFFONI, 1960; DELPHIN, 1963; FREON, 1964; CHALAYE, 1965), chez les Dermap-tères (LHOSTE, 1952), chez les Coléoptères (ARVY et GABE, 1953), chez les Hémip-tères (NAYAR, 1955; JOHANSSON, 1958), chez les Lépidoptères (BOUHNIOL, ARVY et GABE, 1953; KOBAYASHI, 1957), chez les Diptères (KÖPF, 1957; FRASER, 1959).

Pour une espèce donnée, ces cellules sont en nombre constant et ont une localisation bien déterminée.

Elles se répartissent en plusieurs groupes suivant leur taille, leur morphologie,
leurs affinirés tinctoriales. D'une manière générale, on reconnaît:

— des cellules qui présentent des affinties tinctoriales pour l'hématoxyline de
Gomori et la fuchsine paraldéhyde (le plus souvent appelées cellules A).

— des cellules qui montrent une affinité particulière pour les colorants acides
tels que la phloxine et le picro-indigocarmin (le plus souvent appelées cellules B).

— certains auteurs distinguent en plus des cellules qui se colorent uniquement
par l'azocarmin après fixation au Helly et que Raabe, 1965a nomme cellules C.

Le nature histochimique de ces sécrétions est encore peu connue; des auteurs
ont cependant observé que certaines d'entre elles sont riches en groupements sulf-
hydriles et disulfures et ressembleraient par ce caractère, aux cellules neurosécrétrices de la pars intercerebralis (de Besse, 1965; Raabe, 1965a). Selon Fraser,
1959, des cellules des ganglions abdominaux de *Lucilia caesar* sécréteraient un
produit P.A.S. positif qui correspondrait à un glyco- ou un phospholipide ou
encore à un composé lipoprotéique.

Parmi toutes les cellules décrites comme neurosécrétrices, un certain nombre
ont reçu à tort cette qualification. Une des caractéristiques essentielles pour une
cellule sécrétrice est de présenter des cycles d'activité. C'est pourquoi nous insiste-
rons quelque peu sur ceux-ci. Raabe, 1965a, a décrit pour les cellules A de *Clitumnus* différentes étapes de cette activité.

Pour notre part, nous avons examiné la chaîne nerveuse ventrale de *Carausius
morosus*. Les cellules neurosécrétrices, cellules sécrétant une substance qui s'écoule
le long de l'axone pour gagner un organe neurohémal, se répartissent dans le
ganglion infra-oesophagien, les ganglions thoraciques et les quatre premiers
ganglions abdominaux distincts (fig. 2B) (Naisse et Mouton, 1965).

On distingue deux types cellulaires: d'une part, les cellules ventrales (2) du
ganglion infra-oesophagien et d'autre part toutes les autres cellules: cellules latérales du ganglion infra-oesophagien (une paire antérieure et une paire postérieure),
cellules antéro-latérales des ganglions thoraciques (deux paires) et les cellules
latéro-postérieures des ganglions abdominaux (une paire). Les cellules ventrales
du ganglion infra-oesophagien ont une taille de 25 μ environ et le cytoplasme est
régulièrement parsemé de formations golgiennes (fig. 3C). Les cellules latérales des
ganglions sécréteurs sont plus grandes (35 μ environ), leur cytoplasme montre une
zone périnucléaire riche en ergastoplasme et une zone périphérique contenant les
complexes golgiens (fig. 3E). Toutes ces cellules possèdent un cycle d'activité
sécrétoire (Naisse et Mouton, 1965). Pour les latérales, le cycle correspond dans
ses grandes lignes à celui décrit par Raabe, 1965a. Au stade de repos, le cytoplasme
est clair, les dictyosomes sont peu visibles. Au moment de l'élaboration, ces formations s'accusent davantage, l'ergastoplasme se développe (fig. 3E), de petits
grains de sécrétion colorables au bleu alcian après oxydation permanganique
apparaissent alors au contact du Golgi. Ce phénomène débute dans la région
axonale particulièrement riche en dictyosomes et s'étend ultérieúrement à tout le
cytoplasme (fig. 3F). Au moment de l'excrétion, ces granules s'assemblent en
grains plus gros dans le cône axonal et s'écoulent ensuite le long de l'axone. A ce

stade, les zones golgiennes devenues inactives prennent une teinte turquoise au bleu alcian et finissent par s'estomper. La cellule reprend l'aspect du repos.

Les cellules ventrales présentent un cycle semblable dans l'ensemble, mais au moment de l'élaboration, on voit apparaître dans le noyau des gouttes colorables au bleu alcian (fig. 3C). Ces gouttes traversent la membrane nucléaire et gagnent le cytoplasme. A ce moment, apparaissent des granules de sécrétion au niveau des dictyosomes et le cycle se poursuit parallélement à ce que l'on observe pour les latérales. Ici cependant, l'élaboration se produit simultanemént dans tout le péricaryon (fig. 3D). De telles formations ont également été observées par RAABE, 1965c, uniquement chez des phasmes noirs et particulièrement en période de ponte.

Les sécrétats élaborés au niveau des cellules cheminent le long des ramifications des axones qui se dirigent vers la région dorsale du neuropile. A cet endroit, le produit de sécrétion s'accumule de place en place, le long des fibrilles en leur donnant un aspect moniliforme. Ces fibrilles traversent le neurilemme, qui, à cet endroit, recouvre directement le neuropile, et viennent déverser leur sécrétion dans l'hémolymphe. A la fin de l'élimination, il ne reste plus dans le neuropile que des traces turquoises qui finissent par disparaîte à leur tour. Cette région dorsale de chacun des ganglions sécréteurs correspondrait donc à un organe neurohémal. Remarquons également qu'une partie de la neurosécrétion est éliminée par des ramifications axonales dans les connectifs interganglionnaires (NAISSE et MOUTON, 1965). Ce cheminement interganglionnaire a été observé par plusieurs auteurs (GELDIAY, 1959; DELPHIN, 1963; RAABE, 1965c; CHALAYE, 1966).

Quant à savoir dans quel sens ce cheminement s'effectue, une seule expérience a été réalisée en ce sens jusqu'à présent. Ainsi GELDIAY, 1959, ligature la chaîne nerveuse ventrale de *Blaberus craniifer* et observe une accumulation de neuro-sécrétion de part et d'autre de la ligature.

D'autre part, certains auteurs ont observé le transfert des produits de sécrétion le long des nerfs issus du ganglion infra-oesophagien soit vers la glande de mue, soit vers les nerfs allates (ARVY et GABE, 1952; CHALAYE, 1966).

L'élimination des sécrétats dans l'hémocoele au niveau d'organes neuro-hémaux situés sur le trajet des nerfs transverses du système sympathique impair a été également signalée par RAABE, 1965b, et CHALAYE, 1966.

Les cellules neurosécrétrices de la chaîne nerveuse ventrale semblent donc, par leur présence constante et leur activité, avoir un rôle important dans la physiologie des Insectes. Ce rôle est encore peu connu actuellement, bien que diverses observations histophysiologiques et expérimentales aient déjà été faites:

GABE, 1952, suggère l'existence d'un rapport entre le fonctionnement des cellules neurosécrétrices du ganglion infra-oesophagien et celui de la glande ventrale des Ephémères et des Odonates. D'autre part, le ganglion infra-oesophagien pourrait produire un facteur responsable dans la formation d'oeufs diapausants (FUKUDA, 1952). Dans certains cas, les phénomènes de pigmentation seraient sous le contrôle de certaines cellules de la chaîne nerveuse ventrale (HASHIGUSHI, 1965; HIDAKA, 1961), principalement des cellules neurosécrétrices des ganglions thoraciques. Pour RAABE, 1965c, les cellules ventrales du ganglion infra-oesophagien «subissent des modifications importantes en liaison avec la pigmentation des Insectes».

14*

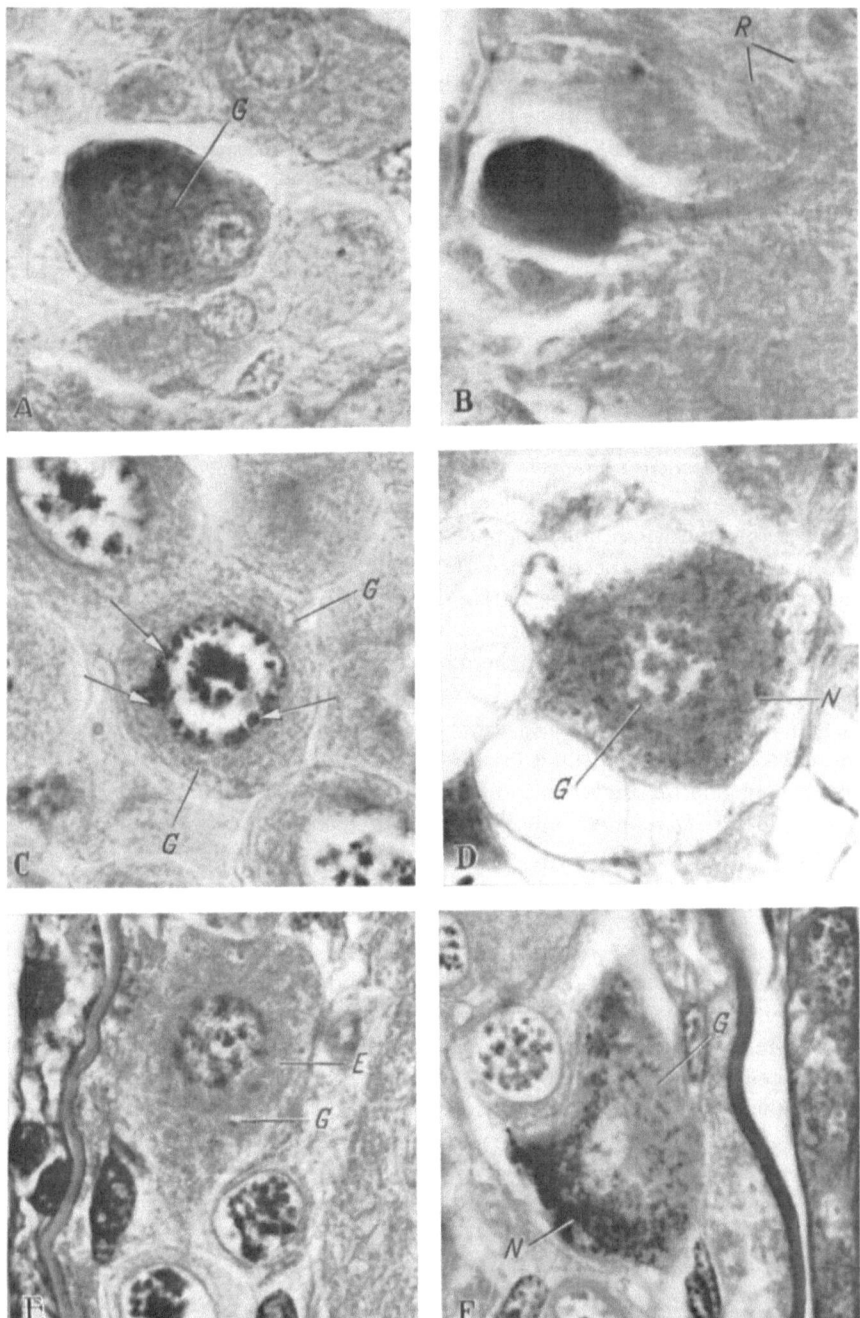

Fig. 3 A—F. Cellules neuro-endocrines de la chaîne nerveuse ventrale d'*Eisenia foetida* (A—B) et de *Carausius morosus* (C—F) (Bleu alcian après oxydation permanganique-hémalun-phloxine). A: cellule phloxinophile antérieure: dictyosomes dans la région supra-nucléaire (G) et produit de sécrétion en croissant périphérique. B: cellule phloxinophile postérieure, 3 h. après la section. Forte phloxinophilie du péricaryon, de l'axone et de ses ramifications (R).

Les cellules neurosécrétrices montreraient également des variations en fonction du degré hygrométrique (RAABE, 1965 c).

Des hypothèses concernant le rôle dans le métabolisme de l'eau ont été également avancées. Ainsi pour DELPHIN, 1963, les cellules neurosécrétrices du ganglion abdominal 2 de *Schistocerca gregaria* libérerait une hormone antidiurétique.

Mais pour de nombreux auteurs, les cellules neurosécrétrices de la chaîne nerveuse ventrale interviendraient principalement dans les phénomènes de reproduction.

B. SCHARRER, en 1955, observe, à la suite d'expériences de castration, des modifications des cellules neurosécrétrices ventrales du ganglion infra-oesophagien de *Leucophaea maderae*. Pour cette raison, B. SCHARRER appelle ces cellules des «castration cells». De tels éléments furent par la suite, observés dans tous les ganglions chez *Corethra* (GERSCH, 1959).

Pour sa part, RAABE, 1965 a, suggère un rapport entre des cellules situées latéralement dans les ganglions abdominaux (B 2) et les phénomènes de reproduction.

FREON, 1964, chez *Locusta migratoria* et HUIGNARD, 1964, chez *Gryllus domesticus* observent, après des expériences de castration et de mise à jeun, une variation du contenu des cellules neurosécrétrices ventrales du ganglion infra-oesophagien.

Ces auteurs mettent en relation le fonctionnement de ces cellules avec les phénomènes de vitellogenèse et de ponte. De plus, THOMAS, 1964 a, b, qui fit des expériences d'implantation du ganglion infra-oesophagien obtint des résultats semblables: il note une action stimulatrice de l'ovogenèse.

L'observation de cycles sécrétoires au niveau des différentes cellules de la chaîne nerveuse ventrale au cours d'expériences de castration et d'allatectomie nous permet d'envisager qu'il existerait des rapports fonctionnels entre les différentes cellules neurosécrétrices et certaines manifestations de la reproduction, notamment le métabolisme ovarien la maturation des œufs et l'oviposition (NAISSE, MOUTON, LAMERS, VAN DEN BERGH inédit). Ces rapports restent à préciser.

Conclusions

Quoiqu'un certain nombre d'auteurs se soient attachés, au cours de ces dernières années, à l'étude de la chaîne nerveuse, les renseignements que nous possédons actuellement concernant son rôle dans les phénomènes neurosécrétoires sont encore fort imprécis. On sait actuellement que chez tous les Invertébrés, il existe des cellules neurosécrétrices, dans les ganglions ventraux, et que ces éléments sont variés, en nombre généralement fixe et parfaitement localisés dans le ganglion. Le plus fréquemment, ces différentes cellules se retrouvent dans tous les ganglions, et dans ce cas, elles réagissent, simultanément et de manière identique à certains stimuli.

Mais il existe également des éléments, tels chez *Eisenia*, les cellules C_4, chez *Lumbricus*, les cellules «u», chez *Carausius*, les cellules ventrales des ganglions

---

C: cellule ventrale du ganglion infra-oesophagien au début de l'activité sécrétoire. Remarquer le passage des gouttelettes nucléaires dans le cytoplasme (flèches). G: Golgi. D: cellule ventrale du ganglion infra-oesophagien en activité sécrétoire. G: Golgi; N: neurosécrétion. E: cellule latérale du ganglion infra-oesophagien au début de l'activité sécrétoire. E: ergastoplasme; G: Golgi. F: cellule latérale du ganglion infra-oesophagien contenant de nombreux grains de neurosécrétion: N; G: Golgi

infra-oesophagiens, qui sont plus strictement localisés dans certains ganglions de la chaîne ventrale.

En ce qui concerne la diversité de ces cellules, de nombreux points restent à élucider, et leur classification est loin d'être établie. S'il est facile de considérer deux catégories d'éléments, les uns qui se colorent par le Gomori et les autres qui sont acidophiles, il devient plus spécieux d'établir des sous-catégories. Le fait que certains produits ne se colorent que par l'azocarmin vient encore compliquer le problème.

Pour qu'un peu de clarté puisse apparaître, il serait indispensable que chaque type cellulaire étudié par les différents auteurs soit soumis aux mêmes critères morphologiques, cytologiques, ultrastructuraux et histophysiologiques et que ces travaux soient coordonnés. Cela permettrait en outre, d'exclure un certain nombre de cellules décrites comme neurosécrétrices sur le seul critère de la coloration mais qui ne répondent pas à cette qualification.

Quant au rôle de ces cellules, on ne le connaît encore que superficiellement, mais il semble fort important. Leur étude plus approfondie permettra certainement de comprendre certains faits qui n'ont pu être expliqués par la seule intervention d'hormones issues du cerveau.

Parmi ces faits, citons l'opposition des Polychètes aux Oligochètes en ce qui concerne le rôle du cerveau dans la reproduction et dans la régénération, opposition sur laquelle une étude plus approfondie de la chaîne nerveuse commence à jeter quelque lumière. Citons aussi, chez les Insectes, la contribution de phénomènes neurosécrétoires autonomes des ganglions ventraux dans différentes manifestations de la reproduction.

Plusieurs auteurs ont parlé d'inhibition de certains centres neurosécréteurs sur d'autres; il est bien certain qu'il existe entre le fonctionnement endocrine des ganglions dorsaux et des ganglions ventraux des corrélations qui assurent l'équilibre physiologique et dont l'étude devrait être approfondie.

Summary

Neurosecretory cells have been observed in the nervous chain of all Invertebrates studied until now.

There cells are various, in constant number, and very well localized in the ganglia. Some are Gomori positive, others acidophilic; for still others, coloration of the secretion can only be obtained with azocarmin. However, the quality of "neurosecretory" cells requires confirmation for some of them.

The role of neurosecretory cells belonging to the ventral nervous chain is not yet precisely established; it is known that some of them present a greatly increased activity during the phenomena of regeneration; also, they can show secretory cycles related to various manifestations of sexual life.

Bibliographie

I. Annelides

Aros, B., and B. Vigh: Neurosecretory activity of the central and peripheral nervous system in the earthworm. Acta biol. Acad. Sci. hung. **12**, 169—186 (1961).

Arvy, L.: Contribution à l'étude de la neurosécrétion chez les Annélides Polychètes sédentaires. Bull. Lab. marit. Dinard **40**, 15—24 (1954).

BERN, H. A., R. S. NISHIOKA, and I. R. HAGADORN: Association of elementary neurosecretory. J. Ultrastruct. Res. 5, 311—320 (1961).

BRANDENBURG, J.: Neurosekretorische Zellen des Regenwurms. Naturwissenschaften 43, 453 (1956).

DE ROBERTIS, E. D. P., and H. S. BENNETT: Some features of fine structure of cytoplasm of cells in the earthworm nerve cord. In: Fine Structure of Cells, Internat. Union Biol. Sci. Symp. (B), 21, p. 261—273 (1954).

DEUSE-ZIMMERMANN, R.: Vergleichende Untersuchungen über Neurosekretion bei Enchytraeidae, Tubificidae und Naididae. Z. Zellforsch. 52, 801—816 (1960).

GERSCH, M., u. K. WOHLRABE: Experimentelle Untersuchungen über die Beziehungen zwischen Neurosekretion und Regeneration bei Enchytraeus. Zool. Jb. Physiol. 71, 393—413 (1965).

HAGADORN, I. R.: Neurosecretion and the brain of the Rhynchobdellid Leech, Theromyzon rude (BAIRD, 1869). J. Morph. 102, 55—89 (1958).

— H. A. BERN, and R. S. NISHIOKA: The fine structure of the supraesophageal ganglion of the Rhynchobdellid Leech, Theromyzon rude, with special reference to neurosecretion. Z. Zellforsch. 58, 714—758 (1963).

HARMS, J. W.: Über ein inkretorisches Cerebralorgan bei Lumbriciden sowie Beschreibung eines verwandten Organs bei drei neuen Lycastis-Arten. Arch. Entwickl.-Mech. Org. 143, 332—346 (1948).

HERLANT-MEEWIS, H.: Regeneration in Annelids. In: Advances in Morphogenesis (M. ABERCROMBIE et J. BRACHET), vol. 4, p. 155—215. London-New York: Academic Press 1965.

— Les cellules neurosécrétrices de la chaîne nerveuse d'Eisenia foetida. Z. Zellforsch. 69, 319—325 (1966).

—, et S. GALLARDO: Phénomènes neurosécrétoires au cours de la régénération postérieure d'Eisenia foetida Sav. Gen. comp. endocr. 5, n° 6 (1965).

—, et N. VAN DAMME: Phénomènes neurosécrétoires chez Nereis diversicolor et Eisenia foetida. C. R. Acad. Sci. (Paris) 255, 2291—2293 (1962).

HUBL, H.: Über die Beziehungen der Neurosekretion zum Regenerationsgeschehen bei Lumbriciden nebst Beschreibung eines neuartigen neurosekretorischen Zelltyps im Unterschlundganglion. Arch. Entwickl.-Mech. Org. 149, 73—87 (1956).

JUBERTHIE, C., et M. MESTROV: Données sur la neurosécrétion d'un Oligochète souterrain, Pelodrilus leruthi Hrabe. C. R. Acad. Sci. (Paris) 255, 394—396 (1962).

— — Régénération postérieure en milieu humide et activité neurosécrétrice de la chaîne nerveuse chez Eophila pyrenaica (Oligochètes Lumbricidae). C. R. Acad. Sci. (Paris) 260, 991—994 (1965).

MICHON, J., et FR. ALAPHILIPPE: Contribution à l'étude de la neurosécrétion chez les Lumbricidae. C. R. Acad. Sci. (Paris) 249, 835—837 (1959).

— J. MAISSIAT et A. ANGEVAIN: Contribution à l'étude de la neurosécrétion chez le Lumbricien Eiseniella tetraedra f. typica. C. R. Acad. Sci. (Paris) 259, 1248—1249 (1964).

MORGAN, T. H.: Experimental Studies of the internal Factors of Regeneration in the Earthworm A. F. Roux' Entw. Mech. Organ. 14, 562—591 (1902).

NAISSE, J.: Elaboration de la neurosécrétion au niveau de vésicules golgi-ergastoplasmiques chez l'Opilion. C. R. Acad. Sci. (Paris) 252, 185 (1961).

OTREMBA, P.: Beobachtungen an neurosekretorischen Zellen des Regenwurmes (Lumbricus spec.). Z. Zellforsch. 54, 421—436 (1961).

SAUSSEY, M.: Contribution à l'étude des phénomènes de diapause et de régénération caudale chez Allolobophora icterica (Savigny) (Oligochète Lombricien). Mem. Soc. Linn. Normandie, Zool. 3, 5—158 (1966).

SCHARRER, B.: Über sekretorisch tätige Nervenzellen bei Wirbellosen Tieren. Naturwissenschaften, 25, 131—138 (1937).

—, and S. BROWN: The formation of neurosecretory granules in the earthworm, Lumbricus terrestris L. Z. Zellforsch. 54, 530—540 (1961).

STIENNON, J. A., and P. DROCHMANS: Electron Microscope Study of Neurosecretory Cells in Phasmidea. Gen. comp. endocr. 1, 286—294 (1961).

TAKEUCHI, N.: Neurosecretory elements in the central nervous system of the earthworm. Sci. Rep. Tôhoku Univ. Ser. IV (Biol. 31, 105—116 (1965).

II. Mollusques

Gabe, M.: Données histologiques sur la neurosécrétion chez les Pterotracheidae (Hétéropodes). Rev. canad. Biol. 10, 391—410 (1951).
— La neurosécrétion chez les Mollusques et ses rapports avec la reproduction. Arch. anat. micr. Morph. exp. 54, 371—385 (1965).
Gorf, A.: Untersuchungen über Neurosekretion bei der Sumpfdeckelschnecke *Vivipara vivipara* L. Zool. Jb. Physiol. 69, 379 (1961).
Herlant-Meewis, H., et J. van Mol: Phénomènes neurosécrétoires chez *Arion rufus* et *Arion subfuscus*. C. R. Acad. Sci. (Paris) 249, 321—322 (1959).
Krause, E.: Untersuchungen über die Neurosekretion im Schlundring von *Helix pomatia* L. Z. Zellforsch. 51, 748 (1960).
Lever, J., J. Jasen, and T. A. de Vlieger: Pleural ganglia and water balance in the fresh water pulmonate *Limnaea stagnalis*. Proc. Kon. ned. Akad. Wet., Ser. C, 64, 532—542 (1961).
Lubet, P.: Effets de l'ablation des centres nerveux sur l'émission des gamètes chez *Mytilus edulis* L. et *Chlamys varia* L. (Mollusques lamellibranches). Ann. Sci. nat., Zool., 11e série, 18, 175—183 (1956).
— Incidences de l'ablation bilatérale des ganglions cérébroïdes sur la gamétogenèse et le développement du tissu conjonctif chez la Moule *Mytilus galloprovincialis Lmk.* (Moll. Lamell.). C. R. Soc. Biol. 159, 397—399 (1965).
Nagabhushanam, R.: Neurosecretory cycle and reproduction in the Bivalve, *Crassostrea virginica*. Indian J. exp. Biol. 1, 161—162 (1963).
Nolte, A.: Neurohämal-„Organe" bei Pulmonaten (Gastropoda). Zool. Jb. Anat. 82, 365—380 (1965).
— H. Breucker u. D. Kuhlmann: Untersuchungen am Schlundring von *Crepidula fornicata* L. (Prosobranchier, gastropoda). Z. Zellforsch. 68, 1—27 (1965).
Rohnisch, S.: Untersuchungen zur Neurosekretion bei *Planorbarius corneus* L. (Basommatophora). Z. Zellforsch. 63, 767—798 (1964).
Simpson, L., H. A. Bern, and R. S. Nishioka: Inclusions in the Neurons of *Aplysia california* (Cooper, 1863) (Gastropoda Opisthobranchiata). J. comp. Neur. 121, 237—258 (1963).
van Mol, J. J.: Phénomènes neurosécrétoires dans les ganglions cérébroïdes d'*Arion rufus*. C. R. Acad. Sci. (Paris) 250, 2280 (1960).

III. Crustacés

Matsumoto, K.: Neurosecretion in the thoracic ganglion of the crab, *Eriocheir japonicus*. Biol. Bull. 106, 60—68 (1954a).
— Chromatophorotropic activity of the neurosecretory cells in the thoracic ganglion of *Eriocheir japonicus*. Biol. J. Okayama Univ. 1, 234—248 (1954b).
— — Morphogical studies on the neurosecretion in crabs. Biol. J. Okayama Univ. 4, 103—176 (1958).
— Neurosecretory cells of an Isopod, *Armadillidium vulgare* (Latreille). Biol. J. Okayama Univ. 5, 43—50 (1959).
— Experimental Studies of the neurosecretory Activities of the thoracic ganglion of a Crab, *Hemigrapsus*. Gen. and comp. Endocr. 2, 4—11 (1962).
Otsu, T.: Precocious development of the ovaries in the crab, *Potamon dehaani*, following implantation of the thoracic ganglion. Annat. Zool. Jap. 33, 90—96 (1960).

IV. Insectes

Arvy, L., et M. Gabe: Données histophysiologiques sur les formations endocrines rétrocérébrales de quelques Odonates. Ann. Sci. Nat., Zool. 14, 11e série, 345—374 (1952).
— — Particularités histophysiologiques des glandes endocrines céphaliques chez *Tenebrio molitor* L. C. R. Acad. Sci. (Paris) 237, 844—846 (1953).
Baffoni, G.: Osservazioni sui neuroni secretori del cerebro e dei gangli ventrali di un Ortottero (*Gryllotalpa gryllotalpa*). Lincei Rend. Sci. Phys. Math. Nat. 29, 400—404 (1960).
Bart, A.: Données histologiques et expérimentales sur le système neurosécréteur de l'Insecte aptérygote *Petrobius maritimus*. Gen. comp. Endocr. 3, 398—411 (1963).

DE BESSE, N.: Recherches histophysiologiques sur la neurosécrétion dans la chaîne nerveuse ventrale d'une blatte *Leucophaea maderae*. C. R. Acad. Sci. (Paris) **260**, 7014—7017 (1965).

BOUNHIOL, J.-J., M. GABE et L. ARVY: Données histophysiologiques sur la neurosécrétion chez *Bombyx mori L.* et sur ses rapports avec les glandes endocrines. Bull. Biol. France-Belgique **87**, 323—333 (1953).

CHALAYE, D.: Recherches histochimiques et histophysiologiques sur la sécrétion dans la chaîne nerveuse ventrale du Criquet migrateur *Locusta migratoria*. C. R. Acad. Sci. (Paris) **260**, 7010—7013 (1965).

— Recherches sur la destination des produits de neurosécrétion de la chaîne nerveuse ventrale du Criquet migrateur *Locusta migratoria*. C. R. Acad. Sci. (Paris) **262**, 161—164 (1966).

DAY, M. F.: Neurosecretory cells in the ganglia of Lepidoptera. Nature (Lond.) **145**, 264 (1940).

DELPHIN, F.: Histology and possible functions of neurosecretory cells in the ventral ganglia of *Schistocerca gregaria*. Nature (Lond.) **200**, 913—915 (1963).

FRASER, A.: Neurosecretory cells in the abdominal ganglia of larvae of *Lucilia caesar* (Diptera). Quart. J. Micr. Sci., **100**, 395—399 (1959).

FREON, G.: Contribution à l'étude de la neurosécrétion dans la chaîne nerveuse ventrale du Criquet migrateur *Locusta migratoria*. Bull. Soc. Zool. France, **89**, 819—830 (1964).

FUKUDA, S.: Function of the pupal brain and suboesophageal ganglion in the production of non-diapause and diapause eggs in the silkworm. Annot. Zool. Jap., **25**, 149—155 (1952).

GELDIAY, S.: Neurosecretory cells in ganglia of the roach *Blaberus craniifer*. Biol. Bull., **117**, 267—274 (1959).

GERSCH, M.: Weitere Untersuchungen über neurohormonale Beziehungen bei Insekten. Acta symposii de evolutione insectorum. Praha 1959. Ontogeny of Insects, 127—132 (1959).

HASHIGUSHI, T.: Hormone determining the black pupal colour in the silkworm *Bombyx mori*. Nature (Lond.) **206**, 215 (1965).

HIDAKA, T.: Recherches sur le mécanisme endocrine de l'adaptation chromatique morphologique chez les Nymphes de *Papilio xuthus L.* J. Fac. Sci. Univ. Tokyo, sec. IV, **9**, 223—261 (1961).

HUIGNARD, J.: Recherches histophysiologiques sur le contrôle hormonal de l'oogenèse chez *Gryllus domesticus*. C. R. Acad. Sci. (Paris) **259**, 1557—1560 (1964).

JOHANSSON, A. S.: Relation of Nutrition to Endocrine-Reproductive Functions in the Milkweed Bug *Oncopeltus fasciatus* (Dallas) (Heteroptera:Lygaeidae). Nytt Mag. Zool., **7**, 1—132 (1958).

KOBAYASHI, M.: Studies on the neurosecretion in the silkworm *Bombyx mori L.* Bull. Ser. exp. Stat. **15**, 263—273 (1957).

KÖPF, H.: Über Neurosekretion bei *Drosophila*. Zur Topographie und Morphologie neurosekretorischer Zentren bei der Imago von Drosophila. Biol. Zbl. **67**, 28—42 (1957).

LHOSTE, J.: Données histophysiologiques sur les cellules neurosécrétrices céphaliques et le complexe rétrocérébral de *Forficula auricularia*. Arch. Zool. exp. gén. **89**, 169—183 (1952).

NAISSE, J., et J. MOUTON: Phénomènes neuro-endocrines au niveau de la chaîne nerveuse ventrale de *Carausius morosus* (Phasmides Orthoptères). C. R. Acad. Sci. (Paris) **261**, 3887—3890 (1965).

NAYAR, K. K.: Studies of the neurosecretory system of *Iphita limbata Stal*. Distribution and structure of the neurosecretory cells of the nerve ring. Biol. Bull. **108**, 296—307 (1955).

NOIROT, C.: Neurosécrétion et sexualité chez le Termite à cou jaune *Calotermes flavicollis F*. C. R. Acad. Sci. (Paris) **245**, 743—745 (1957).

PASTEELS, J. M.: Description d'un système neuro-endocrinien dans le ganglion infra-oesophagien du Phasme *Carausius morosus* (Insecte, Orthoptère). C. R. Acad. Sci. (Paris) **261**, 3884—3886 (1965).

RAABE, M.: Recherche sur la neurosécrétion dans la chaîne nerveuse ventrale du Phasme *Clitumnus extradentatus:* les éléments neurosécréteurs. C. R. Acad. Sci. (Paris) **260**, 6710 ou 6713 (1965a).

Raabe, M.:Recherches sur la neurosécrétion dans la chaîne nerveuse ventrale du Phasme, *Clitumnus extradentatus:* les épaississements des nerfs transverses, organes de signification probable-ment neurohémale. C. R. Acad. Sci. (Paris) **261**, 4240—**4243** (1965b).

— Etude des phénomènes de neurosécrétion au niveau de la chaîne nerveuse ventrals des Phasmides. Bull. Soc. Zool. France **90**, 631—654 (1965c).

Scharrer, B.: Neurosecretion. II. Neurosecretory cells in the central nervous system of cockroaches. J. comp. Neurol. **74**, 93—108 (1941).

— Castration cells in the central nervous system of an Insect (*Leucophaea maderae*, Blattaria). Trans. N. Y. Acad. Sci. **17**, 520—525 (1955).

Thomas, A.: Recherches expérimentales sur le contrôle endocrine de l'ovogenèse chez *Gryllus domesticus L.* C. R. Acad. Sci. (Paris) **259**, 1561—1564 (1964a).

— Etude expérimentale relative au contrôle endocrine de l'ovogenèse chez *Gryllus domesticus L.* Bull. Soc. Zool. France **89**, 835—854 (1964b).

Hormonal Control of Spermatogenesis in Hirudo medicinalis

I. R. HAGADORN

Department of Zoology, University of North Carolina, Chapel Hill, North Carolina, USA.

Introduction

Neurosecretion in the brain of annelids has attracted considerable attention since its first recognition in the supraesophageal ganglion of NEREIS by BERTA SCHARRER in 1936; in the polychetes and oligochetes it has been implicated in the control of reproduction, amongst other functions (see BERN and HAGADORN, 1965 for references). In the Hirudinea, the histology and cytology of the neurosecretory system has been examined by a number of workers, including B. SCHARRER, 1937; HAGADORN, 1958, 1962, 1966; HAGADORN et al., 1963; NAMBUDIRI and VIJAYA-KRISHNAN, 1958; LEGENDRE, 1959; CZECHOWICZ, 1963, and VON TÜMPLING, 1965. Two principal cell types been reported: α-cells, which stain with paraldehyde fuchsin or chrome alum hematoxylin, and β-cells, which stain with orange G or phloxin (HAGADORN, 1958, 1966a). On these, the α-cells are the more prominent, and are consistently present in *Theromyzon rude* (Rhynchobdellida) and *Hirudo medicinalis* (Gnathobdellida). Their secretions have been found to be rich in disulfide groups (BIANCHI, 1964a, b; HAGADORN, 1964, 1966a).

Previous work (HAGADORN, 1962) had indicated that the brain (supra- and sub-esophageal ganglia) in *Theromyzon* is the source of a gonadotropic influence required for completion of spermatogenesis; recently (HAGADORN, 1966b) these observations have been extended to *Hirudo*, with the suggestion that the gonadotropic influence is hormonal in nature. The present paper reports confirmation of these results with respect to spermatogenesis; oögenesis in *Hirudo* has not yet been studied.

Materials and Methods (see also Hagadorn, 1966b)

Hirudo medicinalis were obtained from a commercial supplier. Two experimental series have been carried out (one in 1965, one in 1966) to analyse the role of the brain neurosecretory system in the control of spermatogenesis. The experimental design has included the following groups:

a) *Base line* untreated animals, sacrificed on day zero to evaluate the beginning condition of the testes.

b) *Untreated* animals, maintained in the laboratory during the course of the experiment.

c) *Brain removed* animals, in which the brain was removed on day zero of the experiment.

d) *Operative control* animals, in which all procedures prior to the actual excision of the brain were carried out on day zero of the experiment.

e) *Brain removed, brain injected* animals, in which the brain was removed on day zero and brain injections made immediately under the body wall at regular intervals. In experiment 1 (1965) the injections were made at ten day intervals beginning on day one, for a total of three brains per animal. The brains used were taken at the beginning of the experiment and stored at —20° C until needed. In experiment 2, brains were injected at seven day intervals beginning on day one, for a total of four brains per animal during the course of the experiment. The brains used in experiment 2 were taken the previous July, at the time when the greatest amounts of stainable α-cell secretions are seen in the brain. These brains were lyophilized and stored *in vacuo* at —20° C until required.

Table 1. *Experimental design. The number of animals surviving in each group are indicated for experiments 1 and 2*

Treatment	Exp. 1	Exp. 2
Untreated	11	19
Operative controls	15	10
Brain removed	12	16
Brain removed, brain injections	10	11
Brain removed, muscle Injections	—	7

f) *Brain removed, muscle injected* animals, in which the brain was removed on day zero and fragments of lyophilized body wall (mainly muscle) injected at seven day intervals beginning on day one. This group was include only in experiments 2. Preparation and storage of muscle fragments were identical to that of the brains used in experiment 2; the fragments injected were comparable in size to the brains injected.

Both experiments lasted for a period of one month. The experiments were so timed as to begin just prior to activation of the testis in late winter and to terminate prior to the time when mature sperm would be expected in natural populations (see HAGADORN, 1966 b). Experiment 1 began February 4, 1965, experiment 2 on January 18, 1966. Average mortality in all groups of both experiments amounted to about 40%, due primarily to bacterial infection. Analyses of the effects of treatments were made on Carnoy-fixed smears of testicular contents, on the basis of percent of the total gametes counted which were in each of the following four maturation stages:

Stage 1 (early): small clusters in about the 1—64 cell stage.

Stage 2 (middle): larger clusters of approximately 64—128 or more cells; the developing sperm are rounded, and have relatively abundant cytoplasm. The cytophore is not prominent.

Stage 3 (late): large clusters with elliptical, cytoplasm-poor sperm cells; the cytophore is prominent. The first signs of sperm tail development are evident in some cases.

Stage 4 (mature): large clusters with prominent cytophores and sperm tails fully developed.

In experiment 1 the number of gametes in one evenly-filled 200 diameter microscope field was determined for each animal and the gametes present were classified according to the above criteria; this procedure gave not only information concerning the effects of the experimental procedures upon the ability of the gametes to mature, but also gave an approximate idea of the effects of manipulations upon the total number of developing gametes present per testis. In experiment 2,

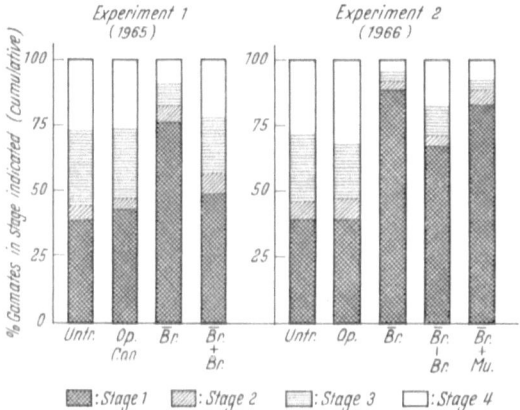

Fig. 1. Results of the several treatments of experiments 1 and 2, portrayed as the cumulative percent of total gametes present which were in each of the four stages of maturation.
▓ : Stage 1   ▨ : Stage 2   ▧ : Stage 3   ▢ : Stage 4

Table 2a—c. *Results of testis smear analysis, expressed in terms of % of total gametes observed which are in each of the four maturation stages. a) experiment 1; b) experiment 2; c) averages of experiments 1 and 2*

a) Experiment 1 (1965)

group	maturation stage			
	1	2	3	4
Untreated	37.8	6.0	28.4	27.8
Op. Cont.	42.9	4.3	25.4	27.4
Br.	76.1	5.5	8.0	10.4
Br. + Br.	49.1	6.4	21.8	22.7

b) Experiment 2 (1966)

group	1	2	3	4
Untreated	38.7	7.3	24.6	29.4
Op. Cont.	39.8	7.2	20.4	32.6
Br.	88.2	2.5	4.0	5.3
Br. + Br.	66.6	4.3	11.1	18.0
Br. + Mu.	82.6	4.9	4.3	8.2

c) Averages of Experiments 1 and 2

group	1	2	3	4
Untreated	38.3	6.6	26.5	28.6
Op. Cont.	41.4	5.7	22.9	30.0
Br.	82.2	4.0	6.0	7.8
Br. + Br.	57.9	5.3	16.5	20.3
Br. + Mu.	82.6	4.9	4.3	8.2

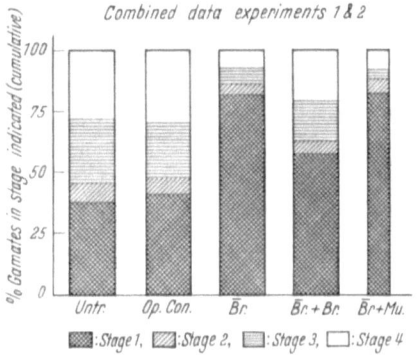

Fig. 2. Combined results of the several treatments of experiments 1 and 2, portrayed as the average cumulative percent of total gametes present which were in each of the four stages of maturation
▓ : Stage 1   ▨ :Stage 2   ▧ : Stage 3   ▢ : Stage 4

sperm clusters were classified by stage as they were encountered on the slide, until a total of one hundred clusters per animal had been categorized. In either case, the scores obtained for each of the several maturation classes in each animal were summed within groups for each experiment, and the totals tested for significance between groups by the X² method. For purposes of this test only, the number of animals per group was equalized at ten for experiment 1 and seven for experiment 2, these being the sizes of the smallest remaining group in each experiment; the percentage figures in Table 2 are based upon the full groups. Selection of animals to be included in each group used for statistics was done with a table of random numbers. Complete details of statistical analyses of experiment 1 are given in Hagadorn, 1966 b.

Results

The results of evaluation of sperm clusters in the testis smears of the several groups are indicated, in terms of percent of total gametes observed which were in each of the four maturation stages, in Table 2 and Fig. 1 and 2. Since the results of the two experiments were similar in character, they will be described mainly in terms of the averages of the data of the combined experiments. Fig. 1 illustrates the results of the two experiments separately; Fig. 2 illustrates the combined data.

a) *Base line untreated animals.* Analysis of testis smears from animals sacrificed on day zero disclosed that in both experiments the most advanced stage found in the testis at the beginning of the experiment was stage 2. No late or mature stages were observed.

b) *Untreated animals* (Fig. 1, 2 and 3). Those untreated animals maintained in the laboratory during the one month duration of the experiment had attained maturity by the end of both experiments, an average of about 55% of the gametes present being in stages 3 or 4. In nature, only about 10% of the sperm clusters present would be expected to be in stage 3 at this time, none in stage 4. Results of experiment 1 (see also Hagadorn, 1966 b) indicate an average of about seventy sperm clusters per 200 × field in smears from untreated animals.

c) *Operative controls* (Fig. 1, 2 and 4). In those animals subjected to a sham operation, the overall average of gametes in stages 3 and 4 at the end of both experiments was about 53%. The slight decrease compared to the untreated groups was mainly due to the increase of stage 1 (early) at the expense of stage 3 (late) clusters. It was statistically insignificant in experiment 1, and significant at the 0.01% level in experiment 2. Results of experiment 1 indicate an average of about fifty-six sperm clusters per 200 × field, also a slight decrease as compared to the untreated groups.

d) *Brain removed animals* (Fig. 1, 2, and 5). Brain removal usually resulted in a severe depletion both of total numbers of developing gametes, and of the proportion of those gametes present which were in advanced stages of maturation. The proportion of clusters in stages 3 and 4 is reduced to a noverall average of about 14% in the two experiments, fully 82% of the gametes being in stage 1. This deviation from the ratios observed in the untreated groups is significant at much better than the 0.1% level in both experiments. The results of experiment 1 indicate an average of about thiry-eight clusters per 200 × microscope field in brainless animals, a marked decrease from the untreated level.

There is some suggestion of an all or none effect of brain removal: in four of the twenty-eight animals surviving in the two experiments the effect of brain removal had an effect little more severe than that of the sham operation, as judged by the proportions of gametes in the several maturation stages. In the remaining animals

the depletion of advanced stages was strong, nine of the twenty-eight having 95%
or more of the gametes present in stage 1. The depression of the total number of
gametes present was in all cases marked.

  e) *Brain removed, brain injected animals* (Fig. 1, 2, and 6). Repeated injection
of frozen or lyophilized brains into brainless animals caused a definite, although

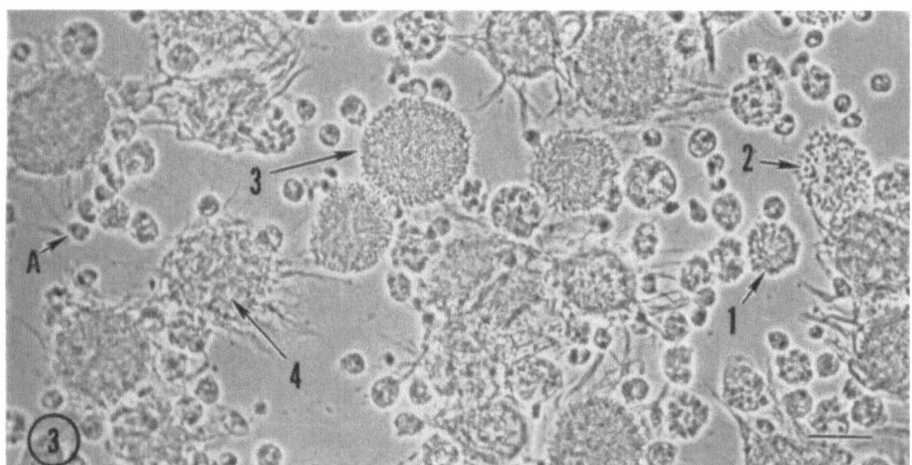

Fig. 3. Normal (untreated) testis smears from *Hirudo*. Phase contrast. Observe numerous
maturing (stage 3 and 4) sperm clusters. *1:* stage 1, early; *2:* stage 2, middle; *3:* stage 3, late;
4: stage 4, mature; *A:* amoebocytes. Marker represents 50 μ

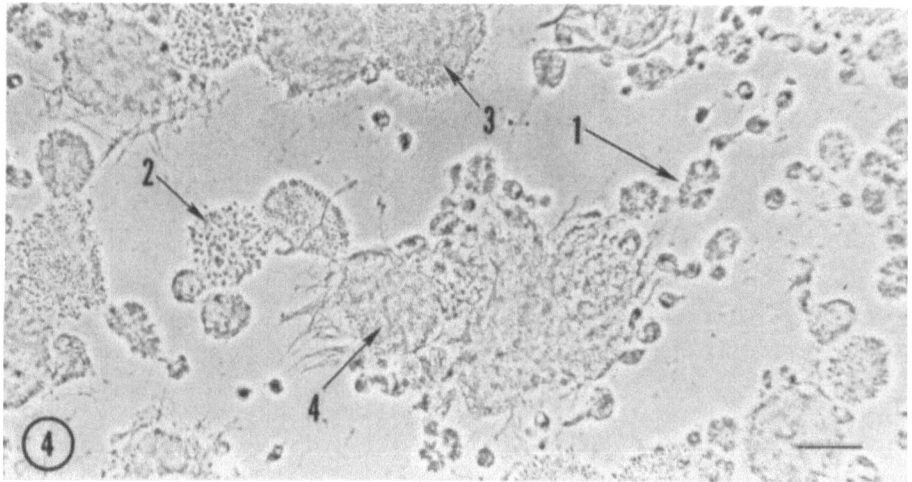

Fig. 4. Testis smear from a sham-operated *Hirudo*. Phase contrast. Note maturing (stage 3
and 4) sperm clusters. The general appearance is similar to that of smears from untreated
animals (figure 3). Labels as in figure 3

not complete, return both of the total number of gametes present and of the proportion of gametes observed in each of the four maturation stages, toward the
values observed for the untreated animals. The proportion of gametes present

which are in late or mature stages of spermatogenesis attains 37%, while the results of experiment 1 indicate an average of about fifty-three sperm clusters per 200 × field. The alteration towards normal of the maturation stage ratios observed are significant in both experiments at better than the 0.1% level.

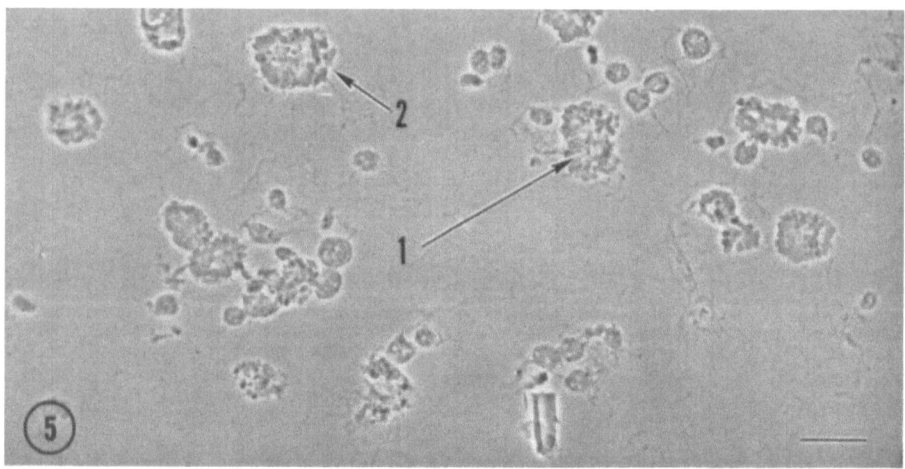

Fig. 5. Testis smear from a *Hirudo* with the brain excised one month prior to sacrifice. Phase contrast. Note marked decrease both in total number of gametes, and in numbers of maturing (stage 3 and 4) sperm clusters. Labels as in figure 3

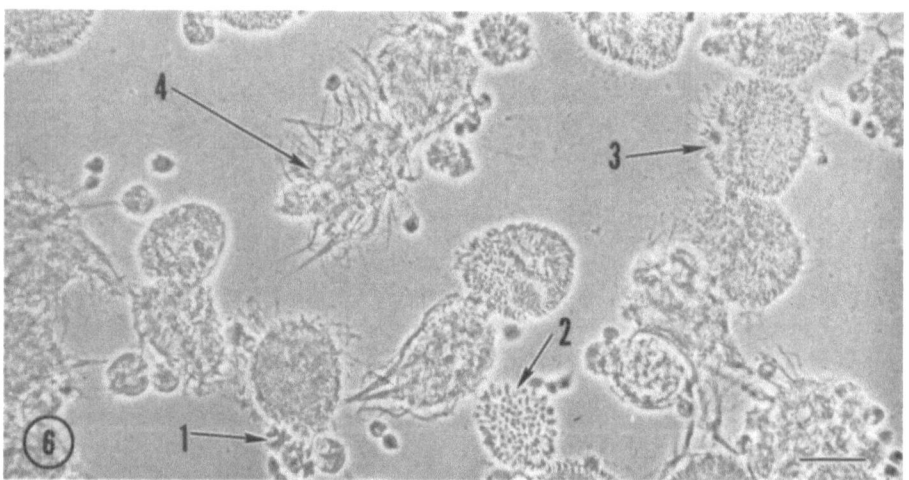

Fig. 6. Testis smear from a *Hirudo* with brain removed and injections of lyophilized brain (for a total of four) over a one month period. Phase contrast. Note the increase in number of maturing (stage 3 and 4) sperm clusters. Labels as in figure 3

f) *Brain removed, muscle injected animals* (Fig. 1, 2 and 7). This group was included only in experiment 2, hence observations of effects upon total number of gametes present are not available. Determination of the proportion of gametes present which are in each of the four stages of maturation shows that about 13% of the gametes are in stages 3 and 4. This compares with 9% of the gametes in comparable stages in the brainless animals of experiment 2, and an overall average of 14% of the total gametes present in brainless animals being in stages 3 and 4 in both experiments combined. The maturation stage ratio observed for brainless animals given injections of muscle is significantly different (p <0.01) when compared to that of the brainless animals of experiment 2 only, but is in fact almost identical to the overall maturation stage ratio obtained for the brainless, uninjected animals of both experiments combined (Fig. 2).

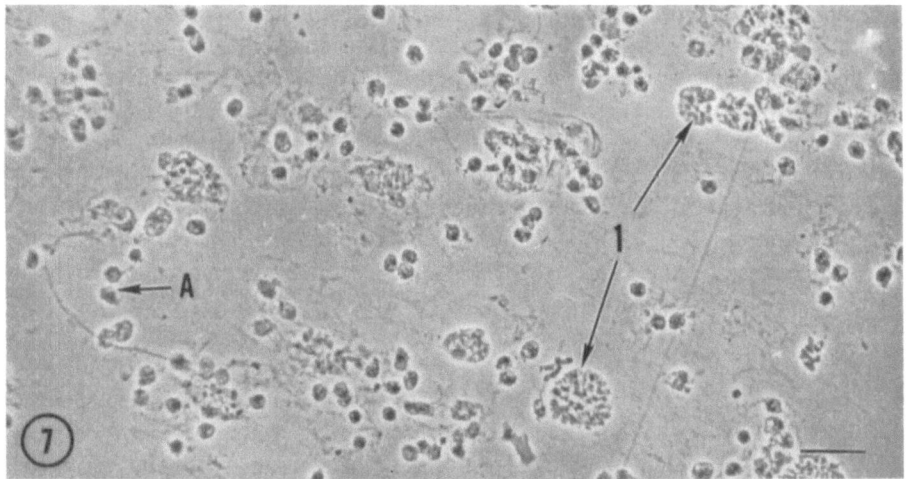

Fig. 7. Testis smear from a *Hirudo* with brain removed and four injections of lyophilized body wall over a one month period. Phase contrast. Note similarity to testis smear of brain removed, uninjected animal (figure 5). Labels as in figure 3

Discussion

The effects of comparable treatments are uniformly consistent between experiments 1 and 2: brain removal results in a severe depression both in total number of gametes present and in the ability of those gametes present to mature; injection of frozen or lyophilized brains partially corrects both of these deficiencies. There is a slight but significant adverse effect of the sham operation on spermatogenesis in both experiments. Since there is this consistency in the results of the two experiments, it seems legitimate to compare the data from the brain removed, muscle injected group of experiment 2 to the combined data for the brain removed, uninjected groups for both experiments 1 and 2. If this is done it can be said that injection of lyophilized muscle into brainless animals has no restorative effect on gametogenesis (Fig. 2); if the brainless, muscle injected group is compared to the brainless group of experiment 2 only, the effect is at best slight (Fig. 1).

The strongly deleterious effect of brain removal upon spermatogenesis indicates the origin in the brain of a gonadotropic influence required for maintenance and successful maturation of the sperm. That this effect is specifically due to brain removal is demonstrated by the results of the operative control group, in which the observed effects, although statistically significant, are minor in magni tude by comparison to those of brain removal. That the sham operation should have a slight adverse effect is not surprising, since there is a real possibility of damaging the brain during this control procedure. The results of brain removal in *Hirudo* confirm for spermatogenesis previous observations in *Theromyzon* (HAGADORN, 1962) which indicated that the brain of that species is the source of a gonadotropic influence required for the successful completion of both spermatogenesis and oögenesis. In the work on *Theromyzon*, as well as in the present observation, it was noted that a certain proportion of the experimental animals (three of thirty-six *Theromyzon* reported in 1962, four of twenty-eight brainless *Hirudo* reported in this paper) could complete spermatogenesis in more or less normal fashion even though lacking a brain. In *Theromyzon* this was interpreted as one line of evidence favoring the hypothesis that the brain gonadotropic factor is required only at some critical stage in sperm maturation, sperm clusters which had already passed this stage at the time of brain removal being no longer dependent on stimulation by the brain factor. Although the evidence in *Hirudo* is not conclusive, it is in agreement with this idea; such an hypothesis would explain the presence of mature sperm clusters in the testes of the brainless groups as being derived from clusters which had already passed the critical stage prior to the beginning of the experiments. The point requires further study.

The partial restoration of spermatogenesis resulting from brain injections indicates that the brain gonadotropin is hormonal in nature; the relative or complete ineffectiveness of muscle injections in this regard suggests that the effect is specific to the brain. In experiment 1, the brain-injected animals closely approached the sham-operated animals in the observed percentage of cell clusters in the several stages of maturation; the brain injections were somewhat less effective in experiment 2. It is possible that the lyophilization and length of storage (six months) of the brains used in the second experiment lowered their potency; it is also possible that the assumption that July brains would contain more of the active principal than brains taken in January is erroneous. This was assumed since the peak of the amount of stainable α-cell secretions occurs in July, which is also just prior to the time when the peak numbers of mature sperm clusters are normally observed in *Hirudo* (see HAGADORN, 1866b).

The demonstration of a hormonal stimulation of spermatogenesis by the brain of *Hirudo* suggests that the pattern of reproductive control in leeches parallels that observed in oligochetes by HERLANT-MEEWIS, 1956, 1959, and by RUDE and LINDER, 1964, and in the Arenicolidae amongst the polychetes by HOWIE, 1963. It contrasts with the inhibitory pattern of control reported in the Nereidae (DURCHON, 1952; HAUENSCHILD, 1956), Syllidae (DURCHON, 1959; HAUENSCHILD, 1959) and Nephtyidae (CLARK, 1956).

Summary and Conclusions

The results of experiments carried out in *Hirudo* over a two year period indicate that:

1. Brain removal in January or February (at a time just prior to or during testicular activation) severely depresses the process of gametogenesis. This indicates the origin of a gonadotropic influence in the brain. It confirms previous observations in *Theromyzon*.

2. The results of brain injections into brainless *Hirudo* support the view that this brain gonadotropic influence is hormonal in nature.

3. The results of injections of muscle into brainless *Hirudo* support the view that the effect is specific to the brain.

4. The proposed method of control of spermatogenesis in *Hirudo* is similar to that observed in the earthworm and in the polychete *Arenicola* in that it involves a stimulatory factor rather than an inhibitory influence as seen in the nereid, syllid, and nephtyid polychetes.

Acknowledgements. The competent technical assistance of Mrs. PAMELA RHODES is gratefully acknowledged. Mr. BARRY SILER aided in the preparation of Tables 1 and 2. Much of the work reported here was supported by grant No. GB-1113 from the National Science Foundation.

References

BERN, H. A., and I. R. HAGADORN (1965): Neurosecretion. In: Structure and Function in the Nervous System of Invertebrates. T. H. BULLOCK, and G. A. HORRIDGE. Vol. I, pp. 353—429. San Francisco: Freeman and Company.

BIANCHI, S. (1964a): Neurosecrezione e sostanze fenoliche nei gangli degli anellidi: I.-Ricerche sugli Irudinei (*Hirudo medicinalis* L.) Soc. Pelor. Sci. fis. mat. nat. Atti. **10**, 287—300.

— (1964b): Istochemica del neurosecreto delle cellule nervose di *Hirudo medicinalis* L. Soc. Pelor. Sci. fis. mat. nat. Atti. **10**, 319—325.

CLARK, R. B. (1956): The neurosecretory system of the polychaete *Nephtys* and its role in reproduction. (Abstr.) XX Internat. Physiol. Congr. (Brussels). 178.

CZECHOWICZ, K. (1963): Neurosecretion in leeches and the annual cycle of its changes. Zool. Polon. **13**, 163—184.

DURCHON, M. (1952): Recherches expérimentales sur deux aspects de la reproduction chez les annélides polychètes; l'épitoquie et la stolonisation. Ann. Sci. Nat. (Zool.) **14**, 117—206.

— (1959): Contribution a l'étude de la stolonisation chez les Syllidiens (annélides polychètes): I. Syllinae. Bull. Biol. **93**, 155—219.

HAGADORN, I. R. (1958): Neurosecretion and the brain of the rhynchobdellid leech *Theromyzon rude* (BAIRD, 1869). J. Morphol. **102**, 55—90.

— (1962): Functional correlates of neurosecretion in the rhynchobdellid leech, *Theromyzon rude.* Gen. comp. Endocr. **2**, 516—540.

— (1964): Histology and histochemistry of neurosecretion in the medicinal leech, *Hirudo medicinalis.* Amer. Zool. (Abstr.) **4**, 141.

— (1966a): The histochemistry of the neurosecretory system in *Hirudo medicinalis.* Gen. comp. Endocr. **6**, 288—294.

— (1966b): Neurosecretion in the Hirudinea and its possible role in reproduction. Amer. Zool. **6**, 251—261.

— H. A. BERN, and R. S. NISHIOKA (1963): The fine structure of the supraesophageal ganglion of the rhynchobdellid leech, *Theromyzon rude*, with special reference to neurosecretion. Z. Zellforsch. **58**, 714—758.

HAUENSCHILD, C. (1956): Hormonale Hemmung der Geschlechtsreife und Metamorphose bei dem Polychaeten *Platynereis dumerilii.* Z. Naturforsch. **11B**, 125—132.

— (1959): Hemmender Einfluß der Proventrikelregion auf Stolonisation and Oocyten-Entwicklung bei dem Polychaeten *Autolytus prolifer.* Z. Naturforsch. **14B**, 87—89.

HERLANT-MEEWIS, H. (1956): Reproduction et neurosécrétion chez *Eisenia foetida* (Sav.). Ann. Soc. Zool. Belg. **87**, 151—183.

— (1959): Phénomènes neuro-sécrétoires et sexualité chez *Eisenia foetida.* C. R. Acad. Sci. (Paris) **248**, 1405—1406.

HOWIE, D. I. D. (1963): Experimental evidence for the humoral stimulation of ripening of the gametes and spawning in the polychaete *Arenicola marina* (L.) Gen. comp. Endocr. **3**, 660—668.

LEGENDRE, R. (1959): Sur la présence de cellules neurosécrétrices dans les ganglions sus-
oesophagiens de la sangsue médicinale (*Hirudo medicinalis* L.), suivie de quelques considérations sur la neurosécrétion. Bull. Biol. **93**, 462—471.

NAMBUDIRI, P. N., and K. P. VIJAYAKRISHNAN (1958): Neurosecretory cells of the brain of
the leech *Hirudinaria granulosa* (Sav.). Current Sci. **27**, 350—351.

RUDE, S. S., and H. J. LINDER (1964): The effect of the brain on spermatogenesis in the
oligochete, *Eisenia foetida*. Amer. Zool. **4**, 327.

SCHARRER, B. (1936): Über Drüsen-Nervenzellen im Gehirn von *Nereis virens* Sars. Zool. Anz.
113, 299—302.

— (1937): Über sekretorisch tätige Nervenzellen bei wirbellosen Tieren. Naturwissenschaften.
25, 131—138.

VON TÜMPLING, W. (1965): Untersuchungen über Neurosekretion bei Hirudineen. Z. wissen-
schaftl. Zool. **171**, 1—43.

A Histological and Experimental Approach to Neurosecretion in Daphnia magna

M. V. ANGEL

National Institute of Oceanography, Wormley, Godalming Surrey, England

Introduction

The lower orders of Crustacea have only received attention from invertebrate endocrinologists during the last decade. Despite BERN, 1963, having emphasised the inadequacy of purely histological evidence for neurosecretory function, only in LOCKHEAD and RESNER's, 1958, investigations on *Artemia salina* has histological evidence been supported by experimental evidence. *Daphnia magna* appeared to be suitable for a similar approach since STERBA, 1957, had described possible neurosecretory cells from a histological study, and SCHULZ, 1928, and HARRIS and MASON, 1956, had shown that *Daphnia* spp. would withstand operations.

Methods

A clone of *Daphnia magna*, derived from a wild population found in the pond of the Clifton Zoological Gardens, was cultured in the laboratory. Filtered pond water enriched with baker's yeast was used as a culture medium. Histological examinations were carried out both on animals from the natural population and on specimens individually reared in the laboratory. The animals were cultured in 150 mls of culture medium in conical flasks immersed in an aquarium which was maintained at a constant temperature of 22° C and continuously circulated. A 40 w fluorescent strip light was mounted beneath the aquarium so that the culture flasks could be examined without interrupting the constant illumination.

Animals at all stages of the moult cycle were fixed by decapitating the animals under fixative. Neurosecretory granules were best preserved by HELLY's fluid with 0.6% sodium chloride added as recommended by STERBA, 1957. Schmorl's osmic acid-alcohol mixture gave excellent fixation for examination of morphological detail. Paraffin sections were out at 7 μ and stained in Gomori's chrome haematoxylin and Heidenhain's iron haematoxylin. Other stains giving useful results were Best's carmine (with and without diastase digestion), periodic acid Schiff's, EINARSON's gallocyanin (at pH 1.4) and ALTMANN's fuchsin. Gabe's paraldehyde fuchsin after both acid permanganate and performic oxidation and HUMBERSTONE's Victoria blue 4 R, specific stains for disulphydryl bonds, gave little positive staining.

Operation experiments were carried out on members of single broods of animals reared under identical conditions. Animals were operated either in the pre-maturation intermoult (body length 1.7—1.9 mm) or in the post-maturation intermoult (body length 2.1—2,3 mm). Organs were removed by pricking them out with a fine glass needle while the animals were steadied in the meniscus at the edge of two thicknesses of wet blotting paper. Obvious operational failures were discarded immediately. Survival (i.e. the animals moulting successfully at least twice after the operation) was 80% or more after all but one of the operations. The removal of the ventral region of the supraoesophageal ganglion (the supra-oesophageal ganglion is referred to as the brain in the rest of this paper) was only achieved with just over 50% survival. The use of penicillin and streptomycin reduced survival, but allowing the animals a four hour recovery period at 18° C

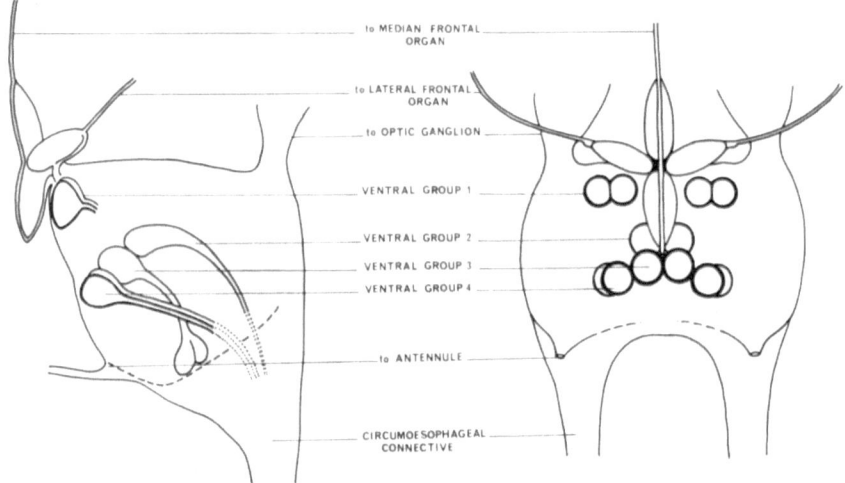

Fig. 1. Diagram showing the relative positions of the four ventral cell groups in the brain viewed laterally and ventrally

improved it. Each animal was reared individually after the operation and the times of the moults were checked to the nearest three hours, and compared with the unoperated controls from the same brood. The young were removed, counted and sexed as soon as they were released. The body length from the top of the head to the base of the tail spine was measured during each intermoult and used as the measure of growth. Culturing conditions were identical for individuals in the same experiment, but were not identical between experiments.

Results

Sterba, 1957, described possible neurosecretory cells in *Daphnia magna* in the ventral region of the brain and in the circum-oesophageal connectives. In this species be found neurosecretory cells neither in the frontal region of the brain nor in the tritrocerebral commissure, positions where they did occur in *Daphnia pulex* and *Simocephalus vetulus*. The present study showed that four distinct cell groups could be found in the ventral region of the brain, distinguished by their positions and the paths of their axons. The cells of all the groups were rich in cytoplasmic basophilia and mitochondria. They showed cyclical changes correlated with the moult cycle in the degree of positive staining with acid chrome haematoxyline and in glycogen content (both were minimal immediately after a moult). These cycles were also described by STERBA. Individual cells of any of the groups were not always strongly positively stained at late stages of the intermoult, sometimes making the cycles difficult to follow. STERBA found that under conditions of cold or starvation the intensity of staining with acid chrome haematoxylin was increased. The increased accumulation of stainable material during stress conditions suggest that the secretions may regulate growth and reproductive rates, rather than the regular moulting rhythm. The growth and reproductive rates are far more sensitive in response to environmental conditions than is the moulting frequency. It was found that after operations there was no increase in the positive staining of these cells with acid chrome haematoxylin. The cycle of glycogen content is a more general cycle shown by many cells of the central nervous system and is,

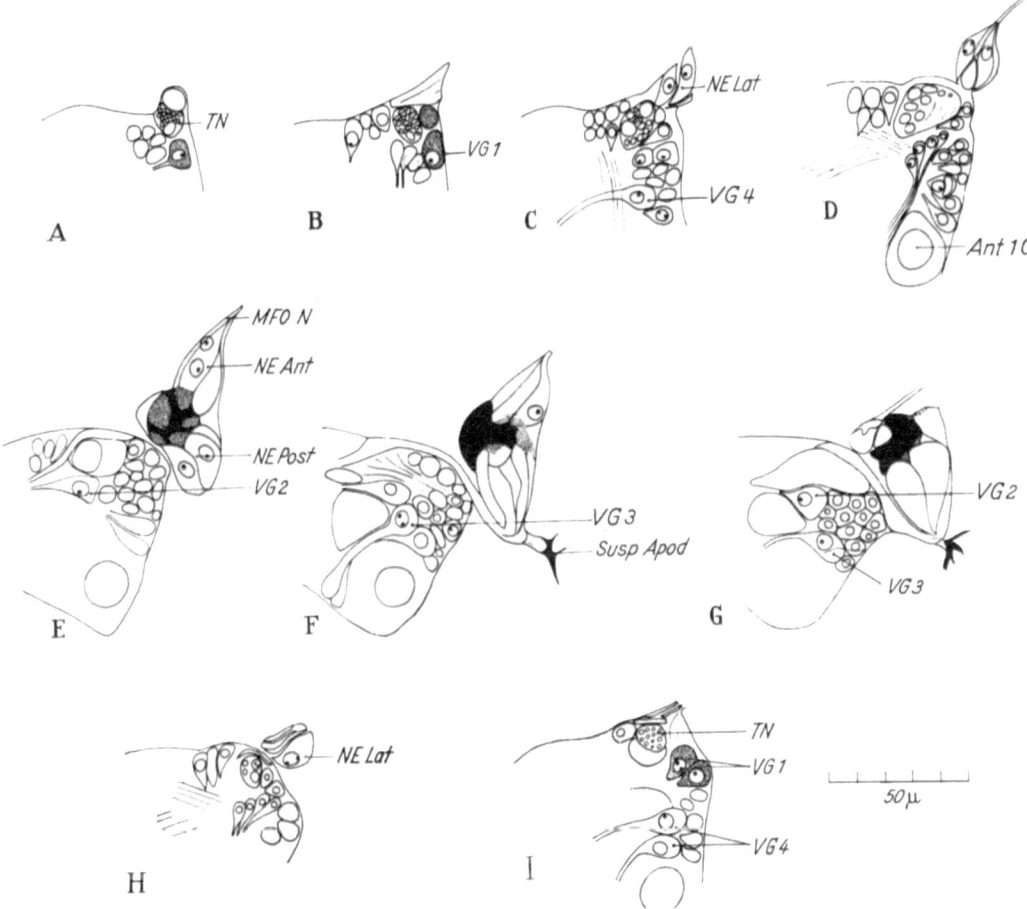

Fig. 2. Camera lucida drawings of consecutive serial sections cut sagittally through the central region of the brain, showing the relative positions and shapes of the cells of the four ventral groups. *TN* Nerve to the lateral frontal organ, *NE Lat* Lateral wing of the naupliar eye, *NE Ant* Anterior wing of the naupliar eye, *NE Post* Posterior wing of the naupliar eye, *MFO N* Nerve to the median frontal organ, *VG 1 to 4* The four ventral groups, *Susp Apod* Suspensory apodeme of the naupliar eye, *Ant 1 C* Brain centre for the antennules

therefore, not indicative of any specialised secretory activity. Fig. 1 shows the relative positions of the cells in the brain. Fig. 2 shows camera lucida drawings of consecutive sagittal sections 7 μ thick through the central region of the brain, illustrating the shape and spatial relationships between the cell groups. Group 1 consists of two pairs of cells lying on the periphery of the brain, just below the origins of the nerves to the lateral frontal organs. Group 2 is a pair of cells lying adjacently on the midline just posterior to the group 1 cells and well within the peripheral layer of nerve cell bodies. Group 3 is another pair of cells immediately posterior to the group 2 cells in the midline. The axons of these two cells are broad and clearly seen to terminate as swollen bulbs on the posterior surface of the brain between the origins of the circum-oesophageal connectives (Fig. 3). Group 4 consists of two pairs of cells just posterior and lateral to the group 3 cells. The axons of all these groups of cells, with the exception of the group 3 cells, could only be followed into the circum-oesophageal connectives and their terminations were not observed.

The frontal region of the brain, the optic ganglia and the lateral and medium frontal organs showed no histological evidence of any neurosecretory tissue. The only other possible neurosecretory cells found were on the dorsal surface of the circum-oesophageal connectives. These cells showed cytological changes for twelve hours after operations or after the animals were placed in various concentrations of sea-water.

Ablation experiments were carried out by removing the following organs: 1) the compound eye, 2) the naupliar eye involving also the cutting of the nerves to the frontal organs, 3) the optic ganglia, 4) the antennules, 5) the head stoare cells, 6) the ventral region of the brain. Fig. 4 shows the positions of these various organs. The results of the operations were assessed by examining a) the moult frequency, b) the growth rate, c) the reproductive rate and the sex of the offspring. Removal of the compound eye had no effect on any of the factors assessed in animals kept in either constant light or in constant darkness (Table 1). Simi-

Table 1. *Operations in all these experiments were carried out on animals in the pre-maturation intermoult*

	Nos animals	Days duration	Moults observed	Average total growth mms.	Average brood size
1. Removal of the compound eye					
Operated constant light	15	29	9	1.68 ± 0.11	17.2 ± 0.92
Controls constant light	15	29	9	1.56 ± 0.08	15.4 ± 0.84
Operated constant darkness	15	29	9	1.66 ± 0.09	16.1 ± 0.46
Controls constant darkness	15	29	9	1.64 ± 0.08	16.2 ± 0.62
2. Removal of the head storage cells					
Operated	14	19	6	0.65 ± 0.05	4.3 ± 0.38
Controls	6	19	6	0.75 ± 0.06	6.0 ± 0.81
3. Removal of optic ganglia					
Operated removal complete	6	18	6	0.90 ± 0.05	8.8 ± 0.85
Operated ganglia damaged	11	18	7	0.89 ± 0.04	9.2 ± 0.96
Controls	7	18	7	0.88 ± 0.06	9.0 ± 0.89
4. Removal of the antennules					
Operated	15	19	6	0.86 ± 0.07	10.2 ± 0.51
Controls	8	19	7	0.92 ± 0.06	11.0 ± 0.62

larly removal of the head storage cells, the optic ganglia, and the antennules had no significant effect (Table 1).

The results obtained after removal of the naupliar eye were inconsistent. In two preliminary experiments several of the animals only produced male offspring and showed reduced longevity, growth and reproductive rates (Table 2). A few of the other animals produced male offspringe and pseudosexual eggs. These animals showed greater longevity, lower growth rates, but higher reproductive rates compared with the animals producing only male offspring. The majority of the operated animals were similar to the unoperated controls, producing only female offspring and with near normal growth and reproductive rates. No histological checks were carried out after these experiments and so it was impossible to assess the damage to the ventral region of the brain. Four full-scale repeats of these experiments were carried out accompanied by full histological examination of all the operated animals. In all these experiments the operated animals showed normal growth and reproduction and moulting behaviour (Table 3). None of them produced any male offspring or pseudosexual eggs. Histological checks showed that in a high proportion (over 60%) of these operated animals there was some damage to the ventral group 1 cells.

The operations on the ventral region of the brain were carried out in conjunction with a further experiment on the effects of extirpating the naupliar eye (Table 4). Once again the animals with only the naupliar eye removed was not significantly different in their growth, moulting, or reproduction from the unoperated controls. Seven out of thirteen animals survived after removal of the whole of the ventral region of the brain, and moulted successfully five times after the operation

Table 2. *Results of the preliminary experiments on the removal of the naupliar eye*

	Nos animals	Moults suryived	Average growth per moult mms.	Average brood size
Operated male broods only	11	3—6 (av. 3.5)	0.15	3.0
Operated males and pseudo-sexual eggs	6	3—8 (av. 5.8)	0.13	4.2 (+ 1 to 3 ephippia)
Operated normal female broods	37	3—8 (av. 6.2)	0.20	16.4
Controls	14	4—8 (av. 7.4)	0.21	19.0

Table 3. *Results of four experiments on the removal of the naupliar eye*
a) Animals operated in the pre-maturation moult

	Numbers	Days duration	Moults observed	Average total growth mms.	Average brood size
1. Operated	29	14	5	0.90 ± 0.03	6.6 ± 0.40
Controls	18	14	5	0.93 ± 0.06	7.1 ± 0.43
2. Operated	29	13	4	1.41 ± 0.03	8.2 ± 0.39
Controls	11	13	4	1.41 ± 0.06	7.9 ± 0.85

b) Animals operated in the post-maturation moult

3. Operated	15	14	5	0.78 ± 0.05	8.8 ± 0.71
Controls	8	14	5	0.70 ± 0.10	9.6 ± 1.20
4. Operated	31	15	5	0.78 ± 0.06	9.9 ± 0.54
Controls	15	15	5	0.81 ± 0.04	9.9 ± 0.43

Table 4. *Results of the experiments on the removal of the ventral region of the brain and of the naupliar eye from animals in the pre-maturation moult*

	Nos animals	Days duration	Moult observed	Average total growth mms.	Average brood size	Maximum body length mms.
Operated naupliar eye	29	15	5	1.17 ± 0.05	5.2 ± 0.42	3.1
Operated ventral region	7	15	5	0.39 ± 0.03	0	2.3
Controls	15	15	5	1.25 ± 0.06	5.3 ± 0.58	3.1

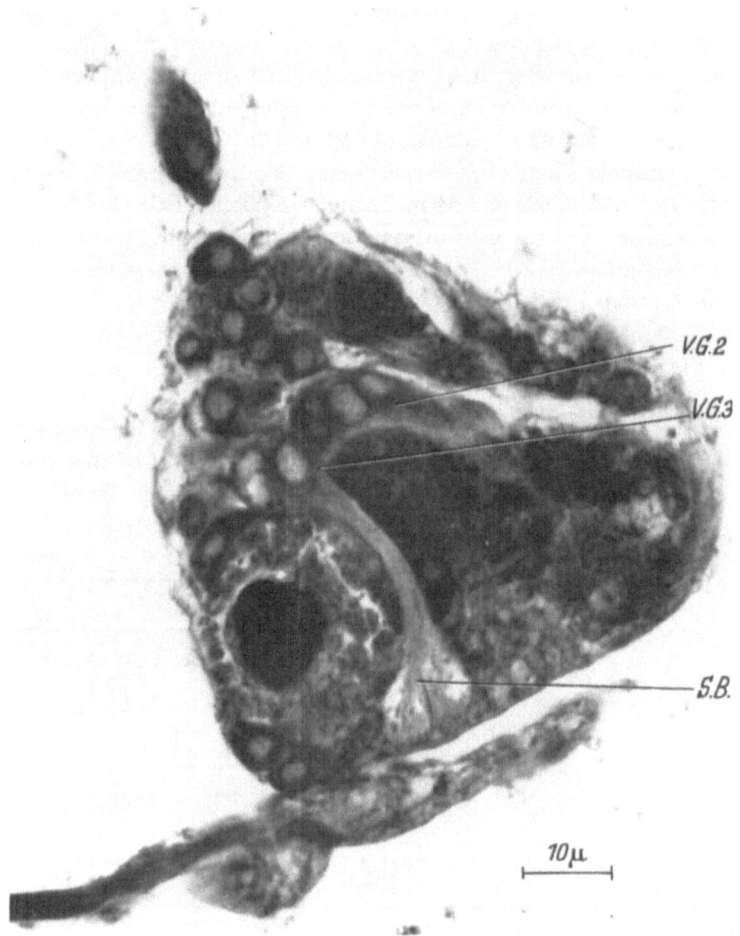

Fig. 3. Sagittal section through the brain showing a ventral group 2 cell (*V.G.2*) and a ventral group 3 cell (*V.G.3*) with its swollen axon ending (*S.B.*) (Schmorl's osmic acid-alcohol, Best's carmine after diatase digestion)

before they were fixed for histological examination. These animals failed to grow beyond the maturation size, and showed no trace of ovarian development. Histological examination showed that all the ventral region had been removed but there were still some connections between the circum-oesophageal connectives and the optic ganglia and antennule ganglia.

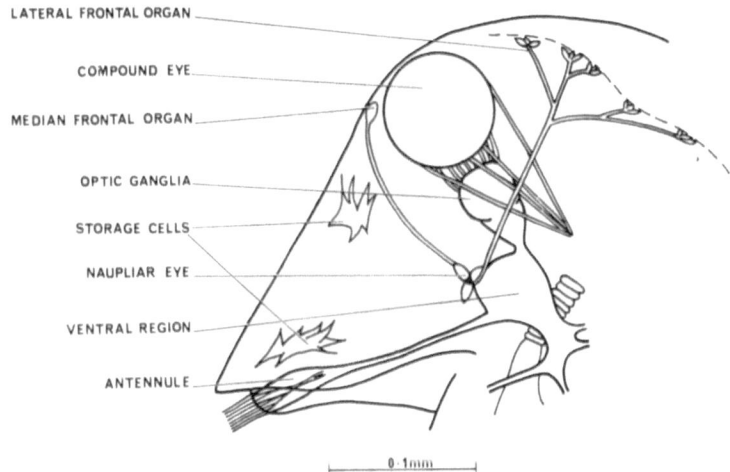

LATERAL FRONTAL ORGAN

COMPOUND EYE

MEDIAN FRONTAL ORGAN

OPTIC GANGLIA

STORAGE CELLS

NAUPLIAR EYE

VENTRAL REGION

ANTENNULE

0·1mm

Fig. 4. Diagram of the head structures based on a camera lucida drawing of a whole mount

Discussion

STERBA, 1957, described the possible neurosecretory cells in the central nervous system of *Daphnia magna*. He did not, however, distinguish the four groups in the ventral region. The group 3 cells can now be termed "probable" neurosecretory cells, according to BERN's criteria (1963), since they have swollen axonal endings that are typical of certain types of neurosecretory cells. The absence of any possible neurosecretory structures in the optic ganglia observed by STERBA was confirmed. Nevertheless, this absence of neurosecretory or neurohaemal tissues is surprising as they have been found in other lower crustacean groups: — Anostrace (MENON, 1962, HENTSCHEL, 1963; 1965) and Ostracoda in *Cypridina chierchiae* (Angel unpublished observation). BARNES and GONOR, 1958a, b, suggested that the absence of storage organs in cirripeds was correlated with their frequent and repeated moulting. The operations on *Daphnia magna* have shown that neither the optic ganglia, nor indeed any of the other structures in the head that were removed, were essential for successful moulting. LOOKHEAD and RESNER, 1958, similarly were unable to detect any physiological disturbance after the removal of the eye-stalks in *Artemia salina*. Their operated animals moulted, copulated and reproduced normally. They were also unable to find any histological evidence of neurosecretory tissue in the optic ganglia. HENTSCHEL, 1963, 1965, has since observed a neurohaemal organ in the eye-stalk of this species. Even in decapods the sinus gland has been shown to be non-functional in *Homarus* until the post-larval fourth stage (PYLE, 1943) and in *Palaemonetes* until the end of the final larval stage (HUBSCHMAN, 1963). Eye-stalk extirpation has no effect on the moulting and maturation of zooeal stages of *Callinectes* (COSTLOW, 1962). Thus even in higher crustacean groups the underlying mechanism controlling moulting is still not completely understood.

The extirpation of all the ventral group cells in *Daphnia magna* prevented post-maturation growth and the development of the ovary. These results are identical to those of MORI, 1933, after castration of female *Daphnia* with X-rays and parallel the results of extirpation of the median brain neurosecretory cells of *Calliophora erythrocephala* (THOMSEN, 1952). Although the results of the two *Daphnia* experiments cannot conclusively be attributed to the interference of endocrine systems, there does seem to be possibility that the median brain cells in arthropods may have the common function of controlling ovarian development and post-maturation growth.

Summary

1. A re-examination of STERBA's, 1957, observations on the histology of neurosecretory cells in *Daphnia magna* revealed four distinct cell groups in the ventral region of the brain (the supra-oesophageal ganglion).

2. One of these ventral cell groups had axons that terminated as swollen bulbs on the posterior face of the brain, between the circumoesophageal connectives.

3. There was no histological evidence for neurosecretory activity in the frontal region of the brain, the optic ganglia, or the lateral and median frontal organs.

4. Extirpation experiments showed that removal of the compound eye, the head storage cells, the antennules, and the optic ganglia had no effect on the moulting behaviour, the reproductive rate, maturation, or on the growth rate.

5. Removal of the naupliar eye gave inconsistent results. In most animals there were no effects on the physiological processes studied, but in two preliminary experiments some animals showed reduction in growth and brood size, and produced either male offspring only, or else male offspring and pseudo-sexual eggs (unfertilised ephippia).

6. Removal of the ventral region of the brain when successful, caused cessation of growth at the maturation size and inhibition of ovarian development. There was no apparent alteration in the moulting behaviour.

Acknowledgments. This work was carried out under the supervision of Professor J. E. HARRIS, and Professor R. B. CLARK during the tenure of a Demonstrationship in the Department of Zoology Bristol University. The author wishes to thank them both for all their helpful advice and criticism during the work, and on reading the manuscript.

References

BARNES, H., and J. J. GONOR (1958a): Neurosecretory cells in the cirriped *Pollicipes polymerus* J. B. SOWERBY. J. mar. Res. **17**, 81—102.
— — (1958b): Neurosecretory cells in some cirripeds. Nature (Lond.) **181**, 194.
BERN, H. (1963): The secretory neuron as a doubly specialized cell. pp. 349—366. of "General Physiology of Cell Specialization" MAZIA, D., and A. TYLER (eds.). New York: McGraw-Hill.
COSTLOW, J. D. (1962): The effect of eye-stalk extirpation on metamorphosis of megalops of the crab, *Callinectes sapidus* Rathbun. Amer. Zool. **2**, 401—402.
HARRIS, J. E., and P. MASON (1956): Vertical migration of eyeless *Daphnia*. Proc. R. Soc. Lond., B, **145**, 280—290.
HENTSCHEL, E. (1963): Zum neurosekretorischen System der Anostraca, Crustacea. Zoll. Anz. **170**, 187—190.
— (1965): Neurosekretion und Neurohämalorgan bei *Chirocephalus grubei* (DYBOWSCI) und *Artemia salina* (LEACH) (Anostraca, Crustacea). Z. wiss. Zool. **171**, 44—79.
HUBSCHMAN, J. H. (1963): Development and function of neurosecretory sites in the eye-stalks of larval *Palaemonetes* (Decapoda, Natantia). Biol. Bull. Woods Hole, **125**, 96—113.
LOCKHEAD, J. H., and R. RESNER (1958): Function of the eyes and neurosecretion in Crustacea, Anostraca. Proc. XV int. Congr. Zool. **4**, 397—399.

MENON, M. (1962): Neurosecretory system of *Streptocephalus sp.* (Anostraca, Branchiopoda). Mem. soc. Endocr. **12**, 275—286.

MORI, Y. (1933): Kastrationversuche bei Cladoceren. 11. Die Entwicklung der sekundären Sexualcharaktere bei radiumbestrahlten Weibchen von *Daphnia magna.* Z. wiss. Zool. **144**, 573—612.

PYLE, R. W. (1943): The histogenesis and cyclic phenomena of the sinus gland and X-organ in Crustacea. Biol. Bull. Woods Hole **85**, 87—102.

SCHULZ, H. (1928): Über die Bedeutung des Lichtes im Leben niederer Krebse (nach Versuchungen an Daphniden). Z. vergl. Physiol. **7**, 488—552.

STERBA, G. (1957): Die neurosekretorischen Zellgruppen einiger Cladoceren (*Daphnia pulex* und *magna, Simocephalus vetulus*). Zool. Jb., Abt. Anat. u. Ontog. **76**, 303—310.

THOMSEN, E. (1952): Functional significance of neurosecretory brain cells and the corpus cardiacum in the female blowfly, *Calliophora erythrocephalus.* J. exp. Biol. **29**, 137—172.

Einige histochemische und elektronenmikroskopische Beobachtungen an den neurosekretorischen Nervenzellen des winterschlafenden Igels (Erinaceus europaeus [L.]).

A. Oksche, M. Vaupel-von Harnack und H. Wolff, Gießen

Im Zentralnervensystem winterschlafender Igel ist im lichtmikroskopischen histochemischen Präparat eine starke Anreicherung von Glykogen (Diastase-Kontrolle) zu beobachten. In der Verteilung dieses paraplasmatischen Stoffes zeigen sich deutliche Prädilektionsorte. So ist das Glykogen sehr stark in den Astrocyten, in den motorischen Neuronen des Rückenmarkes und in den Nuclei originis des Hirnstammes angereichert. Äußerst glykogenreich sind im lichtmikroskopischen Präparat auch die beiden neurosekretorischen Kerngebiete des Hypothalamus — Nucl. supraopticus und Nucl. paraventricularis. Elektronenmikroskopisch konnten wir in den Perikaryen des Nucl. supraopticus in der Nachbarschaft des endoplasmatischen Reticulums typische Glykogengranule beobachten. Häufig finden sie sich auch in der Nähe von 1500—1800 Å großen Neurosekretgranula und cytosomen. In Kontrollstückchen des Nucl. supraopticus, die vorher mit hochgereinigter Diastase digeriert wurden, sind die für Glykogen angesehenen Körnchen nicht mehr nachweisbar. Die funktionelle Bedeutung dieses Befundes wird noch geprüft. (Ein Teil des Materials wurde uns von Prof. Dr. P. Suomalainen, Helsinki, zur Verfügung gestellt.)

Zur Frage neurosekretorischer Elemente im Nervensystem von Archianneliden

G. Ohm und M. Vaupel-von Harnack, Gießen

In der Ordnung der Archiannelida werden sekundär vereinfachte Polychaetenformen zusammengefaßt. Untersucht wurde ein Vertreter der Fam. Protodrilidae, *Protodrilus rubropharyngeus* Jägersten (geschlechtsreife Exemplare). Die getrenntgeschlechtlichen erwachsenen Tiere werden 8—9 mm lang. Das Zentralnervensystem (Gehirn) von *Protodrilus* liegt im Prostomium dicht unter der Epidermis. Es besteht aus einem fibrillären Innenteil (Neuropilem) und einer rindenartigen Zone von Ganglienzellen. In der kaudalen Region des Gehirnes von *Protodrilus*, insbesondere in seinem dorso-lateralen Bereich an der Basis der sog. Nuchalorgane (Riechorgan?) finden sich Zellen, die mit der Paraldehydfuchsin-Methode eine starke Granulation zeigen. Im elektronenmikroskopischen Bild des bis auf 100—200 Å weite Zwischenräume lückenlose Neuropilems sind zahlreiche granulierte Faserprofile zu erkennen. Beobachtet wurden die folgenden Granulatypen: 1. ellipsoide, besonders elektronendichte Granula mit Durchmesserwerten von etwa 1800 zu 800 Å; 2. ellipsoide, elektronendichte Granula mit Durchmesserwerten von 450—800 Å zu 1000—1200 Å; 3. annähernd runde, elektronendichte Elementargranula mit einem Durchmesser von 550—800 Å; 4. elektronenoptisch leere Strukturen von der Größe synaptischer Bläschen, die z. T. auch mit elektronendichten Elementen gepaart sind. Häufig finden sich Perikaryen, die neben konzentrischen Formationen des rauhen endoplasmatischen Reticulums äußerst zahlreiche Elementargranula des 2. Typs enthalten. An der genaueren Diagnose und Klassifizierung der neuroendokrinen Elemente bei den systematisch und ökologisch interessanten Archianneliden wird noch gearbeitet.

(Eingereicht von A. Oksche)

Zur Frage der Gliazellen in den neurosekretorischen Zentren von Lumbricus terrestris L.

P. ZIMMERMANN, Gießen

Nach eingehendem Studium der neurosekretorischen Zentren von *Lumbricus terrestris* in aufgehellten Paraldehydfuchsin-Totalpräparaten und nach Anwendung der Pseudoisocyanin-Reaktion von STERBA (fluorescenzmikroskopische Beobachtungen) wurden neue technische Verfahren zur Darstellung der Neuroglia gesucht. Die filamentreichen Gliazellen von *Lumbricus terrestris* lassen sich in Chromalaunhämatoxylin-Phloxin-Präparaten mit der fluorescenz-mikroskopischen Methode von FLEISCHHAUER erfassen. Noch präzisere Ergebnisse kann man aber beim Regenwurm mit einem eigenen Verfahren erzielen. Die Schnittserien werden mit Orange G-Phosphorwolframsäure (modifiziert nach GOLDNER) behandelt und anschließend im Fluorescenzmikroskop (Ortholux-Orthomat; Filterkombination Blau BG 12, K 530) betrachtet. In einem sonst dunklen Cytoplasma leuchten nur die Gliafilamente auf. Auf Grund der Zellform und der Feinheiten des Astwerks kann man bei *Lumbricus* grundsätzlich drei verschiedene Typen der Faserglia unterscheiden. Die kleinen, stark verzweigten Zellen des Typ I bilden Faserkörbe um die Nervenzellen. Die mit nur 1—2 langen Fortsätzen ausgestatteten, wenig verzweigten Zellen vom Typ II treten bei der Regeneration als erste Gliaform in Erscheinung; sie zeigen zuerst nur sehr zarte Filamente. Typ III umfaßt große, stark verästelte Elemente. Die Gliaarchitektonik der neurosekretorischen Zentren unterscheidet sich vom Gliabild der rein nervösen Areale. So scheint der Glia-Typ IIIc nur im Neuropil des Oberschlundganglions vorzukommen. Aus der Feinstruktur kann auf enge funktionelle Beziehungen zwischen den neurosekretorischen Zellen und der Neuroglia geschlossen werden. Die Neuroglia der Wirbellosen läßt sich mit den neuen Spezialmethoden wesentlich besser darstellen als mit den konventionellen Verfahren. An einer genauen Gliakarte von *Lumbricus terrestris* wird noch gearbeitet.

(Eingereicht von A. OKSCHE)

Conclusions-Schlußwort-Résumé

W. Bargmann, Kiel

Unser Kollege Fred Stutinsky hat mir «une question désagréable» — so jedenfalls meinte er — vorgelegt, indem er mich bat, ein Schlußwort zu sprechen. Da diese Bitte überraschend kam, darf ich das Verständnis der Hörer dafür voraussetzen, daß ich nur einige Teilprobleme aus dem weiten Bereich der Neurosekretionsforschung, der hier erörtert wurde, in unser Gedächtnis zurückrufe.

Zunächst aber sage ich im Namen der Teilnehmer dieses Symposiums allen denen herzlichen Dank, die uns in dieser schönen Stadt, dem Schnittpunkt alter Kulturen, gastlich aufgenommen und unsere Arbeit in jeder Weise erleichtert haben: Herrn Professor Vivien, dem Doyen der Faculté des Sciences und der von ihm vertretenen Fakultät, dem Hausherrn, Herrn Professor Stutinsky, und seinen Mitarbeitern, Herrn Professor Follenius und seinem Stab, auf dem die Sorgen um die Organisation unserer Tagung lasteten, und Herrn Kollegen Benoit, dessen, von seinem Temperament zeugende Eröffnungsansprache einen Rückblick auf die Geschichte dieser internationalen Veranstaltung gab, die nun schon zur Tradition geworden ist. Einen besonderen Dank haben nicht zuletzt die liebenswürdigen jungen Damen verdient, die um den reibungslosen Ablauf des Symposiums erfolgreich bemüht waren.

In diesem Kreise haben sich alte Freunde und Bekannte, aber auch manche Neukömmlinge getroffen. Sie alle vermissen Ernst Scharrer, dessen Herr Benoit bereits am ersten Tage gedachte, schmerzlich. Ich brauche Ihnen, liebe Frau Scharrer, die Sie am Schlußtage die Funktion des Chairman ausüben, nicht zu sagen, daß das Andenken an Ernst Scharrer in uns, mit unserer Arbeit und mit unseren Symposien fortleben wird.

Seit dem ersten Treffen der „Neurosekretionisten" in Neapel (1953) sind neue Wege erschlossen worden, die uns dem Verständnis des Phänomens Neurosekretion stetig näherbringen. Neben die Färbemethoden mit Chromalaunhämatoxylin, Aldehydfuchsin, Alzianblau und Pseudoisocyanin sind die Histochemie, die Fluorescenzmikroskopie, die Autoradiographie, die Elektronenmikroskopie, die Ultrazentrifugation, die Biochemie und die Untersuchung der lebenden Zelle getreten. Aus der Kombination der verschiedenen Verfahren ergeben sich vielfältige, in den nun schon alten Neapeler Zeiten noch nicht bekannte oder genutzte Möglichkeiten zur Lösung der Neurosekretionsprobleme. Als besonders ingeniöse haben wir das methodische Vorgehen von W. W. Douglas empfunden, da es Beobachtungen an der lebenden, Hormone bildenden und abgebenden Markzelle der Nebenniere und an der überlebenden Neurohypophyse mit biochemischen Untersuchungen verknüpft.

Aber nicht nur die Einführung neuer Methoden hat das Gesicht des internationalen Symposiums über Neurosekretion verändert. Auch unsere Vorstellungen von der neurosekretorischen Zelle und ihre Definition haben begonnen, sich zu wandeln. Als sekretorisches Neuron galt noch vor wenigen Jahren eine Nervenzelle, die lichtmikroskopisch faßbare, elektiv färbbare Produkte enthält und an den Endigungen ihres Neuriten Hormone in den Säftestrom abgibt, Hormone, die an eben diese Produkte gebunden sind. So ist hier die Frage aufgeworfen worden, welche Rolle die Dendriten der neurosekretorischen Zelle spielen, ob sie als Receptoren aufzufassen sind oder ob auch sie Wirkstoffe absondern, etwa in den Ventrikelliquor des Gehirns. Ferner wurden Zellen in den Kreis der Betrachtung gezogen, die als Abkömmlinge des Sympathicus Hormone an das Blut abgeben, ohne im ursprünglichen Sinne neurosekretorische Zellen zu sein, ferner die vegetativen Neurone des Sympathicus. Rechnet man die Zellen des vegetativen Systems, die spezifischen Stoffe produzieren und mit ihnen in die inkretorische Regulation eingreifen, zu den Gegenständen unserer Bemühungen, so muß man fragen, ob das Symposion über Neurosekretion nicht besser *Symposion für Neuroendokrinologie* genannt werden sollte.

Trotz der angedeuteten Auflockerung der Grenzen und der Erweiterung des uns interessierenden Gebietes ist in diesen Tagen ein Mangel spürbar geworden, soweit es sich um die neurosekretorischen Systeme von Wirbeltieren handelt. Im Mittelpunkt unserer Diskussionen stand die *sekretorische Nervenzelle des Zentralnervensystems*. Es scheint mir notwendig zu sein, daß das nächste Symposion größeres Gewicht auf die Frage der Neurosekretion *im peripheren autonomen System* legt. Sie wissen, daß es eine Reihe von Untersuchungen gibt, deren Ergebnisse für den Ablauf sekretorischer Prozesse in Sympathicuszellen sprechen. Es sei an Studien von Ernst Scharrer, Lennette und Eichner erinnert, um nur einige Autoren zu erwähnen.

Lassen Sie mich nunmehr zu einigen Einzelfragen kurz Stellung nehmen, deren Problematik uns nach unserer Rückkehr an unsere Arbeitsstätten sicherlich beschäftigen wird. Zunächst sei daran erinnert, daß die Frage der *Beteiligung des Zellkerns* an der Ausarbeitung von Neurosekretpartikeln auch diesmal wieder diskutiert worden ist. Es war die Rede von intranucleär gelegenen Neurosekretkügelchen und ihrer Extrusion. Natürlich soll nicht bestritten werden, daß der Zellkern eine bedeutende Rolle bei der Stoffbildung durch die Zelle insofern spielt, als er messenger-RNA entsendet und auf die Ribosomen einwirkt, damit auf die Proteinsynthese. Für eine Entstehung hormonhaltiger Einschlüsse unmittelbar innerhalb des Kernraumes liegen indessen bis heute — soweit wir dies sehen können — keine unumstößlichen Hinweise vor. Die Elektronenmikroskopie hat wiederholt gezeigt, daß die Existenz von kugeligen Kerneinschlüssen, etwa in der Leberzelle, durch die Invagination charakteristisch differenzierter Cytoplasmabezirke in Kerneinsenkung vorgetäuscht werden kann. Darauf ist schon in Bristol, 1961, aufmerksam gemacht worden. Als Ort der Sekretformung ist nach unseren heutigen Kenntnissen nicht das Karyon, sondern das Perikaryon der sekretorischen, in unserem Falle neurosekretorischen Zelle anzusehen. Hierzu einige Bemerkungen unter dem Stichwort „*Granula und Vesikel*".

Zahlreiche elektronenmikroskopische Untersuchungen haben gezeigt, daß das färbbare Neurosekret aus *Elementargranula* besteht, deren Durchmesser je nach Tierart 1000 bis 3000 Å beträgt. Es handelt sich um elektronendichte kugelige Teilchen, die von einer Membran umhüllt werden. Sie entstehen wie die Sekretgranula anderer Zellen im Golgiapparat und werden durch einen Axoplasmastrom bis in die Endigungen der Nervenzellfortsätze transportiert. Über diese letztere Vorstellung wird noch zu sprechen sein.

Soweit das neurosekretorische Zwischenhirn-Neurohypophysensystem zur Debatte steht, enthalten die Elementargranula die Octapeptide Vasopressin und Oxytocin, Hormone, die bei Bedarf an den Nervenendigungen abgegeben werden. Im Zuge der Abgabe von Wirkstoffen kommt es zur Entleerung der Elementargranula von massendichtem Inhalt, d. h. es entstehen elektronenmikroskopisch leere *Vesikel*. Es dürfte auf diesem Symposion deutlich geworden sein, daß über das weitere Schicksal dieser Vesikel Unklarheit besteht. Sind sie imstande, sich unabhängig vom Golgiapparat, ihrem Kondensationsort, wieder mit elektronendichtem, hormonhaltigem Material zu füllen oder verkleinern und teilen oder fragmentieren sie sich, wie MARC HERLANT ausführte, so daß Vesikel vom Aussehen jener Bläschen entstehen, die wir als synaptic vesicles bezeichnen? Auf welche Weise kann man Mikroformen entleerter Elementargranula von synaptic vesicles unterscheiden?

Diese Fragen sind ebenso offen, wie diejenigen nach der Herkunft der *synaptic vesicles*, deren Inhalt aus Transmittersubstanz besteht und für die Abgabe von Hormonen aus den neurosekretorischen Endigungen notwendig sein soll, eine Ansicht, auf die ich noch einmal zurückkomme. Es ist vorstellbar, daß die synaptischen Bläschen durch Abschnürung aus endoplasmatischem Reticulum entstehen, eine Ansicht, die z. B. ANDRES vertritt, oder von den Enden der Neurotubuli abgegliedert und in die synaptischen Endverbindungen transportiert werden. Die Nennung dieser Frage zeigt, daß die Erforschung der sekretorischen Nervenzelle ebenso Sache der Neuroendokrinologie wie der allgemeinen Neurophysiologie und -cytologie ist.

Da es bisher schwer abzuschätzen ist, ob und inwieweit verkleinerte entleerte Elementargranula mit synaptischen Bläschen deswegen verwechselt werden können, weil sie durch Fixation verändert wurden, scheint mir folgendes wünschenswert zu sein: eine systematische Studie über die Wirkung verschiedener Fixantien und ihrer Applikation auf das Strukturbild der neurosekretorischen Zelle speziell ihrer Elementargranula.

Weiterer Überlegungen bedarf auch die Frage nach den Beziehungen der von ACHER nachgewiesenen und schon lange postulierten Hormon-*Trägersubstanz* zur Ultrastruktur der sekretorischen Nervenzelle. Die fluorescenzmikroskopischen Untersuchungen von STERBA sprechen dafür, daß es bei der Abgabe von Hinterlappenhormonen aus den Elementargranula zu einem Übertritt dieser Wirkstoffe in das Grundplasma kommt, aus dem sie an das Plasmalemm gelangen, um es zu passieren. Wie verhält sich bei diesem Vorgang die Trägersubstanz der Hormone, das Neurophysin? Eine Frage, die insbesondere durch DOUGLAS auf diesem Symposium gestellt wurde. Welche Zellstrukturen sind als Substrat des Neurophysins anzusprechen?

Als besonders wichtige, die weitere Arbeit befruchtende Feststellung müssen die Angaben von DOUGLAS über den *Mechanismus der Hormonabgabe* durch die Nervenendigungen in der Neurohypophyse und die Markzellen der Nebenniere angesehen werden. Allem Anschein nach steht die auf den ersten Blick bestechende Annahme, in "synaptic vesicles" enthaltenes Acetylcholin spiele bei der Hormon-

16*

abgabe eine entscheidende Rolle, auf schwachen Füßen. Vielmehr handelt es sich nach Douglas bei dem release in erster Linie um einen Calcium-abhängigen Prozeß, in der Neurohypophyse wie im Nebennierenmark und in anderen Drüsen.

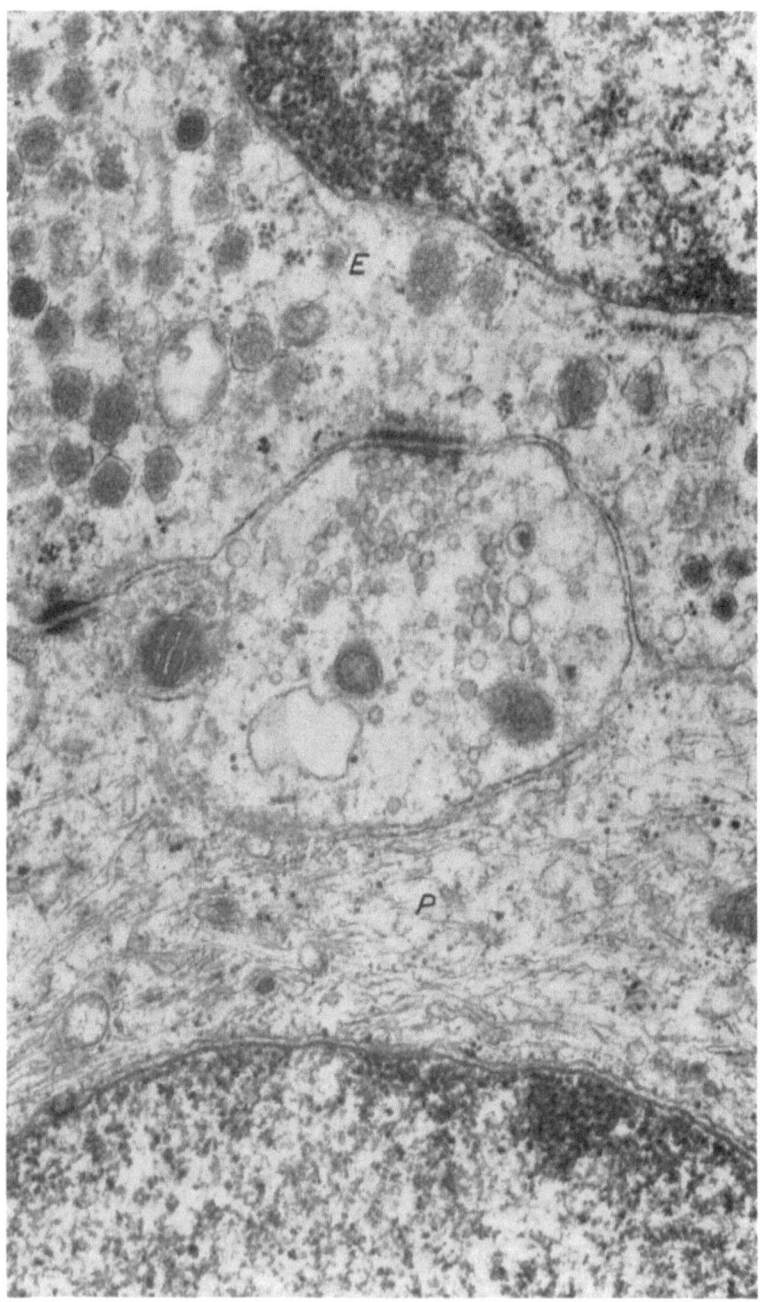

Abb. 1. Synapse an Epithelzelle (*E*) der Pars intermedia. *P* Palisadenzelle, deren Cytoplasma feine Filamente enthält. Vergr. etwa 45000fach

Diese wichtige Beobachtung regt dazu an, der Bedeutung von Calcium, Kalium, Natrium und Magnesium für die Stoffabgabe seitens der neurosekretorischen Zelle weit größere Beachtung zu schenken, als es bisher geschehen ist, und damit einen engeren Anschluß an die Neurophysiologie zu gewinnen. Für die Elektronenmikroskopiker und Biochemiker stellt sich dabei die Frage, welche Bedeutung den oft beschriebenen und abgebildeten synaptic vesicles zukommt, von denen bereits die Rede war.

Wie ich eingangs andeutete, ist die klassische *Definition der neurosekretorischen Zelle* in den letzten Jahren in Frage gestellt worden. Sie besagte, die neurosekretorische Zelle erreiche mit ihren verdickten, sekrethaltigen Endigungen die Wandung von Capillaren in Neurohämalorganen (KNOWLES) verschiedener Art und gebe ihre spezifischen Produkte im Dienst hormonaler Regulationen in den Blutstrom ab, d. h. sie bilde im Gegensatz zu den „banalen" Neuronen keine Synapsen. Abgesehen von einigen elektronenmikroskopischen Untersuchungen der letzten Jahre, die Zweifel an diesem Konzept aufkommen ließen, hat FRANCIS KNOWLES gezeigt, daß es synaptische Verknüpfungen zwischen den neurosekretorischen Endigungen und der Oberfläche hypophysärer Pituicyten gibt. Echte *Synapsen*-Skeptiker mögen zunächst die Bezeichnungen „synaptoide Formation" bevorzugen — sind aber auch an den Epithelzellen des Zwischenlappens der Hypophyse von Säugern ausgebildet, wie aus Untersuchungen von BARGMANN, LINDNER und ANDRES (im Druck) hervorgeht (Abb. 1). Dabei handelt es sich teils um Endformationen mit Granula vom Typus der Katecholaminkörnchen, teils vom Typus neurosekretorischer Elementargranula. Ob und welche dieser Endigungen eine inhibitorische oder excitatorische Wirkung ausüben, wissen wir noch nicht. Ohne Zweifel aber haben wir es mit einem Gegenstand der Neurosekretionsforschung zu tun, dessen morphologische und experimentelle Erforschung intensiver Anstrengungen wert ist. Wir stehen offenbar vor der Notwendigkeit, die bisher übliche Definition der neurosekretorischen Zelle zu überdenken bzw. aufzugeben.

Zu einer Bereicherung unserer Bildes von den Eigenschaften der neurosekretorischen Zelle trägt auch die Feststellung bei, daß es *verschiedene Formen neurosekretorischer Elemente* gibt, die sich sowohl im färberischen Verhalten ihrer Produkte als auch hinsichtlich der Größe ihrer Granula unterscheiden (NAISSE, KNOWLES), d. h. auch verschiedene funktionelle Bedeutung besitzen dürften. Mit dieser Bemerkung rückt die Frage ins Feld der Diskussion, aus welchem Grunde die Katecholamingranula bildenden und entsprechende Wirkstoffe absondernden Neurone nicht zu den neurosekretorischen Zellen gerechnet werden sollen. Man kann sie zwar nicht in ähnlicher Weise färberisch hervorheben wie die peptidbildenden Zellen des Hypothalamus, doch entstehen auch in ihnen Elementargranula, wenngleich von geringerem Kaliber als in den sekretorischen Neuronen des Nucleus supraopticus und paraventricularis, und auch sie geben Hormone ab. Studien von FALCK und FUXE besagen, daß es spezifische Stoffe bildende Neuronensysteme gibt, die Dopaminsysteme, die sich zwar nicht mit Färbeverfahren üblicher Art, wohl aber fluorecenzmikroskopisch charakterisieren lassen. Dieser Hinweis unterstreicht noch einmal das eingangs über eine Ausweitung des Forschungsgebietes Neurosekretion Gesagte.

Da dieses Resumé immer wieder auf die Thematik früherer Symposien abhebt, um Veränderungen in der Situation und Fortschritte in der Erkenntnis zu vergegenwärtigen, wollen wir uns nunmehr daran erinnern, daß zunächst das *hypothalamisch-neurohypophysäre System* im Vordergrund des Interesses stand. Inzwischen ist jedoch außer den neurosekretorischen Systemen für die Regulation des Wasserhaushaltes, des Blutdrucks und der Muskulatur des graviden Uterus ein weiteres System erkannt worden, das *tuber-infundibuläre System*, das mit der Eminentia mediana verknüpft ist. Allem Anschein nach wirkt es über das portale Gefäßsystem am Hypophysenstiel auf gonadotrope Zellen des Vorderlappens ein. Rechnet man katecholaminhaltige Neuronensysteme gleichfalls zu den neurosekretorischen Systemen, dann wird man auch das den Hypothalamus mit dem Zwischenlappen der Hypophyse verbindende System von Nervenzellen in unsere Betrachtung einbeziehen müssen. Es steht zu erwarten, daß sich durch das systematische Studium des Zentralnervensystems und des inkretorischen Apparates verschiedener Wirbeltierklassen bis zu unserem nächsten Symposion weitere neuroendokrine Organisationen herausgeschält haben werden, deren synaptische Verknüpfung mit verschiedenen Abschnitten des Gehirns — beiläufig gesagt — besondere Beachtung verdient.

Es wäre zu begrüßen, wenn bei späterer Gelegenheit auch die *neuroendokrinen Systeme der Wirbellosen* gesichtet und in einem Überblick dargestellt würden. Unzureichende Sachkenntnis läßt mich von dem Versuch Abstand nehmen, in diesem Schlußwort auch die hier vorgetragenen Beobachtungen an Wirbellosen Revue passieren zu lassen. Es ist jedoch für jeden Betrachter offenkundig geworden, in wie hohem Maße Erkenntnisse auf dem einen Gebiet die Arbeit auf einem anderen fördern, da es letztlich um die gleichen Probleme der Biologie sekretorischer Nervenzellen geht.

Ein wesentliches Glied der Neurosekretionslehre, mag es sich um Wirbeltiere oder Wirbellose handeln, ist bis heute die *Transporttheorie*. Sie besagt, daß in den Perikaryen sekretorischer Neurone gebildete Sekretpartikel durch einen "axonal flow", wie er von Paul Weiss und seinen Mitarbeitern an markhaltigen Nervenfasern nachgewiesen wurde, in die Nervenendigungen gelangen, um hier — in storage organs — angereichert zu werden. Es ist zu wünschen, daß den früheren Beobachtungen von Hild an Gewebekulturen und von Carlisle am Hypophysenstiel von Teleostiern (Lund, 1957) weitere Untersuchungen am lebenden oder überlebenden Objekt folgen, die die Richtigkeit der Transporttheorie im wahrsten Sinne des Wortes augenfällig machen. Obwohl neuere Vital- und Supravitalbeobachtungen fehlen, können wir indessen feststellen, daß die Transporttheorie eine gewichtige Stütze erhalten hat, nämlich durch die überzeugenden Untersuchungen von Frau Flament-Durand. Die autoradiographischen, an das Vorgehen von Sloper anschließenden Befunde, der Autorin lassen klar erkennen, daß sich radioaktives Cystein (^{35}S) selektiv zuerst in den neurosekretorischen Zwischenhirnkernen, 10 Std später im Stapelorgan Hinterlappen anreichert. Unter bestimmten biologischen Bedingungen kann es zu einer Beschleunigung des Transportes der markierten Substanz in den Hinterlappen kommen.

Als Arbeiter auf dem Gebiete von Grundlagenwissenschaften, von basic sciences, finden wir uns bereits reich belohnt, wenn es uns gelingt, das eine oder andere Rätsel zu lösen, das uns die neurosekretorische Zelle aufgibt. Dies mag ein Grund dafür sein, daß *medizinische Aspekte* auf unseren Tagungen bisher eine relativ geringe Rolle spielten, obwohl schon vor Jahrzehnten auf die Bedeutung des hypothalamisch-neurohypophysären Systems für das Zustandekommen des Diabetes insipidus des Menschen hingewiesen wurde. Inzwischen hat der Pädiater RODECK (Bristol, 1961) auf die Beziehungen des sich entwickelnden neurosekretorischen Zwischenhirnsystems zum Wasserhaushalt des Neugeborenen mit seinem „physiologischen Diabetes insipidus" hingewiesen und hier in Strasbourg SLOPER das Thema *Diabetes insipidus des Erwachsenen* aufgegriffen. Es ist verdienstvoll, daß SLOPER und seine Mitarbeiter die Erkenntnisse der Neurosekretionsforschung zur Grundlage des Verständnisses der Pathogenese des Diabetes insipidus machen. Vielleicht kann die elektronenmikroskopische und biochemische Untersuchung des *hereditären Diabetes insipidus* der Ratte weitere Beiträge zur Analyse der Erkrankung liefern.

Wenn Sie nun, meine Damen und Herren, die Vorträge und Diskussionen der letzten Tage vor Ihrem geistigen Auge vorüberziehen lassen und überdenken, werden Sie sich ohne Zweifel mancher wichtigen Frage entsinnen, die in diesem improvisierten Resumé nicht wieder auftauchte. Dennoch hoffe ich, wenigstens durch Erwähnung eines Teils der hier behandelten Probleme zu erkennen gegeben zu haben, daß wir reich an Anregungen in unsere Laboratorien zurückkehren. Mögen die Früchte dieses Symposiums in einigen, nicht zu fernen Jahren in einem neuen Treffen geerntet werden, das uns alle in Gesundheit und Schaffenskraft vereinigt.

List of Lecturers — Liste des Rapporteurs

Angel, M. V.: National Institute of Oceanography, Wormley, Godalming Surrey (England).

Bargmann, W.: Anatomisches Institut der Universität Kiel (Bundesrepublik Deutschland).

Barry, J.: Laboratoire d'Histologie, Faculté de Médecine, 59 Lille (France).

Bern, H. A.: Department of Zoology and its Cancer Research Genetis Laboratory, University of California, Berkeley (USA).

Disclos, P.: Laboratoire de Biologie Animale S.P.C.N., Faculté des Sciences, 33 Bordeaux (France).

Douglas, W. W.: Department of Pharmacology, Albert Einstein College of Medicine, Bronx 10461, New York (USA).

Flament-Durand, J.: Laboratoire d'Anatomie Pathologique, Faculté de Médecine de l'Université Libre de Bruxelles et Fondation Médicale de la Reine Elisabeth, Bruxelles (Belgique).

Follenius, E.: Laboratoire de Zoologie et Embryologie Experimentale, Faculté des Sciences, 67 Strasbourg (France).

Fuxe, K.: Department of Histology, Karolinska Institutet, Stockholm (Sweden).

Hagadorn, I. R.: Department of Zoology, University of North Carolina, Chapel Hill, North Carolina (USA).

Herlant-Meewis, H.: Laboratoire de Biologie Animale et d'Histologie Comparée, Faculté des Sciences, 50, avenue F. Roosevelt, Bruxelles 5 (Belgique).

Herlant, M.: Laboratoire d'Histologie, Faculté de Médecine, 97, rue aux Laines, Bruxelles 1 (Belgique).

Jasinski, A.: Hoyer Department of Comparative Anatomy, Jagiellonian University, Cracow, 50 Krupnicza Str. (Poland).

Van De Kamer, J. C.: Zoölogisch Laboratorium, Utrecht (The Netherlands).

Sir Knowles, F.: Department of Anatomy, Medical School, University of Birmingham, Birmingham (England).

Kordon, C.: Laboratoire d'Histophysiologie, Collège de France, 4 avenue Gordon-Bennett Paris XVIe (France).

Lederis, K.: Department of Pharmacology, Medical School, Bristol (England).

Mazzuca, M.: Laboratoire d'Histologie, Faculté de Médecine, Institut Pasteur, 59 Lille (France).

Oksche, A.: Anatomisches Institut der Justus-Liebig Universität Gießen (Deutschland).

Sachs, H.: Department of Physiology, Western Reserve University, School of Medicine, Cleveland, Ohio (USA).

Sloper, J. C.: Pathology Department of Charing Cross Hospital Medical School, London (England).

Taxi, J.: Laboratoire de Cytologie, Faculté des Sciences, Paris (France).

Teichmann-Vigh, I.: Department of Histology Embryology, Tüzolto 58, Budapest IX (Hongrie).

Vigh, B.: Department of Histology and Embryology, Tüzolto 58, Budapest IX (Hongrie).

Subject Index — Table analytique des matières